Neurologic Skills

Neurologic Skills

Examination and Diagnosis

THOMAS H. GLICK MD
Associate Professor of Neurology
Harvard Medical School
Cambridge, Massachusetts

Boston
BLACKWELL SCIENTIFIC PUBLICATIONS
Oxford London Edinburgh
Melbourne Paris Berlin Vienna

Editorial offices:
238 Main Street, Cambridge
Massachusetts 02142, USA
Osney Mead, Oxford OX2 0EL, England
25 John Street, London WC1N 2BL
England
23 Ainslie Place, Edinburgh EH3 6AJ
Scotland
54 University Street, Carlton
Victoria 3053, Australia

Other Editorial Offices:
Librairie Arnette SA
2, rue Casimir-Delavigne
75006 Paris
France

Blackwell Wissenschafts-Verlag GmbH
Meinekestrasse 4
D-1000 Berlin 15
Germany

Blackwell MZV
Feldgasse 13
A.1238 Wien
Austria

First published 1993

Set by Excel Typesetters Company, Hong Kong
Printed and bound in the United States of America by
Maple-Vail, Binghamton, New York

93 94 95 96 5 4 3 2

DISTRIBUTORS

USA
Blackwell Scientific Publications, Inc.
238 Main Street
Cambridge, Massachusetts 02142
(*Orders*: Tel: 617 876-7000
800 759-6102)

Canada
Times Mirror Professional Publishing, Ltd
130 Flaska Drive
Markham, Ontario L6G 1B8
(*Orders*: Tel: 800 268-4178
416 470-6739)

Australia
Blackwell Scientific Publications Pty Ltd
54 University Street
Carlton, Victoria 3053
(*Orders*: Tel: 03 347-5552)

Outside North America and Australia
Marston Book Services Ltd
PO Box 87
Oxford OX2 0DT
(*Orders*: Tel: 0865 791155
Fax: 0865 791927
Telex: 837515)

Library of Congress
Cataloging-in-Publication Data

Glick, Thomas H., 1939–
Neurologic skills: examination and diagnosis / Thomas H. Glick.
p. cm.
Includes bibliographical references and index.
ISBN 0–86542–292–3
1. Nervous system – Examination.
2. Nervous system diseases – Diagnosis.
3. Medical history taking.
I. Title.
[DNLM: 1. Medical History Taking – methods. 2. Nervous System Diseases – diagnosis. 3. Neurologic Examination – methods. WL 141 G559n]
RC348.G55 1993
616.8′0472 – dc20

To my son, Steven, and daughter, Sharon

contents

acknowledgments

I wish to thank a number of physicians, not only from the field of neurology, but also from neuroradiology, ophthalmology, internal medicine, and psychiatry for reviewing parts of the manuscript: Drs Shahram Khoshbin, Carolyn Bernstein, Jonathan Kleefield, Michael Marmor, David Bor, Richard Pels, Andrew Billings, and Alfred Margulies. In particular, I wish to acknowledge, in memoriam, the contributions of the late Dr Camille Draskoczy, my colleague in practice for many years, who graciously reviewed the entire manuscript and offered suggestions despite the afflictions of a terminal illness. She, Dr John Boyd, and Dr Carolyn Bernstein unstintingly helped to meet patient care needs, so that this writing project could move forward. Also at the Cambridge Hospital, the strong personal support and encouragement of Drs Robert Lawrence and David Bor, as well as my many other colleagues in the Department of Medicine, are greatly appreciated. Mr John O'Brien, a remarkable chief executive officer, has done much to create an environment at The Cambridge Hospital in which attention to patient care, scholarship, and community health needs can coexist and thrive.

Edwin Furshpan and David Potter in the Harvard Medical School Department of Neurobiology not only inspired me as a student but continue to do so as my colleagues in the clinically integrated Human Nervous System and Behavior course at Harvard Medical School. I wish again to acknowledge my teachers and mentors in clinical neurology and neuropathology at the Massachusetts General Hospital: Drs Raymond Adams, C Miller Fisher, and EP Richardson Jr. Valuable lessons have also come from the students of Harvard Medical School and the Medical and Psychiatric House Officers of the Cambridge Hospital, as well as my patients there. At Blackwell Scientific Publications, my editors, Dr Vicky Reeders, Coleen Traynor, and Charles Hamlyn, have been generous in their confidence and advice. The medical artist, Clare Williams, contributed greatly with a complete set of new line drawings. Drs Jonathan Kleefield and Jonathan Kramer were most helpful in contributing the neuroimages. Dr Robert Levine tracked down the physics of Weber test lateralization. My Administrative Assistant, Joanne Marchurs, has once again been most skillful and patient in preparation and revisions of the manuscript. Finally, the love and support of my wife, Georgia, encouraged and sustained me throughout the book's long gestation, a process that kept lengthening because I kept learning.

introduction

This book is designed to enable students (and house officers) to learn, understand, and improve essential neurologic clinical skills. These skills involve not only the acquisition of a reliable data base, but also the critical next step: localization, the keystone of diagnostic formulation. To this clinical formulation is then added the interpretation of neuroimaging and laboratory tests. Finally, a series of special topics is included to broaden and extend competence in such important areas as peripheral neurology, eye movements, screening or selective examinations, and dealing with patients who are "difficult to examine." Thus, your use of the book is intended to grow with your development as a clinician.

In going well beyond the neurologic examination sections in general physical diagnosis and neurology texts, this book addresses issues that are essential for continuing growth in neurologic competence: a positive attitude; priority-setting that is sensitive to the many demands confronting students and house officers; and creation of learning frameworks that will enable efficient retrieval of information and diagnostic skills when later needed. Neurologic case studies are used not only for illustration of syndromes, but to provide practice in problem-based learning. (Fictitious names have been used in the case studies to preserve patient anonymity.)

This book is not only for students beginning their study of clinical neurology, but for others whose experience with basic neurologic assessment has been frustrating from the beginning. The purpose is to make neurologic evaluation more accessible and more human – to prevent the negative attitudes and poor performance that arise from two sources: the intimidation of neuroanatomy and the tedium of rote, mindless examinations.

The approach to neurologic assessment presented in this book will help you achieve the following goals.

1 To attain a basic competence in the neurologic evaluation, even for those who have an extremely limited neuroscience background. Drawing upon communication skills, personal insight, and inventiveness will help achieve this.

2 To demystify the neurologic examination by articulating the objectives and adapting techniques to each individual patient.

3 To humanize the neurologic assessment by enabling the patient to become an ally in your evaluation, not just a subject.

4 To facilitate use of neurologic methods within the total medical work-up by using a logical, open-minded approach to neurologic data-gathering and formulation. This will facilitate your performance in neurologic clerkship, medical clerkships, and subsequent house officer rotations.

5 To improve your understanding of the relevance of test results and neuroimages – which can only be achieved by understanding the neurology of the patient's symptoms.

6 To provide a foundation for dealing with neurologic emergencies.

7 To guide your understanding of those neuroanatomic facts that are truly important for diagnostic localization.

8 To articulate the rules and constructs by which neurologists simplify neuroanatomy for clinical diagnostic purposes.

9 To anticipate and respond to frequently asked questions and points of confusion.

Many students come to the neurologic examination discouraged or intimidated by prior encounters with the complexities of neuroanatomy. You cannot learn the basis for all of the normal and abnormal responses to neurologic tests. Truly understanding the anatomy and physiology of just one test, such as "the cop's neurologic" (walking a straight line) would challenge your most learned professor!

Some of you may have wondered whether you could ever be competent in neurology. In actuality, you already know, or can readily acquire, the facts that pave the way to dealing successfully with common diagnostic problems. (Even neurologists use only a tiny core of neuroanatomy in the vast majority of their cases!) Do not let the complexities of the nervous system form a roadblock – a roadblock that causes turn-off. With sound skills in history taking and examination, and a small amount of neuroscientific knowledge, your way will be clear to continue the integrated learning needed to pass subsequent professional milestones.

By concentrating on the basic features of the neurologic evaluation in a common sense way, you will be able to relate the history and examination to your own experiences as a mobile, perceptive, thinking, feeling human being with lots of practice in fact-finding. In so doing, you will draw upon your powers of observation, and your interpersonal skills. Finally, you can build your knowledge of the relevant neuroscience as you go, realizing that this is an open-ended endeavor which will enrich your professional competence and intellectual growth. If you regard the exploration of your patient's neurologic function as a clinical extension of your daily discovery of people, you will make the evaluation more interesting for yourself as well as less frightening for the patient.

Effective neurologic assessment must face the combined challenge of relating to the whole patient, while trying to gather and evaluate technical neurologic information. A good start and continued progress in clinical neurology require a keen awareness of the patient–doctor relationship: which parts of the process are confusing or cause anxiety to the patient? And which parts confuse or worry you as the examiner, diagnostician, and care-giver? Making the most of the neurologic encounter depends upon the rapport you establish with the patient, a rapport that can be thwarted both by heavy-handed techniques (as with pin or hammer) and by failure to appreciate the very personal nature of delving into neurologic functions, especially mental status and behavior. A sensitivity to these issues will pay off in better patient compliance, better data, and improved mutual confidence.

You may ask whether bedside skills are becoming outmoded in an era of high technology. The heart of most neurologic work-ups is still the evaluation of symptoms and signs, especially since many neurologic problems cannot presently be diagnosed (especially at onset) by imaging, blood tests, or electrophysiologic techniques. However, appropriate investigations can confer two types of benefit: the first is obvious – improved diagnosis; the second may be less apparent – liberation of the clinician to pay more attention to the patient, with less fear of missing a lurking lesion, such as a brain tumor. However, the better the sensitivity of imaging is, the greater the problem of knowing what structural abnormalities are actually responsible for symptoms – and which are incidental. This issue of clinical relevancy represents an increasing challenge to neurologic localization and its interpretation.

In the initial phase of the educational process in neurology you should aim to acquire the skills and understanding to do the following:

1 gather and document basic neurologic data from the history and examination of the patient within the context of the bio-psycho-social medical model;

2 approach the formulation of these data in a systematic way, exposing the limitations of the information available;
3 identify the need for more experienced or specialized help – not only as a resource for knowledge and judgment, but as a way to amplify, clarify, or confirm the data base;
4 heighten your awareness of the important interdependence between general health promotion and the prevention of neurologic disease and disability;
5 maintain an open-mindedness that will foster critical questioning and further learning, as you subsequently probe more deeply into the pathophysiology and epidemiology of neurologic disorders.

The case vignettes will help you to understand the process of data gathering in actual clinical situations. While this book is not a text on neurologic disease (or treatment), it includes the typical presenting symptoms and signs of many syndromes and diseases. Further sources, mainly review articles and textbook sources, have been suggested at the end of each chapter. The pediatric examination is not covered: the examination of infants and young children is best approached in a developmental context, provided in the major textbooks of pediatrics; the examination of the older child and adolescent differs little from that of the young adult, if the developmental perspective is maintained and simple observation of behavior is well utilized.

In neurology, as in all areas of medicine, the growth of information requires choices about what to learn and when to learn it. In the following chapters I have endeavored to share my judgment as to what will provide an understandable and helpful basis for learning and improving clinical skills.

part

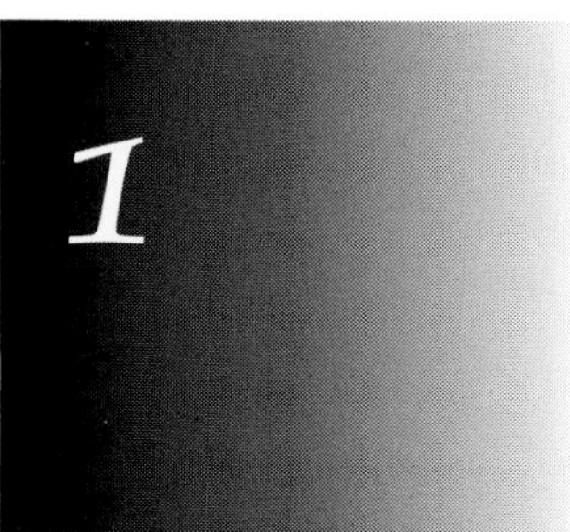

An Approach to the Neurologic Patient: The History

chapter 1

The Neurologic History: Why it is Special

INTRODUCTION TO THE NEUROLOGIC PATIENT

Relating to neurologic illness

First encounters with neurologic illness are often unsettling, if not shocking. Although people commonly experience minor neurologic symptoms, like the uncomfortable tingling that occurs when the "funny bone" (ulnar nerve) is hit, the origin of major neurologic problems usually seems more remote and hence more mysterious: a lesion in the brain or spinal cord typically manifests itself not by local pain or tenderness, but by specific neurologic symptoms affecting another part of the body, such as an arm or leg. Thus, patients find it especially hard to relate to neurologic illness and may react with disbelief.

Responses to disability and deformity

While many neurologic patients behave normally, some others – by the very nature of their disease or injuries – appear helpless, deformed, or irrational. Disturbing manifestations of neurologic dysfunction, such as delirium, incontinence, and convulsion, challenge the very perception of personhood. It is understandable that you may feel frightened or repulsed by some neurologic patients. Especially at a time when you are trying to establish a sense of medical control, it is difficult to encounter patients behaving irrationally. Certain patients are unpredictable in their

Table 1.1 How the history helps diagnostic formulation

Type of data	Aspect of formulation	Example
Character of symptoms	Neurologic or not? (Better to reserve judgment – see Chapter 14)	Itching (rarely a symptom of neurologic disease, but can be)
	Particular neurologic system	Constricted, encased feelings in legs (suggests "posterior column" pathways)
Distribution of symptoms	Anatomic localization	Tingling in first three and a half digits of hand (suggests median neuropathy)
Temporal profile of symptoms	Pathologic process (type of tissue change)	Gradual progression of headaches (suggests an enlarging mass, possibly brain tumor)
	Pathogenesis (mechanism of disease)	Abrupt onset of nonsensical speech with slow improvement in subsequent days (suggestive of embolic mode of infarction)
Risk factors (background conditions)	Etiology (root cause); may also help suggest pathology or pathogenesis	Chronic exposure to old paint suggests that lead encephalopathy might be cause of child's headaches

behavior, and others have disorders of movement and speech so severe that they stymie communication. One of my patients developed such a violent tic of the head and choking of his speech when he tried to talk that I found myself dreading encounters with him. I was afraid that I would cause him more frustration and suffering, and that I would feel frustrated, awkward, and unhelpful. (Yet patients dread this very reaction; to frighten others may lead to abandonment and isolation.)

Conversely, the ravages of neurologic disease need not be physically grotesque or even obvious to casual inspection: how shocking it is to discover that a normal-looking person actually has lost all capacity to form memories. Whether the disability is glaring or veiled, you should heed your own reactions. To evaluate neurologic patients well you need to be able to sit with them and to abide with your feelings in their presence.

History as key

Neurologic diagnosis depends especially heavily on the subjective data base of the history. Most of the nervous system is not visible or palpable (as are skin and bones), and we therefore infer much about its structural integrity from how well it is working. Many disorders are manifest subjectively long before any abnormal signs are detectable on examination. A good neurologic history not only helps diagnostically (Table 1.1), but is also a vehicle for advancing your understanding of the patient as a person. Even a good history will not always crack the case: sometimes the examination will break it open; in other instances "the right laboratory test is worth a roomful of neurologists," as the saying goes. But an understanding of the history-taking process – and its limits – is a key to good neurologic assessment and management.

THE IMPACT OF BRAIN DYSFUNCTION ON THE HISTORY

What is special about the neurologic history? The very neurologic process that is causing symptoms may distort the patient's ability to recognize or communicate them. An historical account depends on witnessing and reporting. How good a witness can a patient be to his or her own experience? And what colors the reporting?

CASE 1A
Loss of control

History

Susan Squires, a 19-year-old college sophomore, came to the emergency room because of an overwhelming feeling that she was losing control. She said that she had been under a great deal of stress, but for the first time that morning she was riveted with a strange vibrating sensation in her head and felt her face contort. As she reached for the telephone with her left arm it shook uncontrollably. Then these feelings drained away and she became aware of herself trembling all over and sobbing in a state of near-panic.

In the emergency room she described her experience, although brief, as being of the most profound sort, as if something had taken ahold of the very core of her being and then relaxed its grip. She also recalled that she had had occasional "blackouts" in the last 2 years that had never been observed by others. The resident physician found no neurologic abnormalities, and wondered whether the episode had been a severe anxiety attack.

She clearly faced a challenge in communicating her "strange, vibrating" symptoms, but could she even perceive them accurately? Might her perceptions be altered by the very pathologic process that was causing them?

Observations

At that point she exclaimed, "It's starting again." The left side of her mouth twisted and began to twitch, her head and eyes turned to the left, her left arm elevated and began to jerk, and she then lost consciousness as her entire body started to convulse in an epileptic seizure.

Diagnosis

Radiologic tests revealed a right frontal arteriovenous malformation (AVM), an abnormal tangle of blood vessels in the brain. The AVM had caused reaction in adjacent tissue that led to abnormal electrical

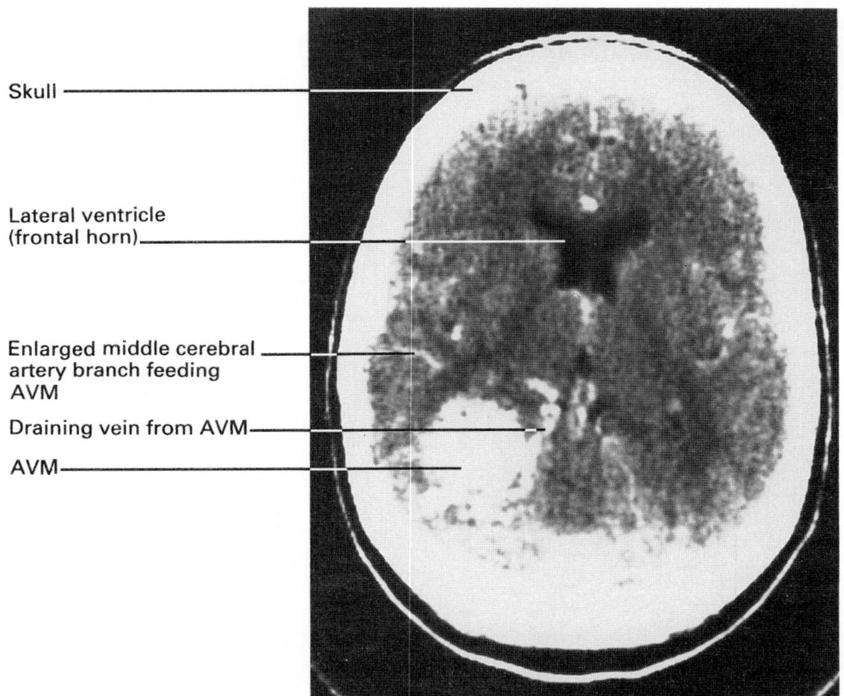

Fig. 1.1 Arteriovenous malformation (AVM). A contrast-enhanced computerized tomography (CT) scan shows the concentration of abnormal vessels as a dense, white lesion in the right occipital lobe. (In CT and magnetic resonance imaging scans the patient's right side is the viewer's left.) Note the adjacent, large, feeding and draining vessels. (Courtesy of Jonathan Kleefield MD.)

discharges. She was treated with anticonvulsant medications. A neurosurgeon successfully obliterated her AVM, but she continued to require medication to prevent seizures (see Fig. 1.1 which shows an AVM in another patient).

Thus, her vibrating feeling turned out to be the aura (first symptom) of an epileptic seizure. When she lost consciousness, she lost any further chance to observe herself. Her capacity to witness and report the critical events of her acute illness was severely limited by their impact on the function of her brain.

In problems involving the brain, the disease processes that can distort the history form a sort of pathologic insulation, obstructing the perception and flow of information within the patient's mind and from the patient to you, the interviewer. Some of the types of neurologic impairment that impact on the history include:

1 memory loss;
2 language impairment (aphasia) in comprehension, expression, or both;
3 confusion, attention deficit;
4 lack of awareness of a particular segment of reality, such as the left side of space;
5 impaired consciousness;
6 psychotic disruption of thought processes.

History mismatch

Suspect a cerebral deficit when you recognize a mismatch between the patient's complaint and the family's complaint. When a patient focuses on symptoms such as indigestion or achy joints (while the family expresses desperation over the patient's wandering off at night), cerebral dysfunction is likely. At other times you will only catch subtle hints of discrepancy. Suspect a failure of insight or communication when the complaint is vague, shifting, tangential to the concerns expressed by others, or grossly at odds with your positive findings. You may not fully appreciate the depth of inadequacy of the patient's history until you have completed the examination or talked with family or friends. The influence of cerebral dysfunction on the chief complaint and present illness is illustrated in the following case examples.

CASE 1B
His complaint and hers

Marcus Landry, a 59-year-old right-handed man, was evaluated because his wife thought that "a screw had come loose" in his head. When asked why he had come to the hospital, he said that he did not know why he was there; his wife stated that he had been alone from 7 p.m. until 8 p.m. On her return he had complained, "When are we going to have supper?" She was taken aback, because they had eaten together earlier. She reminded him of this, but a minute later he again inquired about supper and asked other questions indicating that he had no recollection of the events of that afternoon. She wrote out a series of answers on a piece of paper and told him to keep looking at it.

His neurologic examination was normal, except that he could not form new memories, yet he knew who he was and could remember events further in the past. His memory deficit gradually resolved over the next 24 hours.

Memory loss

In this case Mr Landry did not offer a complaint that would open the door into the relevant area of history, as a chief complaint usually does. Whereas abdominal discomfort would not ordinarily affect one's ability to divulge the pertinent history, Mr Landry's memory deficit negated the subjective account. The physician had to rely mainly on the neurologic history supplied by an independent observer, the patient's wife. The patient was, however, quite capable of reflecting his experience moment by moment, such as the absence of ongoing headache. Mr Landry's diagnosis was the syndrome of transient global amnesia (a self-limited lapse of recent memory capacity, apparently due to a temporary dysfunction of the memory apparatus in the temporal lobes and/or thalamus).

In other cases the reason why cerebral dysfunction interferes with the history-taking process is an inability to communicate rather than a lack of awareness.

CASE 1C
No telling what happened

Miriam Jones, an 81-year-old widow, was brought to the hospital by her landlord because of "trouble talking" and a bruise on her head, which was the result of a fall. She could not express herself, except for a few habitual phrases such as, "Oh, my goodness," or "Isn't that the limit," and was able to follow only the simplest commands (like sticking out her tongue). Had she fallen before a cerebral event or as the result of such an event?

Aphasia

In this case the block to access of historical information was due to an aphasic episode (which recalls the lyrics of Ol'Man River: "He must know somethin', but don't say nuthin'"). It was subsequently reconstructed that she had answered the telephone, been unable to communicate (due to a stroke) and then jumped out of bed too quickly, resulting in a fall and a slight bump on her head. (The stroke was a left middle cerebral artery territory infarct produced by an embolus).

More startling, but quite common, are cases in which the patient's world view, so to speak, is truncated by a neurologic lesion.

CASE 1D
A one-sided world view

Marlene Fair, a 67-year-old right-handed woman, was admitted because of the sudden onset of left-sided weakness noted by her husband. Examination revealed that she had not only a moderate left hemiparesis, but also a left visual deficit (homonymous hemianopia) and partial left-sided sensory deficits. Yet when asked, both before and after the examination, what was bothering her – what, if any, trouble she was having – she denied any problem at all. When asked why she could not walk, she said that her knees had been giving her trouble. Instructed to hold out both her arms, she held up only the right one, but insisted that both arms were out. When her physician picked up her limp left arm and presented it in front of her, she asked him to please get his hand out of her face. Later, she referred to her left arm as an artificial limb that the doctors had given her, but she could not imagine why.

Lack of "insight"

Not only was this patient unable to supply a history, she could not relate to the major deficits that were so obvious to others on inspection. Because of the parietal lobe involvement from her large right hemispheric stroke, her schema of her own body and of the external world no longer included the left side. In conjunction with this left-sided neglect, she remained unaware of any deficit on her left side, and, hence, "lacked insight" into the fact of any deficit at all (anosognosia). Again, as in the case of Marcus Landry with transient memory loss, the medical care team had to rely entirely on the observations of others to piece together her history. But unlike Marcus Landry, who was a good witness to ongoing events at the moment they occurred, Marlene Fair could not even provide current symptomatic information: anything happening to her left side was beyond her ken. Both "insight" and "outlook" were distorted.

FORMAT OF THE HISTORY

Informant: patient, family member, care-giver, etc.

Chief complaint/main symptom: note the patient's own words, but assess whether the first complaint is really the main or underlying issue in the patient's mind; also, whether the patient is aware of, and able to communicate this leading symptom that ordinarily opens the door to the present illness.

Present illness: characterization of symptoms and self-observation; neurologic symptoms like "numbness" are notoriously hard to represent faithfully.

Chronology—temporal profile. The minute details of onset and progression enable inferences as to the pathologic process and pathogenesis (see Table 1.1).

Accounts from third parties (family, friends, etc.). The patient's history, which may be distorted, must be matched against other data.

Past medical, social, occupational, environmental, and family histories: see Chapter 2.

Review of neurologic symptoms: see Chapter 2.

THE PRESENT ILLNESS: SYMPTOMS, SELF-OBSERVATION, AND WITNESSED EVENTS

Subjective and objective

The patient's history intertwines information from different sources (Table 1.2). Distinguish among these, since you will weigh them differently. Just as the neurologic examination contains many subjective elements, the historical data base includes not only degrees of subjectivity, but much information that is quite objective. Observations appear in the history, and the history helps guide the examination (see Chapter 19). While we search for congruity of information from different sources, we should recall that symptoms are not directly subject to verification. No one can truly know another person's pain (even though behavior may

Table 1.2 Types of historical input: example of a patient with "blackouts"

Types of input	Ways of eliciting	Comments
Open, nondirective questioning	"How can I try to be of help?" "What is troubling you?" "What brought you here?"	Clarify and amplify: "Please describe your blackout experience"
Directed questioning about symptoms	Further characterize symptoms, distribution, temporal profile, etc.	Try to relate to medical model (loss of consciousness vs loss of vision?)
Review of neurologic symptoms	A systematic review (see Chapter 2) that jogs recollection (nausea, double vision, taste hallucination?)	This may "suggest" new, somaticizing complaints (see text)
Patient's observation of own behavior, appearance, or function	"Have you noticed any twitching of your muscles?"	Emphasize what patient actually saw, heard, etc. – not what patient was later told about
Patient's report of the observations of family or friends ("third parties")	"Did your wife say that she saw any twitching or staring?"	Patient's report may be distorted (like patient's own symptoms)
Direct third party reports	Ask patient's spouse to describe his or her observations	Compare to professional observations, if warranted

partially reflect it). "Soft" subjective data may be consistent and reliable, whereas objective findings are often subject to dispute among different examiners!

The following additional aspects of the history deserve particular attention at this point:

1 unexpressed concerns (a "hidden agenda");
2 description of function;
3 data from third parties (family, friends, etc.);
4 diagnostic attributions by patient or family.

Unexpressed-concerns

By eliciting the history in a nondirective fashion initially, you may discover important issues that are not reflected in the "chief complaint." Such problems often need some "time and space" to emerge. A headache may be just a headache, plain and simple, but it may serve as a façade, behind which lies another somatic or psychiatric problem. Sexual dysfunction, suicidal ideation, and alcohol and drug abuse are often neglected because of exclusive attention to the first complaint which may not turn out to be the chief complaint. Headache and dizziness are two of the most common presenting problems – symptoms that may seem to patients (perhaps unconsciously) to lend legitimacy to their seeking medical attention.

Description of function

Keeping in mind the interplay between subjective and objective elements in the history of the patient's illness and the present physical condition, we compare what the patient says with what the patient does, and how the patient feels with how the patient functions. We assess whether the facial expression, the animation, the tone of voice – in short, the affect and behavior – match the complaint (allowing, of course, for individual and cultural differences of style). To know that a patient feels stiff and weak is important, but to know when he last walked (how far, with how much assistance) better portrays the disability. We learn something from a patient's complaint of spotty memory, but knowledge of how he or she is functioning as an executive or teacher adds another important facet. Insist on concrete descriptions of what the patient actually does, how this has changed, and what is the best that the patient is currently able to do. (The better the peak performance, the more the patient is structurally capable of doing.) While patterns of activity may reflect changes of interest, beware of rationalization: the change in interest sometimes follows the change in functional capacities.

Third party history

Patients often divulge to intimate care-givers (nurses, aides, physical therapists) certain items of information that they do not share directly with the doctor. Actively seek data from such sources. While you may have the advantage of a growing professional skill in observation, the family member or friend typically has the advantage of seeing the patient *in situ* – dealing with everyday life situations – and often in continuity. On the other hand, third party accounts are just as subject to the influence of attribution as the patient's own story.

Attributions

The chief complaint is often skewed by the significance that the patient (or family) attributes to the symptom: a patient has headaches and fears a possible brain tumor. He complains that "my migraine is getting a lot worse." This conveys the descriptive information that the headaches are increasing, but the diagnostic attribution of "migraine" tends to dispel any more ominous implication. The complaint is the product of a tremendous ambivalence – wanting to know the answer, but wanting the news to be good. At the same time, monitor yourself for intrusion of your own hopes and fears for the patient. Wishing the patient well may subtly be transformed into wishful thinking. A very likeable young patient reported a brief respite in a pattern of progressively severe headaches. The physician seized upon this favorable morsel of history and delayed tests that would have revealed a large benign brain tumor. (Even expanding mass lesions typically show some fluctuation in symptomatic expression.) Thus, when you recognize that emotional investment (either the patient's or your own) is coloring the history, pause to sort out the feelings involved, pursue the history afresh, and reassess the management plan.

CLARIFYING NEUROLOGIC SYMPTOMS

Heed the patient's own words

The recorded data base that emerges from the history is a mutual creation: you will attempt to express the essence of the patient's story in medically meaningful terms, but not obscure it in jargon or glib translation. One patient complained of "head pain," but the physician later recorded it as "headache." You might regard this difference as trivial; however, the patient purposely tried to convey the fact that this was a different sort of discomfort, unlike previously experienced headaches. Patients often use terms like "seizure" loosely. To a doctor a seizure is epileptic, but to the patient it may be a "heart seizure." Some patients call any bad headache a "migraine."

"Images"

"Stereotypic" pattern?

Clarifying events through dramatic "images" can be helpful, if the patient does not already display a histrionic bent. We often ask the patient to explain whether the onset of a headache was like a "hammer blow" or a "thunder clap," or whether it built up over many seconds or minutes. Similarly, did a limb sensation feel like electricity, a "zap" (which is a very characteristic nerve symptom)? It is very helpful when such a characterization "clicks": "That's just the way it felt—I haven't been able to put it in words." Look for a stereotypic character of recurrent symptoms. Qualitative similarity is often more important than variations based on severity. When asked whether he had had previous headaches like this one, a patient said, "No, not like this"—meaning "never this bad"—but, in fact, past headaches were otherwise very similar. Focal neurologic lesions tend to produce at least a stereotypic core of symptoms that will help you to localize the neurologic dysfunction. Neurologists often imagine that they can predict the examination from a good history. This is by no means always possible, but the boast makes a point.

In the case of a patient who complains of "head pain," you would attempt to elicit the following aspects of the presenting symptoms:

1 temporal profile (steady, progressive, waxing and waning, maximal at onset, intermittent, etc.);

2 warnings of onset—any premonition (sparkling lights or jagged lines in one field of vision);

3 character of the pain (burning, throbbing, pressing, sharp, etc.);

4 distribution of the pain (side, front or back, deep or superficial, spreading or radiating);

5 exacerbating or triggering factors (coughing, bending down, medication effects);

6 relieving factors (lying down, darkening room);

7 degree of similarity with prior headaches or pains—how stereotyped, qualitatively and quantitatively? (Do the symptoms have a "stamp" of their own—"It's that same feeling again");

8 associated symptoms (nausea, tingling numbness in one hand);

9 epidemiologic associations (occurrence at the workplace, in other family members, during a particular season, etc.);
10 additional background information from the past medical, social, and family histories (see Chapter 2) may be highly pertinent as well.

Elaboration of symptoms

You will encounter some patients who seem to thrive on neurologic or other symptoms – the more you inquire about particular symptoms, the more they report. Such patients, who may be unusually suggestive, attention-seeking, or preoccupied with bodily symptoms ("somaticizers"), will tax not only your forbearance but your judgment: how long should you let the process continue? A patient walks in with a headache and walks out with numbness and tingling, weakness, unsteadiness, blurred vision, etc. This problem is not unique to neurology, but is especially difficult: there is no test for a tired mind or tired muscles equivalent to the serum iron or vitamin B_{12} tests for "tired blood" (anemia). In cases of suspected elaboration of symptoms, you should carefully note the exact wording of the chief complaint and list the other symptoms precisely. Schedule a return visit at which time you will retake the history with a fresh slate: ask the patient to explain to you the most concerning symptoms and the most troublesome changes in function. Rely most on the consistent core of symptoms, if such exists.

Take a fresh history

Temporal profile

The temporal profile – the graphic line of the onset and course of symptoms and events – provides your first and often best clues to the type of pathology and pathogenesis of symptoms (see Table 1.1). Determine whether the symptoms have been progressively severe, waxing and waning, or truly episodic. With symptoms of "sudden" onset, ask yourself what were the moment by moment events of that time? No detail of this phase is to be ignored.

Points of reference

The temporal profile that you trace may also, in retrospect, include misleading demarcations. In one instance, a change in personality was dated to the time of a family gathering at Thanksgiving. Rather than starting then, the change was simply first noticed at that time by relatives who had not seen the patient recently. Thus, an artificial impression of sudden onset resulted in concern about a stroke, rather than a tumor or other gradually progressive process.

DETERRENTS TO A GOOD NEUROLOGIC HISTORY

As you work-up patients, you will encounter a variety of deterrents to a good neurologic history. Some of these will originate with the patient, some with "the system," and some directly with you! (Table 1.3).

Discomfort

I sometimes find myself merely going through the motions of a history, rushing to escape the discomfort of the encounter or to get on with other pressing tasks. Even patients who command your greatest empathy may have speech defects, hearing impairments, or other disabilities that

Table 1.3 Deterrents to a good history

Issues	Examples
Patient	
Inconsistent or vague account	Impaired memory or attention (Alzheimer's disease)
Continual elaboration of more symptoms	Suggestible; somaticizing disorders
Psychotic thought processes	Paranoid delusions – will not reveal data
Speech or hearing disability	Dysarthria; aphasia; deafness
Inappropriate behavior	Inebriated; delirious; frontal lobe lesion
Language barrier	Refugee – no adequate interpreter immediately available
Physician	
Time pressure	Physician over-extended; unrealistic scheduling; emergencies
Fatigue	Up the night before with gastrointestinal bleeder
Anger	Perception of patient as manipulative
Distraction from other pressing or worrisome issues	Professional or family crisis
Reactions to off-putting appearance of patient	Impulse to withdraw from severely disfigured patient, e.g. old craniofacial trauma

result in long and arduous history-taking sessions. This is not to say that you must suffer through the interminable histories of garrulous or somaticizing patients, but at least be aware of the effect on yourself: plan limit-setting and other strategies rationally rather than emotionally. A perfunctory history rarely solves the problem.

"Poor historians"

A challenge for you as a history taker is not to blame or short-change the victim. The patient may find the neurologic encounter intimidating; the flustered patient is less likely to provide the detail and consistency that you expect. You will hear physicians speaking of patients as "poor historians," but the reason for the poor quality of the patient's account is usually no one's fault. Nonetheless, a poor history may represent a diagnostic clue in itself (see Table 1.3). A repeat history is usually far more productive than a repeat laboratory test. On the other hand, defining the limits of the available history will better enable you to plan your examination and laboratory evaluation. History and testing occupy the ends of a seesaw; as a rule, the lower the quality of one type of data, the greater the need for other types.

SUMMARY

1 A patient's cerebral dysfunction may limit or distort the account of symptoms. When this is suspected, rely more on third-party sources.
2 The key to diagnosis is often found in the temporal profile, especially in the minute details of the onset of symptoms (for example, whether a severe, acute headache began instantaneously like a hammer blow or whether it built up gradually over 10 minutes).
3 Look for a stereotypic character of recurrent symptoms. Changing symptoms should not be minimized, but consistent ones facilitate diagnosis.
4 What are the effects of symptoms on function? Analyze how the patient's practical function has changed in relation to the way the patient feels, and how symptoms and reported function match up with deficits on examination.
5 Pursue an initially confusing or inadequate history by starting afresh. Frequently, the first round of questioning jogs memories or stimulates an awareness that only later proves informative.
6 Subjective data, whether from the history or from the examination, are vital to neurologic diagnosis. Such "soft" data may be as consistent and reliable as more objective examination findings.
7 In "wishing the patient well," beware of "wishful thinking" (which can color the history you record, as well as the diagnostic interpretation you subsequently formulate).
8 Explicitly recognize when the history is not good. ("If you don't have the right history, you don't have the history.") The poorer the historical data in a case, the higher the quality of the data from the examination or laboratory tests must be.

FURTHER READING

Brown, M.M., Hachinski, V.C. Acute confusional states, amnesia, and dementia. In: Wilson, J.D., Braunwald, E., Isselbacher, K.J., *et al.* (eds) *Harrison's Principles of Internal Medicine*. 12th edn. McGraw-Hill, New York (NY), 1991. The syndrome of transient global amnesia and other disorders of memory and attention are summarized, and references provided.

Creditor, M.C. Me and migraine. *N Engl J Med* 1982; 307:1029–32. A physician's personal description of neurologic (classic) migraine symptoms and their changing pattern over four decades.

Glick, T.H. *The Process of Neurologic Care in Medical Practice*. Harvard University Press, Cambridge (MA), 1984, pp. 6–20. Further discussion of pitfalls in neurologic history taking and interpretation of subjective data.

Lancet 1990; 365:93–6, 161–4, 231–4, 291–6, 350–4, 423–7, 486–91, 551–5. (Epilepsy Octet). With reference to the seizure case presented in this chapter, the series on epilepsy appearing in eight issues of the *Lancet* provides readable and concise background information – virtually a microtextbook.

Luria, A.R. *The Man with a Shattered World. The History of a Brain Wound*. Basic Books, New York (NY), 1972. A long collaboration between an eminent neuropsychologist and a brain wound patient produced this personal account of living and learning with major malfunctions.

Sacks, O. *The Man Who Mistook His Wife for a Hat*. Summit Books, New York (NY), 1985, pp. 7–41, 53–5. Cases of visual misunderstanding, memory loss from the Wernicke–Korsakoff syndrome, and loss of "insight" from the nondominant parietal syndrome exemplify ways in which cerebral disorders can affect provision of accurate information.

chapter 2

Background to the Present Illness

Overview: the roots of the present illness

Digging into the past history will often disclose the roots of the present illness. These roots may extend through a genetic lineage (traced in the family history) or may arise from other familial, environmental, social, and past personal sources. The roots may tap the water supply, the food chain, street drugs, and the side effects of medicines prescribed therapeutically. The origins of the present illness may be in the mechanics of an occupational task or in a remote, accidental trauma. A large burden of neurologic disability results from, or is strongly influenced by, trauma, substance abuse, and environmental toxins (see Further reading section).

RISK FACTORS AND EPIDEMIOLOGY

Inapparent epidemics

Good neurologic history taking seeks to uncover these antecedents to the present illness, but even the best individual history will often miss factors unknown to the individual patient. From the perspective of the bedside, most patients appear to be sporadic cases.

CASE 2A
An epidemic of "isolated" cases

A 14-year-old Japanese boy Kenichi Hirano developed gait ataxia, slurred speech, and visual blurring over a 2-week period. Neither the physician in his seaside village nor the specialist at a major referral center found any clue in the history of examination as to the cause of the cerebellar and visual syndrome. Cerebellar tumor with raised intracranial pressure was suspected, but not found.

Only over ensuing weeks and months did it become known that other similar cases were occurring in nearby villages and that, in retrospect, there had been scattered cases in previous months. Eventually, the origin of what turned out to be a large epidemic was traced to the industrial discharge of a methyl mercury compound into Minamata Bay. The toxic organic mercurial reached humans by way of fish and shellfish ingestion.

This composite but representative case illustrates one individual component of the Minamata epidemic of the 1950s, a landmark in the modern annals of epidemiology and neurotoxicity. More recently, sophisticated tools of molecular biology and analytic chemistry have been increasingly applied to genetics and epidemiology to augment the patient and family encounter.

FORMAT OF THE HISTORY

The following issues deserve special emphasis in neurologic cases.

Past medical history: cardiovascular, hematologic, diabetic, "autoimmune" disorders; psychiatric disorders (including suicidality); prior neurologic diseases and trauma, medications, allergies; pre- and perinatal problems, trauma.

Family history: seizures, stroke, tumors; "psychiatric" disorders; movement and gait disorders; signs of neurocutaneous disorders (e.g. birthmarks).

Social history: level of schooling, occupation, domestic situation, environmental exposures, travel, sexual practices, habits (substance abuse), stress.

Review of neurologic symptoms: checklist review of possible neurologic symptoms not elicited in present illness or past medical history (pp. 23–4).

PAST NEUROLOGIC HISTORY

Risk factors: at risk of what?

If you have not yet diagnosed the patient's disease, how can you know whether a given prior condition is a relevant risk factor? You cannot, but

Table 2.1 Risk factors for neurologic disorders

Risk factors, illustrated by:	Acute disorders	Subacute or chronic disorders
Past history		
Hypertension	Stroke (infarct or hemorrhage)	"Subcortical encephalopathy" (periventricular white matter ischemia)
Bleeding disorder/ anticoagulation	Stroke (intracranial hemorrhage)	Subdural hematoma (even without obvious trauma)
Medications (antipsychotic)	Dystonic reaction (such as inability to open mouth)	Parkinsonism; dyskinesias
Atrial fibrillation	Stroke (embolic)	
Myocardial infarction	Anoxic encephalopathy from cardiac arrest; embolic stroke	
Diabetes	Coma (ketoacidosis, hyperosmolar); hypoglycemia	Neuropathies
Family history		
Huntington's disease	Suicide attempt	Movement disorder (chorea); dementia
Social history		
Alcohol abuse	Seizure (withdrawal); trauma	Polyneuropathy (alcoholic–nutritional)
Drug abuse	Seizure; hypoxia from overdose	AIDS (encephalopathy, CNS toxoplasmosis, tumors)
Smoking		CNS metastases from lung
Homelessness	Coma (hypothermia)	Polyneuropathy (malnutrition)
Environmental/ occupational	Trauma; acute intoxications	Nerve entrapment (from repetitive motion); toxic polyneuropathies

CNS, central nervous system.

knowledge of common neurologic risk factors can suggest diagnostic avenues and shift the priorities of your work-up (Table 2.1).

Old labels/new thinking

An unproven diagnostic label in a medical record can actually constitute a risk as well. Unless there is reasonable certainty, carry forward the symptom complex or syndrome that constitutes the patient's problem into your data base (Table 2.2): conditions like multiple sclerosis, tuberculosis, and neurosyphilis provide classic examples of misdiagnosis. AIDS and Lyme disease have joined this family of mimics more recently.

Table 2.2 Pitfalls in the background history

Pitfall	Case
Incomplete data base: history not known to be negative (key: differentiate "unknown," "denied," "documented negative")	A 66-year-old man with a seizure; no known history of alcoholism (but no independent source and no medical records). Cause of seizure suspected when patient developed withdrawal syndrome
Buried past history: (key: a good problem list, computerized data base)	A 38-year-old woman with headaches and blurred vision, but "no past medical problems." Buried in her record of routine visits was a report of a pigmented mole removed 8 years previously. Diagnosis: melanoma metastatic to brain
Over-reliance on past diagnostic labels: an assumption that an unconfirmed impression is, in fact, an established diagnosis. (key: list the symptoms or syndromes as the problem, not the presumed cause)	A 24-year-old man with episodic double vision, dizziness, and limb numbness was treated for multiple sclerosis; reevaluation (demanded by the family 5 years later) revealed a small pontine AVM that was successfully treated by microsurgery
Hidden family history: (key: interview/examine family members; obtain past medical and autopsy records; genetic analysis)	See Case 2C
Social history: risky habits masked by "respectability." (key: open-mindedness, thoroughness)	A prominent suburban businesswoman was admitted for seizures; a work-up for tumor was negative, but it was finally learned that she used cocaine heavily
Environmental and occupational history: pseudo-isolated cases. (key: computerized case data bases and registries)	See Case 2A

AVM, arteriovenous malformation.

CASE 2B
The headaches of a doctor's wife

Olga Balnakoff, a 32-year-old left-handed woman, wife of a general surgeon, had suffered intermittent headaches since late adolescence. Her mother had been treated for migraine. The headaches were pounding and at times more in the right temple, but unaccompanied by other symptoms until the last year when she experienced some associated nausea and vague visual blurring. The headaches had been diagnosed as migraine and treated with limited success until they became much more severe and her menses ceased. This factor eventually prompted a new diagnostic appraisal. Work-up demonstrated a large pituitary tumor that was successfully removed, and she then remained headache free through 5 years of follow-up.

It is not very unlikely that a patient may contract one uncommon disease in the face of another very common one (like migraine).

FAMILIAL NEUROLOGIC DISEASE

Overview

A good family history helps to identify not only genetic problems, but other familial diseases as well. Epilepsy may run in a family on a hereditary basis, but it may also appear in several members in the same or successive generations for other reasons: head injuries from child abuse, a pattern of violent activities, or alcoholism. Toxic environmental exposures, such as lead poisoning, typically affect more than one sibling.

A really searching family history is often necessary to uncover a dominant pattern of inheritance that can be traced from one generation to the next. Because of variations in phenotypic expression, the existence of the disease may not be apparent in certain affected family members. Alternatively, the forebearer at risk may have died before the symptoms manifested themselves or were sufficiently developed to permit a clinical diagnosis. Some hereditary diseases are so stigmatized that their existence in a family member is hidden. The disease is literally "unmentionable." Obtain medical or autopsy records, examine living relatives, and ascertain the availability of genetic and metabolic analyses.

CASE 2C
The uncle nobody knew

John Claridge, a 33-year-old father with two children, was evaluated for personality changes noted by his wife. The examining psychiatrist noted a unique degree of restlessness and a suggestion of involuntary twitching movements. A family history revealed that the patient's father had died at the age of 25 in a motor accident, when the patient was a young child. The father's older brother was said to have been injured in another vehicular accident in a distant state. It was known that he had required prolonged hospitalization, but further reference to him was never made and Claridge grew up without any knowledge of him. Eventually, inquiries established the fact that the uncle had remained chronically institutionalized with a progressive course of mental deterioration and uncontrollable movements, ending in his death at the age of 55. Review of the autopsy record disclosed typical findings of Huntington's disease (Huntington's chorea), a dominantly inherited disease causing personality changes, a movement disorder, and dementia.

The psychiatrist concluded that Claridge might very likely be at risk of Huntington's disease and was probably showing early manifestations. A neurologic referral was made and work-up, including an offer of genetic analysis and counselling, was belatedly initiated.

SOCIAL DETERMINANTS OF NEUROLOGIC ILLNESS

Psychosocial information is sometimes overused in neurologic diagnosis, but more often it is overlooked. Initially show an interest in the patient as a person by asking open-ended questions about daily interests and activities, home, friends, etc. Naïve assumptions about the patient's personal habits will undermine your history. Especially with alcohol, drugs, and sexually related issues, you can afford no presumptions, positive or negative.

ENVIRONMENTAL AND OCCUPATIONAL RISK FACTORS

Overview

Work and environment related diseases and injuries deserve special emphasis because they represent a large proportion of neurologic and other disorders and disabilities. In fact, most diseases and all injuries have an environmental component, but some factors are more obvious than others. In our society trauma is the major cause of loss of economically productive livelihood from neurologic disability. Travel and immigration bring globally common diseases with major neurologic manifestations, such as Hansen's disease (leprosy), cysticercosis, and malaria, to the thresholds of our clinics, but not necessarily to the thresholds of our awareness.

Table 2.3 History taking and preventive neurology (data base and patient education)

Item of history	Example of preventable neurologic damage
Auto safety belt use (and protective headgear for cycling, etc.)	Cranial and spinal fracture; intracranial hemorrhage; brain and cord contusion
Water safety; boating and alcohol; diving in unsafe areas or when inebriated	Quadriplegia, paraplegia, due to neck injury; head injury; drowning and brain damage due to near-drowning
Protective eye gear for racquet sports, chopping, metal work, etc.	Blindness (usually one eye)
Protection against excessive noise	Hearing impairment (usually starts with high-frequency loss)
Smoking	Nervous system metastases from lung and other cancers; hypoxic effects of chronic lung disease
Alcohol and substance abuse	Nervous system trauma; metabolic encephalopathies; polyneuropathy; memory loss; AIDS from contaminated needles
Unsafe sex	AIDS encephalopathy, brain infections, tumors (e.g. toxoplasmosis; lymphoma)
Prescribed medications	Side effects: confusion, myopathies (steroids); neuropathies (chemotherapy); parkinsonism (antipsychotics)

In taking a neurologic history we can do the following.

1 Document a known agent, such as a toxin or dangerous activity, to which the patient is exposed. (Does the patient know "what is in the barrel" at work or on the shelf at home? For example, is there a hydrocarbon solvent that might cause neuropathy?)

Exposure to specific toxin

2 Inquire about types or locations of activities that might bring the individual into contact with harmful factors. Is there a context for environmentally induced disease or injury? For example, did the patient with confusing neurologic symptoms spend a vacation in an area endemic for Lyme disease (a tick-borne spirochetal infection)?

Risky environment

3 Determine whether other family members, co-workers, or companions have had any unusual or unexplained illnesses.

Similar symptoms in companions

You obviously cannot launch major inquiries on every patient with unexplained neurologic symptoms. However, computer technology has enabled greater use of registries and environmental profiles. In addition, public health agencies can undertake investigations once a suspected index case is identified and reported.

The opportunity to take a history is also an opportunity to educate (Table 2.3). As you begin to learn clinical neurology, there is no better time to reaffirm your commitment to prevention.

History and patient education

REVIEW OF NEUROLOGIC SYMPTOMS

In contrast to the initially open-ended and nondirective inquiry of the present illness, this review consists of leading questions that screen for any additional neurologic symptoms or events not already mentioned.

To remember what items to review, follow the general format of the neurologic examination: think about the head and ask about headache and head injury; the eyes bring to mind dim or double vision; the motor examination stimulates questions about weakness or involuntary movements; mental status evaluation reminds you to ask about episodes of loss of consciousness, confusion, forgetfulness, mood, etc. Always use common language, not jargon. A list of symptoms follows.

Symptom screening

Head, neck, cranial nerves	Headaches, head injury
	Abnormal smells or tastes
	Loss or blurring of vision
	Bumping into things on right or left; trouble reading
	Double vision (with right or left eye covered?)
	Numbness of face
	Difficulty chewing or swallowing
	Slurring of speech, twisting or pulling of face, drooling
	Difficulty hearing, dizziness, ringing in the ears
	Change of voice, coughing on food or drink, loss of taste

Motor, coordination	Weakness, inability to use an arm or leg normally Thinning, melting away of muscles Involuntary movements such as shaking, tremors, twitching, jerking Poor balance, trouble walking, staggering, difficulty getting into or out of a chair, bed, or up or down stairs Reeling to one side, sense of being pushed Trouble getting started walking, "freezing" in one's steps Difficulty controlling arms or legs; trouble writing, bringing a cup to one's lips Tightness of muscles or joints, pain with stretching, cramping
Sensory	Numbness, pins and needles, sense of constriction in arms, legs, or body Alteration in sense of hot or cold, burning or hurting body parts without realizing it, unexplained sores Pain, burning Other sensations, spontaneous or induced by touching, rubbing, etc.
Mental status	Fainting, passing out, convulsions Forgetfulness, change of mood, personality, ability to do daily work, sports, or hobbies Depression, suicidal ideation (name specific symptoms) Trouble with speech, comprehending commands, reading, trouble with numbers Getting lost, difficulty following directions Delusions, hallucinations Mind playing "tricks"
Other	Difficulty with urination or bowel movements, sexual difficulties (such as impotence)

In performing a neurologic review of symptoms you will necessarily need to exercise your judgment as to the appropriate degree of thoroughness. In general, the less articulate and forthcoming the patient is regarding the present illness and past medical history, the more meticulous your symptom review should be. Of course, you need not repeat questions already asked in taking the earlier parts of the history.

PROBLEMS FOR SELF-STUDY

Problems

1 A 25-year-old man who works in a motor repair shop has complained of increasing headaches and fatigue over the course of a year. He has also noted episodic tingling in his fingers. What items of additional history would you wish to pursue in particular?

2 A 28-year-old man with no past history of neurologic disease is seen in a mental hospital where he has been admitted in a "catatonic state," not speaking, very stiff, and barely able to move. If you were to investigate his history, what aspects might you emphasize?

Comments

1 While his occupational history might represent a red herring, a full picture of his potential occupational exposures should certainly be obtained, concurrent with a general and neurologic work-up for his symptoms. Many motor shop workers (especially those dealing with batteries, radiators, etc.) are subject to lead exposure which can cause not only headaches but anemia and peripheral neuropathy. Depending on the working conditions, there may be carbon monoxide exposure. In this case the physician determined from family members that the patient's facial appearance had thickened and that his hands seemed "heavier." An old photograph documented the change that had occurred in the last 5 years. He was found to have acromegaly, due to excessive growth hormone from a pituitary tumor which causes gigantism in the growth years. Subsequently, thickening of soft tissues occurs, sometimes with nerve compression at the wrists or elsewhere. His tumor was successfully treated by surgery. Interestingly, however, the work-place investigation initiated at the motor shop revealed significantly elevated lead levels in several workers who did not have headaches or tingling; they were treated and the work safety conditions improved to meet standards.

2 Any prior psychiatric history requires careful review. Clearly, you would want to know exact details of the mode of onset of the condition. Since you would not be able to obtain a verbal or written history from the patient, you would need to determine whether he or she could reply appropriately using some type of yes/no signal to a series of leading questions. A detailed family and environmental/occupational history would be invaluable. Suspicion of an unusual toxin would be pursued by toxicologic testing, not only for the most common agents in routine hospital screening tests, but also by sophisticated chromatographic analyses of body fluids and other tissues, if indicated. Concern about toxic effects would naturally extend to issues of substance abuse. This case represents a "composite" (from the literature) stemming from a landmark epidemic; the patient was found to have used a home-made "designer drug" containing a by-product, MPTP. A toxic metabolite of MPTP caused a dramatic, acute parkinsonism, and has provided the basis for extraordinarily valuable animal models of this condition. This human case turned out to be but one of a number of cases in the area that appeared to be sporadic until epidemiologic case finding was undertaken (Langston *et al.* 1983).

FURTHER READING

Bateman, D., Boughey, A.M., Scaravilli, F., *et al.* A follow-up study of isolated cases of suspected Huntington's disease. *Ann Neurol* 1992; 31:293–8. An approach to diagnosis when the family history is "negative" for a suspected dominant genetic disease and there is no absolute, confirmatory test; compare to the Grafton *et al.* study cited below which evaluates preclinical predictors in patients known to be at risk.

Black, P.McL. Brain tumors. *N Engl J Med* 1991; 324:1471–6, 1555–64. If the case of a pituitary tumor growing amidst a forest of migraine headaches piqued your interest in brain tumors, this review will acquaint you with current concepts and detailed references.

Charness, M.E., Simon, R.P., Greenberg, D.A. Ethanol and the nervous system. *N Engl J Med* 1989; 321:442–54. As a leading risk factor for neurologic disability, alcoholism must be in the forefront of our attention: the multiple alcoholic or alcoholic–nutritional syndromes are reviewed in this article.

Grafton, S.T., Mazziotta, J.C., Pahl, J.J., *et al.* A comparison of neurological, metabolic, structural, and genetic evaluations in persons at risk for Huntington's disease. *Ann Neurol* 1990; 28:614–21. Positron emission tomography (PET) produces evidence of caudate hypometabolism that predicts the development of Huntington's disease in persons at risk better than other methods. Functional neuroimaging is becoming a useful tool for case ascertainment.

Kurtzke, J.F. The current neurologic burden of illness and injury in the United States. *Neurology* 1982; 32:1207–14. This compilation of neurologic disabilities reveals the potential for primary prevention and the need for strong partnerships between specialists and generalists.

Langston, J.W., Ballard, P., Tetrud, J.W., *et al.* Chronic parkinsonism in humans due to a product of meperidine-analog synthesis. *Science* 1983; 219:979–80. Initial report of the landmark epidemiologic investigation that led to the MPTP model of Parkinson's disease.

Rowland, L.P. (ed.) *Merritt's Textbook of Neurology*. 8th edn. Lea and Febiger, Philadelphia (PA), 1989. The importance of environmental neurology (including neurotoxicology) is evidenced by section 22 accorded to this subject.

part 2

Neurologic Examination

chapter 3

An Approach to Neurologic Examination

Introduction

The following chapters are designed to help you learn and improve your neurologic examination skills in a way that makes sense and therefore will be more memorable. Some techniques are best taught by demonstration – by instructors in person or on videotapes. However, demonstrations typically omit nonmechanical aspects of the examination, which will be emphasized here.

1 Understand the goal and rationale for each part of the examination. (What is the point of the Romberg test?)

2 Keep the patient, as a person, in the examination. Take advantage of the participatory, interactive, character of the neurologic examination by working with the patient as an ally.

3 Rely on your powers of observation, your common sense, and your own ingenuity. If a neurologic examination did not exist already you could invent it – and indeed your examination will continue to benefit from on-the-spot innovation.

4 Do not be intimidated by the complexities of the nervous system. (If a true and comprehensive understanding of the nervous system were

required, no one could master the examination. Approach the examination empirically, like a "systems analyst," testing inputs and outputs.
5 Think about prioritizing your examination time, even as you develop a full range of examination skills. The following chapters, including Chapter 19, are designed to help with this.

Neurology comprises behavior and inner experience, motion and emotion, perception and thought. A good neurologic evaluation is inseparable from your approach to the patient as a whole. The neurologic assessment touches on the patient's sense of self. At the same time, the process of evaluation will touch you as a person. You will feel the impact of encountering deformity, disability, and decline. You will also encounter patients who appear normal, and it will be hard to accept the fact that their lives are threatening to come apart because of intermittent events (that you may never witness), like epileptic seizures. Your ability to respond empathetically will help to determine the success of the neurologic assessment, and the therapeutic relationship to follow.

THE MYSTIQUE OF THE NEUROLOGIC EXAMINATION

The neurologic examination has acquired a mystique. Its potential length and apparent complexity often provoke negative reactions, such as avoiding or short-changing it. In fact, the examination is often regarded as an unwanted stepchild of the general physical examination – an offspring that only a neurologist could love!

Empiric and accessible

You may question the adequacy of your preparation to gather and interpret data. "I don't know enough neuroanatomy to understand what I'm doing." By approaching the examination empirically, within a framework of specific goals, you will be able to elicit the findings that are the essential raw material for subsequent interpretation. As you proceed, increasing pathophysiologic understanding will enable not only better interpretation, but also a better sense of priority. (A guide to clinical–anatomic correlations can be found in Chapter 13.)

The neurologic examination is not a monolith. Neurologic assessment is in fact the most open-ended and flexible of all parts of the physical examination. You will notice that your instructors display individual styles as they examine patients. There is no right or wrong method *per se*, only more or less successful ways of eliciting the relevant data within the context of a good clinical relationship.

AN INTERACTIVE EXAMINATION: HELPING THE PATIENT TO HELP YOU

Trust

The creation of mutual trust between examiner and patient is a vital link in the examination process. The more the patient trusts you and understands the purpose of the examination, the better the information that you will obtain. The more you are able to trust the patient's cooperation, the more importance can be attributed to subtle and subjective responses. Your role is not simply to extract, but to enable.

Vulnerability

Patients may be especially guarded about examiners probing their minds, often more so than the so-called "private parts" of their bodies. Feelings are hurt even more easily than flesh. However, a gentle manner, along with some explanation of what you are doing, helps enormously.

Educational value of the examination

Simply being a patient is already an alien experience for many people. The mystifying succession of tests in the neurologic examination often contributes even more to this bewilderment. "Why should the doctor be scratching the bottom of my feet when my head is doing the hurting?" Since patients often find parts of the examination strange, silly, or seemingly irrelevant, some explanation of the purpose of neurologic tests makes them less confusing to the patient, and there will be less chance of erratic responses confusing the examiner. I often explain to new patients that "neurology has to do with the brain and all its connections and functions: the examination will test strength, coordination, and feeling, as well as hearing, eyesight, reflexes, memory, and so on." Patients learn not only from what they are told, but from what they observe during the examination; for example, when are they tense and when do they relax?

FORMAT OF THE CONVENTIONAL EXAMINATION

The standard neurologic examination is understood to include at least some elements of each of the following categories:

1 pertinent parts of the head, neck, and general examination;
2 cranial nerve functions;
3 motor (excluding coordination);
4 sensory (including primary and discriminative modalities);
5 coordination;
6 reflexes (tendon, superficial, and "pathologic");
7 mental status, behavior, and other higher cortical functions (special examinations appropriate to particular problems).

Order of the examination

I suggest starting with a conventional sequence, as given above. This order, which will be adhered to in the following chapters, is quite arbitrary and can be altered at will. The placement of the mental status and behavioral examinations last does not diminish their importance. In fact, as you will see, much of this evaluation is intertwined with history taking and earlier parts of the examination. Strategies for adapting the order of the examination to your immediate needs and for integrating the neurologic with the general examination will be outlined in Chapter 11.

Tools

The following is a checklist of basic instruments and disposable items you will need in the course of the examination.

Ophthalmoscope–otoscope
Stethoscope

Reflex hammer
Pocket screening card for visual acuity
Scent for testing smell (e.g. cloves or other spice)
Pocket flashlight
Tuning forks (128 Hz for vibratory testing; 512 Hz for testing hearing – alternatively, a 256 Hz tuning fork can serve both purposes, but neither as well)
A cloth or paper tape measure
Supplies of disposables (safety pins – see Chapter 7; tongue blades; throat swabs)

Before starting your examination, lay out your tools, so that you will not need to search for them. After using a tool, put it away. Thus, any remaining tools at the end will remind you of omissions!

Positioning

Each of the following chapters will describe how to position the patient for a neurologic test. However, most tests can be done in any position: lying, sitting, standing. Which position you choose should depend upon the patient's comfort and your efficiency. In general, I prefer the patient to be sitting, legs dangling over the edge of the bed or examination table.

AN EMPIRICAL APPROACH TO NEUROLOGIC TESTING

A good place to start is to confront a patient who cannot be examined in the usual way.

CASE 3A
An exploration

A 21-year-old man, Alfred Peers, was brought to me for an updated neurologic evaluation. Since early childhood he carried the diagnosis of autism (a condition or group of conditions in which there is failure, to a variable degree, of development of speech and social behavior). Alfred would not sit still for any of the usual maneuvers of the examination. For every (unsuccessful) attempt I would make to look in his eyes or test a reflex, he would examine some part of my clothing, such as my socks.

In the course of these interactions I found that I was able to learn quite a lot about this neurologic function simply by observing his activity (just as pediatricians learn by observation much of what they need to know neurologically about young children). I could tell that his arms and legs were quite well coordinated, he had good balance, and he possessed sharp eyesight and hearing. In fact, he was also able to communicate swiftly, but to a limited extent, by a somewhat exclusive sign language known to an attendant who accompanied him from his institutional residence. At the end of the session I felt that I had acquired significant data relevant to his physical neurologic functions without ever completing most of the standard tests. I had learned a very modest amount about his mental and behavioral status (in addition to the wealth of observations that his attendant could relate from prolonged experience), but his autism remained largely enigmatic. I wonder how much Alfred Peers learned about me?

Just as I met my match in trying to do a formal examination on Alfred, you may feel overmatched in undertaking a neurologic examination on certain patients (see also pp. 397–416). Rely on your own powers of observation. As mentioned earlier, you could construct most of the neurologic examination yourself. With no background knowledge, you could set out to learn as much as possible about the structure and function of your patient. As in my improvised approach to Alfred Peers, you might rely, first of all, on observing spontaneous activity and behavior. Then you would go on to apply simple stimuli and measure responses to them. To describe the patient's reaction to a pinprick does not require an understanding of the physiologic connection between stimulus and response. For beginning purposes, you can regard the nervous system as the proverbial "black box": its performance can be characterized even if you cannot see within it or diagram its operational pathways. Create and analyze an exchange of inputs and outputs oriented to empiric discovery. Put yourself in the role of a systems analyst, applying your powers of observation, initiative, common sense, and analytical capacities, rather than relying only upon a time-honored set of tests.

Inventing an examination

Systems analyst

THE TEST SYSTEM: CHAINS OF FUNCTION

The goal of examination is to help expose and characterize abnormal function in order to predict lesions, particularly their location. But abnormalities observed in the neurologic examination, while always signifying something wrong within the test system, do not always represent neurologic dysfunction. The test system encompasses not only the patient but the examiner.

Let us take mobility as an example. We know that the physical activities of daily life require the use not only of muscles, but of bones, joints, tendons, etc. Mobility also depends upon motivation, effort, coordination, and balance. Thus, abnormal motor activity may be in the mind as well as the muscle, in a tendon as well as a tract. Moreover, how well a patient moves sometimes depends on outside stimuli (such as your attitude or behavior) that influence the patient's conscious or unconscious mental input to movement.

Components of performance

Any test system involves:

1 the examiner/observer as a part of an interactive test situation;

2 the patient as a human being, with ideas, feelings, motivation, etc., that influence responses;

3 extraneurologic factors such as joint mechanics, that may affect the function being tested;

4 a neurologic chain of function.

Inputs and outputs

Most tests involve a sequence of interactions, often beginning with the input of the examiner to the patient and ending with the observation or measurement by the examiner of the patient's output. Experiment with a variety of inputs: for example, if you wish to demonstrate that a patient can identify a bell, the input stimulus might be visual, auditory, or tactile. Or, discover what outputs a patient can utilize to respond to just one of the above inputs: can the patient name, spell, match, or show how to use it? When an abnormality of output (performance) is recognized, we then aim to isolate and expose the specific deficits within the chain of function.

Testing a system

Even a relatively simple, uncomplicated test, such as measuring hearing with a tuning fork, depends upon more than just the patient's auditory perception.

1 The examiner must communicate the task ("signal when the sound is heard, and when it is no longer heard").

2 The patient must have adequate hearing capacity to pick up the sound (which depends on the structures of the middle and inner ears, acoustic nerves, etc.).

3 The patient must be aware of hearing the sound in order to generate an output. (A sound can be physiologically registered in brainstem and subcortical structures and can be electronically detectable, or cause autonomic responses, and yet it may not be consciously recognized by the patient.)

4 The patient must be able to communicate to the examiner an accurate response.

Chain of function

The test may fail at any link in the chain of function. (Of course, a linear chain represents an oversimplification in many instances, but is useful conceptually.) In the hearing test, a deaf patient might miss the instruction! A confused patient might not concentrate well enough to keep the task in mind. When you test hearing as part of the neurologic examination, do not just think "neurologically," or you will one day forget about checking for wax, fluid, or a foreign body in the ear!

The following process applies to each part of the examination.

1 State the goal as a specific question. (Knowing that your hearing is normal, ask yourself whether the patient can hear with each ear as soft a sound as you can.)

2 Choose a method of testing appropriate to the goal and to the patient's situation. (Strike a 512 Hz tuning fork, hold it to each ear, determining when the patient can no longer hear the sound and whether, at that point, you still can.)

3 Isolate the link in the chain of function that is under scrutiny. Try to check for other variables, ensuring that the room is quiet, the ear canals

are clear, the eardrums are normal in appearance, and the patient is attentive and understands the instruction. Then, if the hearing threshold is increased, you know that the problem is internal to the eardrums. Additional tests can localize further.

Experienced clinicians do not, of course, formally outline this sequence every time they perform and interpret a neurologic test, since the method becomes ingrained. But until this is second nature, articulate the rationale of the tests you are conducting.

STANDARDS OF NORMAL FUNCTION

"I've examined the patient, but how do I know whether these findings are normal?" Unfortunately, there are no easy answers. Since you cannot yet rely on your personal experience, you will need to make the most of comparisons with certain standards or benchmarks. Does the patient's performance show any deviation from the following points?

Benchmarks

1 General expectations (is there a full range of eye movements from side to side?).
2 Standards appropriate to the patient's subgroup of the population, such as age group (is the shortened stride and decreased fluidity of gait normal for an 80-year-old?).
3 The patient's own standard of normal, as judged by past performance (has handwriting changed?) or by comparison with another part of the patient's body?

Patient as own control

As a practical approach, you will find it easiest to start by employing the patient as his or her own control. Compare performance on a given test with the criteria listed below.

1 Subjective assessment of past abilities ("I was always a whiz with numbers"; "I was always kind of clumsy – in typing class I was slower than anyone else").
2 Descriptive assessments from other observers. ("His memory amazed people – he was able to recall telephone numbers or people's names, but now he is forgetful").
3 Past neurologic examinations ("2 years ago all her tendon reflexes were recorded as 3+ on a scale of 0–4+; now they are absent.)

Compare one part of the body with another:

1 right vs. left;
2 arms vs. legs;
3 proximal limbs vs. distal;
4 upper trunk vs. lower;
5 head vs. body;
6 axial (head, neck, and trunk) vs. appendicular (limb and limb girdle);
7 extensor muscles vs. flexors.

Comparison of different body parts is very helpful, but the interpretation of results needs to be tempered by recognition of pitfalls.

1 Lack of equivalence: right vs. left, because of handedness; topographic differences, as from distal to proximal (sensory discrimination is better on the hand than the upper arm); regional differences, as between legs and arms (the major muscle groups of the thighs are larger and stronger than those of the arms).
2 Bilaterial dysfunction (a mild weakness of both sides of the face can be missed if there is no asymmetry).

THE EVOLVING EXAMINATION

Since a single examination represents only a static or cross-sectional view of structure and function, you will typically need to extend your findings by ongoing observations – a kind of examination over time.

Seizure case revisited

In Case 1A, the patient's subjective experience of a focal seizure was not reflected initially in any abnormalities of examination. Subsequently, the physician actually witnessed another seizure episode. What the initial examination did not reveal, further observation made plain. The witnessed convulsion established a clear connection between her profound subjective experience, which had been so difficult for her to explain in the history, and events that her physician could observe. Her inner experiences could not be shared, but her own symptoms and her physician's observations were now on common ground.

Two points deserve emphasis.
1 Think of the neurologic examination not as a static group of tests, but as one frame in a moving picture.
2 As you examine patients, your findings will not confirm or contradict symptoms, but rather supplement them as ways to understand the patient's problem.

EXAMINATION DISCOMFORT AND INJURY

In the neurologic examination, as in other parts of the physical examination, the need for great care and gentleness is obvious, but sometimes slighted. The pin and hammer may seem like benign tools to you, but they may be threatening to some patients, especially those who are paralyzed, unable to communicate, or just feeling vulnerable. While sick patients are especially susceptible, even healthy individuals may be hurt when physical or mental probing reveals a sore spot on the skin or psyche.

Anticipating discomfort

Before starting the examination, inquire for areas of pain or tenderness. Reassure the patient that you will be careful and protective. Conduct all potentially painful testing in a graded fashion, increasing its intensity only in accordance with the patient's abilits to tolerate it. If pain is anticipated, let the patient exercise as much control over testing as possible. (For example, in testing strength, let the patient push against you rather than vice versa.)

Protecting yourself

Conversely, you also run a small risk of being hurt in your role as examiner, although this occurs infrequently and most instances are unintended. A patient's grip may be unexpectedly powerful. A knee jerk will occasionally explode as a sudden, swift kick! You should always be alert to disinhibited or simply overexuberant patients who might, for example, unexpectedly move during funduscopic examination or wrench your hand or fingers during strength testing. Take sensible precautions, but remember that your own calm manner will have an important calming effect. For your protection as well as the patient's, pins for pain sensation testing should never be reused (see Chapter 7).

PRACTICING THE EXAMINATION AND EXAMINING IN PRACTICE

A repertoire of tests

How comprehensive should a neurologic examination be? How much of this will be applicable in medical practice? As already implied, the neurologic examination is never complete; some further angle of testing can always be imagined, especially in the realms of mental status and behavior. In fact, most seasoned clinicians adopt a problem-oriented approach: omit parts of the examination (such as smell, gag, etc.) if these functions do not seem pertinent. Augment the examination when indicated (such as more detailed cognitive testing in a patient with suspected dementia). For learning purposes, I believe that it is important to try out all parts of the basic, comprehensive examination, but not all of its elaborations. For example, only after you have tested corneal reflexes a number of times will you have confidence in your ability to do so reliably when needed. In your later training and practice you will probably not test corneal reflexes routinely, but you should have this test in your repertoire in case you recognize an indication for it. Thus, in presenting the basic neurologic examination I will not omit standard parts, even though they may be somewhat less useful than others. (In Chapter 19 suggestions are made for a rational and pragmatic approach to screening, selective, and augmented examinations that can be fit to the needs of routine practice.)

Screening and selective examinations

Relying on basics

By the same token, many embellishments on the basic examination (often sanctified by eponyms) will not be presented (see Further reading section). When I carry out a neurologic examination I stick to basics in the vast majority of cases and use straightforward methods to meet my objectives. When I alter a technique it is not usually a fancy refinement, but a modification that makes common sense in terms of the particular patient I am seeing.

A NOTE ON THE EXAMINATION OF INFANTS AND YOUNG CHILDREN

This book does not include the pediatric neurologic examination for several reasons. Most importantly, this examination is best learned and makes most sense within the context of pre- and postnatal growth and development. Since this context is at the heart of pediatric experience of the medical student, it is quite pointless to discuss the examination without relating to these issues in some detail. Secondly, many specific findings depend upon a substantive knowledge of pediatric diseases that represent a special data base that is well beyond the present scope. Finally, the examination of the neonate and infant cannot capitalize upon the kind of interactive skills that represent a major emphasis in this book. Nonetheless, a key to the pediatric neurologic examination is the ability to observe behavior – motor, affective, communicative, etc. The ability to observe, not only freely but also in a planned fashion directly linked to specific examination goals, constitutes a major thrust of the following chapters.

SUMMARY

1. Memorize the standard format of the neurologic examination (more detail is given in subsequent chapters and is laid out and illustrated in Chapter 11). The order of the examination or write-up may be altered.
2. As you learn more about the examination think about how each test relates to your everyday experience of human function. How do you manifest strength and coordination? What is your awareness of sensory experience? How can the examination be supplemented to improve the profile of the patient's true physical and mental capability?
3. If you ever underwent neurologic tests as part of a physical examination, reflect on what it was like for you, or ask friends or family about their own experiences.
4. Think about what parts of the general physical examination require responses from the patient. Compare these with the interactions that will enable testing of motor and sensory functions, mental status, etc.
5. As you improve your examination skills, assess the usefulness of the data you obtain from each part of the neurologic examination. What are the high-yield components? Compare your ideas with the priorities highlighted in chapter summaries and the suggestions for screening and selective examinations in Chapter 19.

PROBLEMS FOR SELF-STUDY

Problems

1 A 44-year-old man complains of shadows in his vision in the right eye. What steps of evaluation would you propose (realizing that you may not have learned a formal eye examination as yet, but utilizing a general, systematic approach)?

2 A 31-year-old woman complains of pain and trouble moving her arm after a fall. What capabilities would you evaluate?

Comments

1 After obtaining a history of the characteristics and time course, it would be important to ascertain whether the symptoms really arise from the right eye (and only the right eye) by covering each eye in turn. Once established as a monocular problem, one systematic approach might follow the path of light from the outside in. Assuming there is no problem with a contact lens, could there be a problem in the cornea, the lens, or in the fluid chambers of the eyeball? Could it be a retinal or optic nerve problem? The next step would be to assess your own capabilities for evaluating each segment of the visual path that might be involved. For example, if skilled with the ophthalmoscope, you could examine each visible part of the eye, but would need to recognize the severe limitations of your examination, vis-à-vis what an expert could see with a slit lamp, etc. At the least, you could shine a flashlight and look for gross opacification of the cornea. Shifting to the patient's point of view, you should test his or her ability to see out of each eye separately, reading newsprint, and describing objects at a distance.

Thus, the most important skills are to approach a problem systematically, to recognize one's own limitations, and to find the right help. Not even very experienced generalists or neurologists should feel confident that their examination with a direct ophthalmoscope would be sufficient to rule out a partial or incipient retinal detachment, which would be a significant possibility in this case example. An ophthalmologist is needed, not only for experience but because of the technology commanded.

2 The history should emphasize any preexisting conditions, especially neck or shoulder problems, as well as the exact circumstances of the fall. An accidental fall may be the cause of a nonneurologic deficit, or result from a neurologic event, such as a stroke or seizure. Whether the fall was primary or secondary, you would want to determine whether there is pain, tenderness to palpation, and a full range of motion at the neck, shoulder, elbow, and wrist joints. Check pulses, then test the power of all the major muscular actions of the right arm and shoulder. Even in the presence of pain and tenderness, ascertain how much strength can be exerted, realizing that pain limits effective effort. By lightly stroking the skin of the arm ascertain whether any

areas feel different (numb). If so, map out the boundaries. In this particular case example, the fall resulted from a convulsive seizure (of which the patient had no direct knowledge). The convulsion also caused a dislocation of the shoulder (with secondary peripheral nerve damage).

FURTHER READING

Haerer, A.F. *De Jong's The Neurologic Examination*. 5th edn. Lippincott, Philadelphia (PA), 1992. A recently revised edition of this encyclopedic reference on the examination.

Katzman, R., Rowe, J.W. *Principles of Geriatric Neurology*. F.A. Davis, Philadelphia (PA), 1992. What is normal? A difficult question in general, but especially in the elderly. In this volume you will find normative data on aging, the neurologic examination in the patient over 80, and other relevant topics.

chapter 4

General Neurologic Examination of the Head and Neck

Introduction

The general and neurologic physical examinations are closely intertwined. In regard to the head and neck, the distinction is quite arbitrary, and testing can occur as part of either the general or neurologic examination. This chapter will emphasize three aspects of the general head and neck examination that are especially important neurologically.

Vascular

1 The vascular examination of the head and neck (Table 4.1). The main purpose is to find signs of disease in the aortocranial vessels (principally the carotid arteries) that might cause stroke. Although noninvasive laboratory tests (ultrasonic imaging and Doppler or magnetic resonance angiograms) can define arterial patency better, these tests are not presently appropriate for general medical screening purposes. Palpation and auscultation can quickly pick up signs of trouble that may warrant further investigation. A normal examination does not rule out disease, however.

Cervical spine

2 Mobility, posture, and tenderness of the neck. Neck stiffness is potentially a very serious complaint, since it may be a sign of meningitis. Neck disorders that cause impingement on the spinal canal threaten the cervical spinal cord and hence all neurologic functions below the neck.

Table 4.1 Vascular examination of the neck

Technique	Comment
Palpation	
Assess pulse along course of vessel, low to mid to upper neck; scale of 0–4+	Pulse cut-off in upper neck: ?Internal carotid disease; correlate with facial/temporal pulses
Auscultation	
Listen for arterial bruit (use diaphragm and/or bell); specify timing, duration (e.g. early systolic); pitch; localization (e.g. low neck); identify origin and extent by "inching" (see text); record localization	Mid to high neck, long duration, high pitch, soft bruits are most ominous (see Table 4.2). A bruit over the carotid artery that is similar to and continuous with a radiating cardiac murmur or bruit heard over the upper chest is not of internal carotid origin
Jugular venous hum? Light compression of upper neck with finger, occluding venous return, obliterates hum	Jugular hum: AVM of brain? Auscultate orbits, cranium; other hums: hyperdynamic circulation (e.g. pregnancy) and thyroid origin
Auscultate (with bell) over supraclavicular fossae; correlate bruit with BP in both arms; check synchrony and symmetry of radial pulses	Bruit may be from subclavian, innominate, or common carotid arteries; decreased BP or pulse or delayed pulses on one side: ?subclavian disease

AVM, arteriovenous malformation; BP, blood pressure.

Ocular fundi

3 The eye is a window to the brain and the vascular system: examination of the eye can help identify systemic conditions (such as hypertension) that can be treated, preventing or minimizing visual and neurologic loss. The optic disc may show a variety of important changes, including papilledema, which usually indicate nonacute, increased intracranial pressure. (The fundus examination could well be included in the section on CN 2 in Chapter 5, but is presented here because of its broad relevance to the general examination.)

Work-up of the following case depended on data from the general and vascular examination of the neck and from observation of the ocular fundus.

CASE 4A
Fiddler's transient ischemic attack (TIA)

Bruit: turbulent arterial flow sound

Mel Branch, a 66-year-old right-handed amateur violinist, experienced two episodes of right hand tingling and weakness, each related to playing his fiddle. Fifteen years previously he had been successfully treated for a thyroid tumor by radical neck surgery and irradiation.

Palpation of the left side of the neck revealed a surgical scar, lack of underlying muscle, and pulsation of the carotid artery lying just beneath the skin. Auscultation at this site revealed a bruit (pronounced "brew-ee"). With placement of his violin in playing position, the chin rest pressed back on the carotid artery. His physician diagnosed TIAs in the left cerebral hemisphere, due to carotid artery narrowing (stenosis) and extrinsic compression (confirmed by imaging tests). He switched from the violin to the cello.

TIA

Two years later he had an episode of visual blurring in his left eye. Prompt examination revealed an occlusion of a small branch of the central retinal artery (CRA), which arises from the ophthalmic artery, a branch of the internal carotid artery. The retinal ischemic episode was due to embolism, presumably from the atherosclerotic plaque at the origin of the left internal carotid artery. Surgery (endarterectomy) to remove the atherosclerotic plaque, thereby opening up the severe stenosis of the internal carotid artery, was elected and successfully performed.

The methods of examination of the vessels of the neck and fundi will be presented in the next two sections.

VASCULAR EXAMINATION OF THE NECK: CAROTID ARTERIES

As in Case 4A, the status of the internal carotid artery is usually the object of greatest concern:

Goals

1 identification of bruits and pulse changes suggestive of vascular stenosis (see Fig. 4.1);

2 detection of pulse changes (without bruits) suggestive of complete arterial occlusion.

Before studying the techniques of palpation and auscultation, be forewarned: you often cannot be sure from which vessel a pulsation or bruit is emanating – the internal carotid, the external carotid, or the common carotid artery. The exact position and strength of pulsation of these arteries in the neck differ from patient to patient. Some arteries have congenital loops or kinks and some develop tortuosity later in life; the precise level of the common carotid bifurcation varies. Describe first what you feel and hear, and only secondarily draw inferences as to the origin and meaning of these findings. If you recognize local abnormalities, weigh the benefits, risks, and costs of laboratory/radiographic tests to characterize the suspected lesion.

Carotid palpation technique

After explaining that you are going to feel the pulse in the neck, palpate the carotid artery with one or two fingers. Do so lightly in order not to compress it or activate the carotid sinus reflex. Never palpate the right and left sides simultaneously. After identifying the pulse, follow it upward and downward through its full extent in the neck (see Table 4.1). Occasionally, you may feel a "thrill," the palpable counterpart of a bruit.

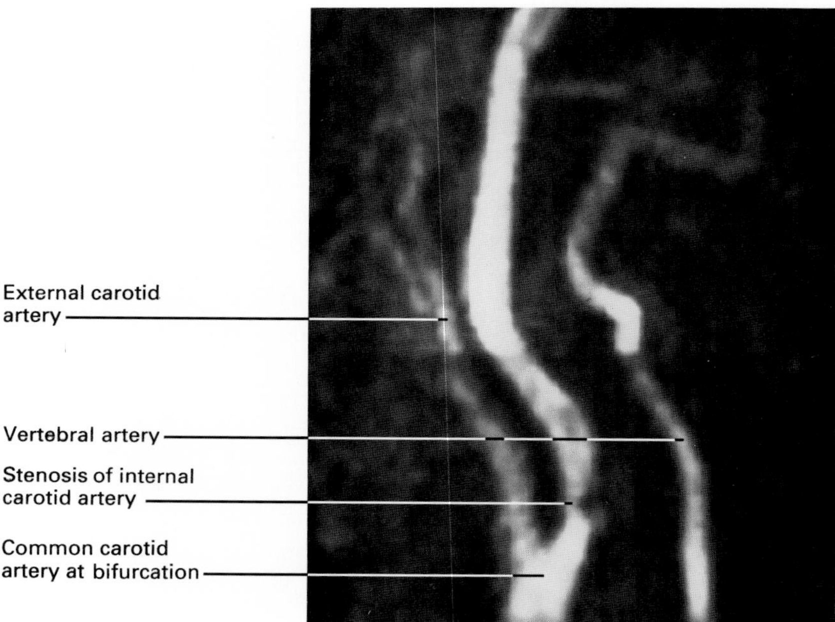

Fig. 4.1 Carotid artery in the neck. A magnetic resonance angiogram noninvasively reveals the bifurcation of the common carotid artery into the external carotid branch and the stenotic internal carotid. The vertebral artery is also seen. (Courtesy of Jonathan Kramer MD.)

Auscultation technique

As in listening to the heart, the stethoscope bell is better for low frequencies and the diaphragm better for high-pitched sounds. The fact that high-frequency bruits are harder to hear and generally more significant favors use of the diaphragm. However, you may succeed in getting a better fit against the tissues of the neck with your bell. As in cardiac auscultation, listen consciously for sounds through a wide range of frequencies.

Localization of a bruit

To help distinguish the origin of a bruit do the following:

1 establish the lowest, most proximal, point where you can hear the bruit (or transmitted murmur) over the neck or chest;

2 define the continuity of the bruit from its origin up to the angle of the jaw. Are there changes in pitch or amplitude?

Bruits originating from the take-off of subclavian or brachiocephalic arteries are usually best heard in the supraclavicular fossae, but may radiate widely into the neck. Bruits that arise from the origin of the common carotid artery are of maximum amplitude low in the neck and usually diminish toward the angle of the jaw. Loud bruits of this type sometimes mask softer (but more significant) bruits arising from the carotid bifurcation.

Table 4.2 Clinical correlations of carotid examination

	Internal carotid stenosis: moderate-grade (moderate narrowing)	Internal carotid stenosis: high-grade (severe narrowing)	Internal carotid stenosis: complete occlusion
Palpable pulse	Usually normal	May feel cut-off above stenosis	May feel cut-off above occlusion
Bruit			Absent (see text)
Frequency (pitch)	Low (gruff)	High (blowing, whispery)	
Duration	Short, early systolic	Long systolic, or systolic–diastolic	
Amplitude	Often loud	Often soft, occasionally inaudible	
Origin (site of detection)	Upper neck (loud, harsh bruit may radiate widely)	Upper neck (under angle of jaw)	Transmitted murmurs and common carotid bruits still audible in neck

Clinical correlation

Gruffer, lower-frequency, but sometimes very loud, early systolic bruits typically have "more bark than bite," whereas long, high-pitched, blowing or whispery bruits are more likely to correlate with tight stenosis (see Table 4.2).

Bruits vs. venous hums

A low-pitched hum of venous origin can be mistaken for a bruit (see Table 4.1). A venous hum of jugular origin can be diminished or obliterated by more rostral pressure against the vascular bundle that is sufficient to occlude the jugular vein but not the carotid artery. While a jugular venous hum may not have pathologic significance, it can provide a clue to major intracranial arteriovenous shunting, as exists in vascular malformations (see Case 1A).

Example of vascular examination

In the examination of Mel Branch (see Case 4A) the left carotid pulse (felt just under the skin) was 4+ (scale 0, 1+, 2+, 3+, 4+) from the base of the neck to the upper neck where it suddenly diminished, as did the transmitted heart sounds. At that point, and radiating upward, there was a soft, almost pansystolic, moderately high-pitched "blowing" bruit, without a thrill. No radiating cardiac murmur or supraclavicular bruit was heard. The superficial temporal pulses were 2+ bilaterally. The right carotid was 2+ with no bruit.

The external carotid artery branches

The palpable branches of the external carotid artery (Fig. 4.2) are of importance to the neurologic examination in two main respects.

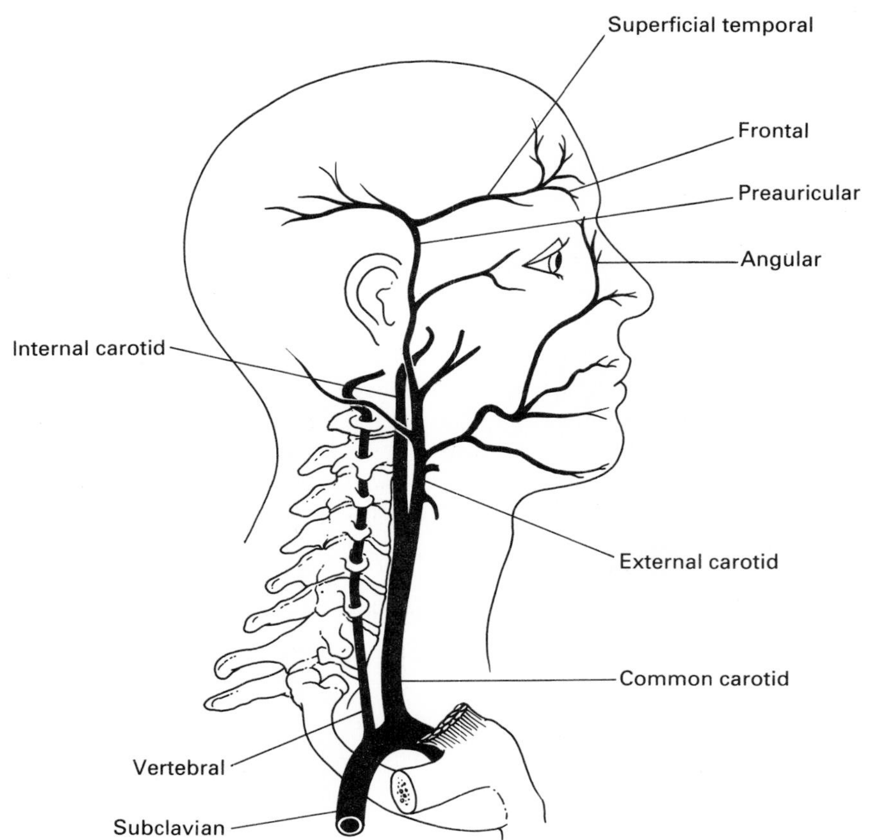

Fig. 4.2 External carotid artery with superficial branches in the face and scalp. Note the superficial temporal, preauricular, and other palpable branches. The right common carotid artery is shown arising from the brachiocephalic trunk, and then bifurcating in the mid neck. The internal carotid has no branches in the neck. The vertebral artery originates from the subclavian.

Pulse changes

1 A decreased pulse in the face or temple usually signifies common or external carotid disease. An increased pulse may reflect increased collateral flow (via the orbit) to a compromised internal carotid.

2 Signs of inflammation provide clues to local or systemic arteritis, as in the syndrome of temporal arteritis which may cause headache, visual loss, etc. Suspicion of temporal arteritis requires emergency work-up and treatment (usually corticosteroids).

Signs of temporal arteritis

To identify signs of inflammation in the superficial temporal artery, look for any redness of the overlying skin of the temple. Palpate for tenderness and for reduced compressibility; the inflammatory changes of arteritis make the artery less pliant.

THE SUBCLAVIAN ARTERIES AND BRANCHES

The subclavian arteries give rise to the vertebral arteries (see Fig. 4.2) that channel blood to the posterior fossa and posterior parts of the cerebral hemispheres. The subclavians are indirectly tested as follows.

Testing

1 Palpate the brachial or radial pulses, checking for symmetry and synchrony; a weaker or delayed pulse suggests stenosis proximally, often at the subclavian origin.
2 Compare the blood pressure in the two arms.
3 Listen for bruits in the supraclavicular fossae (just posterior to the clavicles).

Clinical correlations

Narrowing or occlusion of the proximal subclavian or even the proximal vertebral arteries does not necessarily produce any brainstem signs or symptoms. More distal cervical branches of the vertebrals can receive collateral blood supply. Subclavian disease causing insufficiency of blood supply to the arm produces muscular fatigue, sometimes pain, numbness, and even pallor, as well as pulse and blood pressure deficits. Be sure to distinguish this peripheral vascular syndrome from central nervous system ischemia. (Intracranial occlusion of one or both vertebral arteries often leads to stroke. One of the most notable types is the lateral medullary syndrome; see Chapter 14.)

THE CERVICAL SPINE

Objectives

The general approach to the spinal examination can be summarized with three questions.
1 Is there abnormal posture?
2 Is there a full range of motion?
3 Is there tenderness, or pain with motion?

Testing

Before starting any examination, determine whether there has been any trauma that might have caused a fracture or dislocation. If so, or if there is severe pain, protect the neck and avoid manipulating it until imaging is done. To begin the examination, observe whether the neck is held in an unnatural posture – held stiffly, tilted, or drooping? Can the patient turn, flex, and extend the head through a full range of motion? Is there palpable muscle tightening, resistance, and pain with motion? If the patient's active movement reveals any limitations or guarding against pain, gently move the head in all planes to feel the character and degree of resistance. On palpating the soft tissues of the neck, is there tenderness or swelling?

When examining the bony spine posteriorly, you can press the vertebrae (the spinous processes) and also percuss over each bone, down the spine, with a couple of fingers or carefully with your fist. The jarring of percussion may elicit pain not discovered by palpation.

Clinical correlation

If head posture is abnormal and painful, the usual cause is muscle spasm, either because of local inflammation or because of irritation of the nerve supply. Other mechanisms include pathology of a vertebra or intervertebral joints (such as dislocation, fracture, or arthritis), weakness of supporting muscle groups, and dystonias (abnormal muscle contraction usually associated with medication reactions or other "extrapyramidal" disorders; see Chapter 14). Focal tenderness to percussion of the spinous processes is an important finding in cases of spinal abscess (especially epidural), injury to the bone, and sometimes tumor.

Pitfall

The most difficult problem in interpreting the examination arises from "guarding," a mainly involuntary reaction to pain or anticipated pain. Guarding limits range of motion and muscular effort and is perceived by the examiner as abnormal resistance. Guarding serves as an important sign of pain, but is nonspecific as to cause. Since guarding frustrates a thorough examination, you should place more reliance on imaging and other tests. The "stiff neck" (resistance to flexion) that occurs in meningitis, is an example of involuntary guarding and should be distinguished from generalized rigidity in all planes of movement.

The same general methods and issues apply to the lower spine. Observe sitting and standing posture, as well as bending and turning at the waist in all directions. With forward bending, look for scoliosis (lateral curvature of the spine) by noting any curve in the line formed by the visible spinous processes.

In Chapter 19 a general approach to neurologic examination in cases of spine pain is offered, as well as additional methods for the examination of the patient with low back and leg pain. For more information on the general examination of the spine and other skeletal structures, consult your physical diagnosis text, or medical, neurologic, or orthopedic texts.

Meningeal and nerve root irritation

The signs of meningeal irritation are produced by inflammatory processes, usually due to infection. The cardinal sign is a limitation of head flexion resulting from spasm of the posterior neck muscles. This occurs in response to the inflamed state of the two inner meningeal layers (the pia–arachnoid) and the contiguous nerve roots. Patients may prefer to lie with their legs partially flexed to diminish traction on the spinal meninges and nerve roots.

Testing for meningeal irritation

After observing the patient's neck and leg posture, as well as general behavior (see below), the first test is to ask the patient to bend his or her head forward and down, so that the chin will touch the chest. If the patient experiences any difficulty with this at all (or is unable to participate actively), gently flex the patient's head in this fashion, so that you can feel any resistance. Meningitis usually produces less resistance to extension or sideways deviation or rotation of the head than to forward flexion.

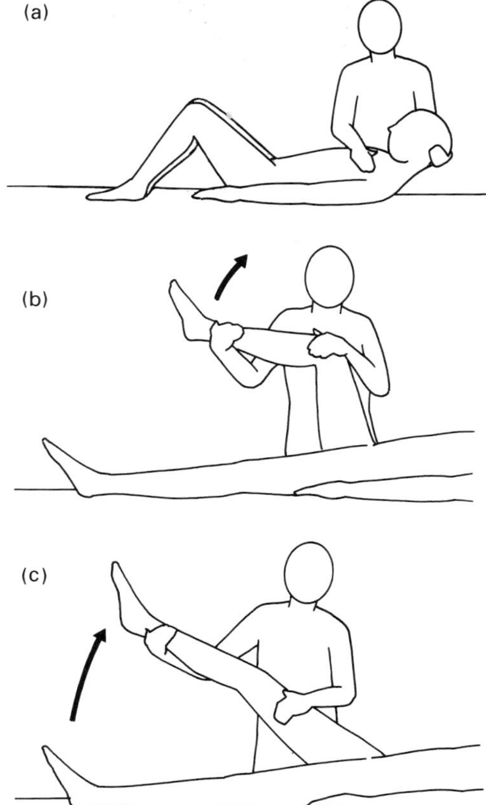

Fig. 4.3 Tests for meningeal irritation. (a) Flexing the neck to demonstrate rigidity; flexion of the knees in reaction to head flexion is the Brudzinski sign. (b) Extending the knee with the thigh flexed at the hip causes resistance and pain (the Kernig sign). (c) Flexing the thigh with the knee extended (straight leg raising) is countered by resistance and pain (another way of eliciting the Kernig sign). Straight leg raising is also used to evaluate irritation of a lower lumbosacral root (as from a herniated disc); see Chapter 19.

Kernig and Brudzinski signs

The other principal meningeal signs follow from the responses described above (Fig. 4.3). Since there is a tendency for the legs to be flexed for greater comfort, it is not surprising that an attempt to flex the thigh with the leg straight at the knee might cause pain, resistance, and involuntary flexion at the knee. Similarly, if both the thigh and knee are flexed, an attempt to extend the leg at the knee will meet resistance and cause pain along the leg or spine. These reactions are called the Kernig sign. In similar fashion, if you flex the neck of the patient with meningeal irritation, the thighs and legs will show a tendency to flex. This is called the Brudzinski sign. Rather than making a point of remembering these eponyms, you should simply be aware of the characteristic responses of the neck and legs to stretching of inflamed meninges and nerve roots by means of the maneuvers described. All of these reactions occur bilaterally, although they may be asymmetric. In Chapter 19 you will encounter similar tests performed to evaluate focal nerve root irritation, as produced by disc disease in the lower back. One of these is the straight leg raising test (see Fig. 4.3c).

Clinical correlation

Meningeal signs due to a generalized meningeal inflammation, such as a bacterial or viral meningitis, will typically be accompanied by headache, fever, sensitivity of the eyes to light (photophobia), and often delirium or lethargy. The latter may advance to stupor or coma. (Some patients experience more pain in the spine than in the head, but the lay term "spinal meningitis" should not suggest an infection limited to the meninges of the spine.)

Meningeal signs usually indicate a widespread meningitis, but are occasionally found with local inflammatory conditions. Much more commonly, you will need to distinguish neck rigidity due to arthritis or parkinsonism from meningitis. In meningeal inflammation the predominance of limitation and guarding upon head flexion, the presence of other meningeal signs, and the behavioral characteristics that accompany symptoms of meningitis will be helpful. In early meningitis, you cannot count on the full array of characteristic physical signs. At the other end of the spectrum of severity, patients in coma may not evidence a stiff neck, as guarding mechanisms are blunted.

FUNDUSCOPIC EXAMINATION

We shine lights in a patient's eyes, but in turn the "light in a person's eyes" reflects something of the inner state. Our clinical aim is not only to examine the eye itself, but also to obtain a reflection of intracranial events, such as increased pressure. The optic disc or nerve head is the only central nervous system tissue that we can directly visualize, eye-to-eye.

Fundus: back of the eye

This section will provide explanations in two areas that are important to the basic funduscopic examination.

1 Hints for getting a good look at the fundus (Table 4.3).

2 Key terms, findings, and correlations for neurologic diagnosis.

In examining the back of the eye via the pupil the main objects of attention are the retinal background including the macula (the area within which the retinal cells for central vision and greatest acuity are located in the foveola); the optic disc (optic nerve head); and the retinal vessels. For the patient, the state of the cornea and lens is of great importance, but these structures, as well as eye findings in systemic disease, are beyond the scope of this discussion. Refer to ophthalmology, general medical, and general physical diagnosis textbooks.

Hints

Make yourself comfortable! This applies to any examination or procedure. You will serve the patient much better if you perform efficiently and with maximum concentration, not distracted by balancing, bending, and backache. Darkening the environment to dilate the pupils seems obvious, but is underused. If this cannot be done, ask the patient to cover the eye not being examined. Since this prevents visual fixation, ask the patient to point the eyes in a fixed direction or towards the thumb

Table 4.3 A better look at the fundus: some basic dos and don'ts

Problem	Dos	Don'ts
Pupils "too small"	Dilate the pupils by darkening the room or move to a darkened area	Do not use dilating (mydriatic) eye drops routinely: (risk of narrow-angle glaucoma; patient inconvenienced from blurry vision; in emergencies, pupils needed for neurologic monitoring)
Difficulty holding the ophthalmoscope steady enough	Make yourself comfortable at same level as patient; brace 4th and 5th fingers of ophthalmoscope hand against patient's cheek	Do not hold the ophthalmoscope with both hands. Especially if the patient is frightened, agitated, or tremulous you should steady the patient's head with your free hand
Patient fixes poorly – moves head or eyes	Decrease ophthalmoscope light intensity; have patient point the eyes towards a distant object (see text)	Do not emphasize necessarily seeing the point of fixation – your head or poor vision in the other eye may cause patient to "look" around you, thereby shifting gaze
Cannot see enough of the fundus at once – too small a field of view	Move ophthalmoscope closer to patient's eye, not quite touching eyelashes	Do not be afraid of hurting the eye, if you move closer cautiously; touching the eyelashes does no harm, just pull back a little
Difficulty getting oriented – cannot find the disc	Approach from temporal side, as the disc is about 15° nasal; follow vessels in to disc	Do not (at first) follow the visual axis straight in towards the macula; patient may blink or withdraw from the brightness
You cannot use one eye, e.g. your right eye	With patient lying down, approach from above the head, facing the feet; examine the patient's right eye with your left eye	Do not try to examine the patient's right eye with your left eye in the usual facing position – you will bump noses and not get close enough

of an outstretched arm, the location of which is known to the patient by internal spatial sensation (proprioception).

The optic discs

Your main job is to observe carefully, without bias as to expected pathologic findings. Beware of "seeing" early or subtle signs that fit your preconceived diagnosis. It is easy to imagine a "slight pallor" in a normal disc. Interpretation of disc changes is difficult and it is therefore advisable to seek help.

Neurologically, the two main items to look for are pallor, as seen in optic atrophy, and the swelling of papilledema or papillitis (Table 4.4). (The important subject of glaucomatous changes is beyond the scope of this book.) Do not mistake the normal whiteness of the optic cup for pathologic pallor. Your best way to gain an idea of normal appearance is to look at many eyes (friends, family, and colleagues, as well as patients). For comparison with abnormals, study the color photos that are included in many of the major medicine or eye texts.

Table 4.4 The fundus: looking in and seeing out

Condition	Appearance of disc	Retina/vessels	Patient's acuity
Papilledema (because of raised ICP)	"Choked," swollen; loss of physiologic cup (early finding); disc margins blurred	Veins engorged; loss of spontaneous venous pulsations; ?hemorrhages	Acutely, preserved; chronically, progressive loss
Optic neuritis (inflammation of optic nerve) or other optic neuropathies	Chronically, pallor of optic disc (due to optic atrophy)	Vessels relatively normal in optic neuritis (refer to optic papillitis)	Acutely and chronically, typically decreased (central scotoma, see text)
Optic papillitis (optic neuritis involving optic disc) (papilla)	Acutely, disc is swollen; similar to papilledema	Vessels relatively normal, may see subtle changes, such as "sheathing"	Acutely and chronically, typically decreased (central scotoma)
Retrobulbar neuritis (optic neuritis involving nerve behind the bulb) (eyeball)	Acutely, normal; chronically (optic atrophy), pale disc	Normal (inflammatory process is posterior to the disc)	Acutely and chronically, typically decreased (central scotoma)
Occlusion of CRA or CRA branches	Arterial attenuation; segmentation of blood column ("boxcar" effect)	Retina (or sector) blanched, without filled arterial branches; ± edema	Decreased if macula involved; monocular field deficits
Venous occlusion	Often normal	Blotchy hemorrhages	Decreased if macula involved (scotomas)

CRA, central retinal artery; ICP, intracranial pressure.

Papilledema

Swelling (edema) of the optic disc (papilla) occurs either because of increased intracranial pressure (ICP) (which the term papilledema connotes) or because of local inflammation (papillitis). Papilledema does not appear immediately with a pathologic increase in ICP, but may become visible in days or weeks, rarely hours, depending on its degree and time course. As pressure from within the cranium causes congestion of the disc, an early change is loss of the physiologic cup (the indentation in the disc where the vessels "enter"); also, the demarcation of the disc from the surrounding retina becomes indistinct ("blurred margins").

As the disc swells above the surface of the surrounding retina, the blood vessels start to show a humping effect as they cross the margin of the disc and then regain the plane of the retina nearby. You should try to measure this difference in elevation between the disc and the normal retina with your ophthalmoscope. Focus on a vessel on the disc near the margin, and then again on the vessels on the retina one to two disc diameters away, noting the difference in diopters as you refocus. A difference between +1 (black) and −2 (red) would be a 3-diopter elevation. Precise quantitation is not so important for you as the sharpening of your powers of observation that comes with measurement.

Since papilledema does not ensue immediately upon a sudden increase in ICP, you should look for earlier funduscopic changes. The presence of spontaneous pulsation of the large veins at the disc virtually excludes venous congestion and therefore any major increase in ICP. Because venous pulsations may be absent normally, their lack is only significant if it represents a documented change. With increased ICP the retinal veins may appear engorged. Hemorrhages (described subsequently) may appear.

Suspicion of papilledema often arises from variations of normal, such as reduced visual demarcation of the disc from the surrounding retina, especially in people of very light complexion. No elevation of the disc will be evident, nor any of the other signs of increased pressure.

Observing retinal arteries

When surveying the fundus for vascular changes, follow the paired artery and vein that extend out into each quadrant of the retina. To describe the location of an abnormality, note its relation to a landmark, such as the second division point of the superior nasal branch in the right eye. Draw and label what you see. Locations can also be specified in terms of the numbers on a clock (the disc being the center). Thus, an occlusion might be described as being "in an arterial branch at 2 o'clock, about three disc diameters out from the disc margin" (Fig. 4.4).

Retinal artery occlusions often result from emboli, either blood clots (as from the heart) or material made up of platelet aggregations, calcific

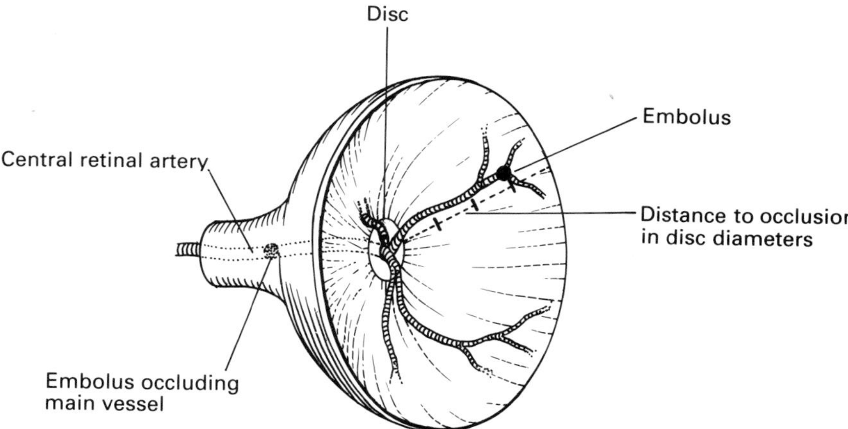

Fig. 4.4 Schematic of the ocular fundus (right eye) with the central retinal artery and major branches. Sites of two vascular occlusions are indicated: in the main artery behind the disc, and at a branch point, three disc diameters out from the disc at "2 o'clock" in the superior nasal branch (right eye). (The posterior retina can be viewed as a clock face with the disc at the center, for the purpose of indicating directions.)

material, or cholesterol crystals, usually originating from an atheromatous plaque in a proximal artery, such as the internal or common carotid (see Table 4.4 for retinal vascular changes).

Retinal findings in Case 4A

In the case of Mel Branch (see Case 4A), a small branch occlusion was visualized, but the examiner did not detect any ischemic signs, perhaps due to the small size of the vessel. (When the symptom of blurring occurred, the embolus was probably lodged temporarily in a larger, more central branch.)

The macula

The macula is the area of the retina at the back of the eye that receives light coming straight in along the visual axis. It contains the fovea and foveola which contain the highest concentration of cone cells and enable maximum visual acuity. Try to practice visualizing the macula by asking the patient to look directly at your ophthalmoscope light (which may need to be turned down somewhat in intensity). Having formed a general idea of the normal macular appearance, you may then be able to suspect an abnormality and seek specialized help in describing and interpreting what you see.

Retinal background: hemorrhages

In surveying the general retinal background you may see yellowish exudates (proteinaceous material from vascular leakage) or "cotton wool" (ischemic) patches associated with systemic pathology. Of more immediate concern neurologically is the presence of hemorrhages. So-called flame-shaped hemorrhages (which may actually be streaks or sharply jagged blotches) take their shape from their spread within the nerve fiber layer of the retina. They occur in severe hypertension (especially in the extreme degree that produces hypertensive encephalopathy). They may also be found with marked increases in ICP, and thus precede or accompany papilledema.

Preretinal (subhyaloid) hemorrhages are located between the retina and the vitreous humor and result from a very sudden, extreme increase in intracranial (and hence venous) pressure. Because they occur in the preretinal potential space they have a more globular appearance. If the patient remains in one position, the hemorrhage will tend to settle according to gravity. Although relatively rare, these are important because of their particular association with subarachnoid hemorrhage from a ruptured cerebral aneurysm.

SUMMARY

Vascular examination

Signs elicited by careful palpation and auscultation provide positive clues to the presence of aortocranial vascular disease. Whether or not this is symptomatic, it alerts you to the existence of potential vascular problems, a knowledge of which will alter your response to future complaints. Priorities in the examination are: listening well for soft and high-pitched bruits; and inching along the course of an artery to establish where an abnormality starts and where it is maximal. The following constellation of signs suggests advanced internal carotid stenosis (indicating a particular need to consider laboratory testing on a case by case basis):

1 a bruit of high pitch and long duration;
2 a bruit heard in the mid to upper neck;
3 a sharp decrease in the pulse felt in the upper neck.

Cervical spine

The evaluation of meningeal irritation causing a stiff neck and its distinction from other forms of rigidity is especially important neurologically. In the case of meningitis you can observe the following symptoms:

1 pain and resistance are greater with head flexion than with rotation or extension;
2 coexistent sensitivity to maneuvers that stretch the lumbosacral meningeal roots suggests a widespread meningeal inflammation rather than a local arthritic or neuromuscular basis for cervical rigidity;
3 systemic symptoms (such as headache), specific signs (such as fever), and behavioral characteristics (like listlessness and photophobia) increase the likelihood that a stiff neck is due to meningitis.

In any case, maintain a high index of clinical suspicion of meningitis even with rather mild or equivocal signs (see Chapter 15 for lumbar puncture technique, and Table 15.3).

For assessment of focal neck (or neck–shoulder–upper extremity) pain or numbness, check for:

1 abnormal head and neck posture and limitation of range of motion (usually due to joint disease vs. primary or secondary muscle spasm);
2 aggravation of pain or numbness in cervical root distributions with change of head position;
3 focal tenderness, especially percussion tenderness, over the spinous processes.

Funduscopic examination

Develop a systematic approach to observing the optic discs, vessels, and retinal background. Your main task is to make the initial observations – to raise the question of abnormality – not to provide the final interpretation for which expert consultation can be obtained. In the funduscopic diagnosis of raised ICP:

1 do not rule out increased ICP because of lack of papilledema, in the acute setting;
2 look for venous engorgement, hemorrhages, and the disappearance of venous pulsations;
3 compare your funduscopic findings with the patient's visual acuity (and peripheral vision). Recently developed papilledema affects acuity little, if at all.

PROBLEMS FOR SELF-STUDY

Problems

1 A 51-year-old right-handed man is examined for routine health maintenance. On viewing the left ocular fundus, the intern sees several bright spots within two of the retinal branch arteries, which

appear to represent clumps of cholesterol crystals. This is confirmed by the attending physician. What further testing might be appropriate?

2 A 30-year-old left-hended baseball pitcher complains of a "tired arm" towards the end of the season. His fast ball is not what it had been, especially after a few innings. If you were the physician, what aspects of the examination would you emphasize?

Comments

1 Pieces of cholesterol plaque have broken off from some proximal vessel and embolized into branches of the central retinal artery. Aside from a general cardiovascular and lipid evaluation, the physical examination should focus on the following. (a) Vision: any alteration of acuity or visual field scotomas (blind spots), or deficits in the peripheral fields. This should be checked in the right eye as well, since the same process might have occurred there, without leaving tell-tale retinal signs. (b) Vascular examination of the neck: are there pulse deficits or bruits to implicate the common or internal carotid arteries in a stenotic or occlusive process? Noninvasive carotid laboratory testing should be done to detect major intravascular lesions. In this case, a 20% narrowing of the proximal left internal carotid artery, by rough plaque, is found. No one can say whether the cholesterol emboli emanated from this site or some other site in the common carotid or ascending aorta. The patient is placed on an antiplatelet agent to try to prevent larger platelet-containing emboli, and will be followed clinically on an anti-atherogenic medical regimen.

2 After taking further history regarding general health and habits, systemic, cardiovascular, neurologic, and emotional symptoms, the examination should emphasize local range of motion, pain, and tenderness in the neck and shoulder; the neurologic examination of the left upper extremity and shoulder girdle should focus on any signs of weakness, atrophy, fasciculations, sensory loss, or reflex changes; and, last but not least, the vascular examination of the chest, neck, and fundus should look for evidence of impaired blood flow to the left arm, which might be suggested by a left supraclavicular (?subclavian) bruit, a decreased blood pressure in the left arm, and a decreased or delayed brachial or radial pulse. Does exercise of the left arm cause symptoms of claudication (pain, fatigue, weakness) or any neurologic symptoms elsewhere? Is there evidence of carotid stenotic or occlusive disease (pulse deficit, bruit, etc.) especially on the right? Has there been any right hemispheric ischemic injury causing subtle left arm dysfunction, or any monocular symptoms or findings in the right eye? In this case, a left subclavian stenosis was detected and surgically corrected with relief of symptoms. A medical program to prevent accelerated atherosclerosis was instituted.

FURTHER READING

Lancet 1992; 339:342–7, 400–5, 473–7, 533–9, 653–8, 791–5. (Stroke Octet). Problems like carotid artery occlusive disease are included in this multiauthored, eight-article review of stroke, the third-ranked, overall killer and a major cause of morbidity and disability.

Mayo Clinic. *Clinical Examinations in Neurology*. 6th edn. Mosby, St. Louis (MO), 1991. Provides further helpful details on the neurovascular, funduscopic, and spinal examinations.

Posner, J.B. Mechanical lesions of the spine and related structures. In: Wyngaarden, J.B., Smith, L.H., Bennett, J.C., (eds) *Cecil Textbook of Medicine*. 19th edn. WB Saunders, Philadelphia (PA), 1992. Pains in the neck, creaky backs, and much worse. Spine problems account for an enormous burden of neurologic suffering and disability that virtually all practitioners must confront.

Quagliarello, V., Scheld, W.M. Bacterial meningitis: pathogenesis, pathophysiology, and progress. *N Engl J Med* 1992; 327:864–72. This review of current concepts starts where most standard medical texts leave off. Consult the latter for symptoms and signs; this article deals with how the meninges and brain are injured.

Reich, K.A., Giansiracusa, D.F., Strongwater, S.L. Neurologic manifestations of giant cell arteritis. *Am J Med* 1990; 89:67–72. Temporal arteritis, one manifestation of this type of inflammatory arterial disease, may cause headache, blindness, and other treatable or preventable neurologic symptoms and signs.

Tyler, K.L., Martin, J.B. *Infectious Diseases of the Central Nervous System*. F.A. Davis, Philadelphia (PA), 1983. A valuable survey of meningitis and other infections, such as encephalitis and abscess (which also usually cause meningeal reactions).

Whitley, R.J. Viral encephalitis. *N Engl J Med* 1990; 323:242–50. Viral infections of the brain usually display some mengineal signs (meningoencephalitis), as well as features referrable to the parenchyma. This article succinctly reviews the panoply of manifestations, as well as causes and mechanisms.

chapter 5

Examination of Cranial Nerve Functions

Overview

The examination of cranial nerve functions occupies a special place in the neurologic evaluation. The structures they serve, such as the face, ears, and eyes, are intimately associated with the patient's sense of self. Many of the functions mediated by cranial nerves are vital to interaction with the outside world and to life itself.

Some cranial functions, like olfaction, are entirely perceptual (although a good sniff helps you to smell), whereas chewing is clearly motor (although feedback regarding jaw position helps you avoid biting your tongue!). The close relationship between looking and seeing epitomizes the integration of motor and sensory functions.

The cranial nerve examination is actually a microcosm of physical neurologic testing as a whole. However, the cranial nerve examination differs from the other main parts of the neurologic assessment because of a regional approach: the format follows an orderly rostrocaudal progression which reflects (excepting CN 1 and 2) the order of exit of cranial nerves from the brainstem. (As you see, I use numerals 1–12 to specify the cranial nerves, rather than the more traditional and cumbersome Roman numerals. Some of your instructors may be aghast!)

Cranial nerves and their principal functions that are tested:

CN 1: olfactory	Sense of smell
CN 2: optic	Funduscopic examination: optic nerves and retina Visual acuity (V/A) Visual fields (pupillary reactions with CN 3)
CN 3: oculomotor *CN 4: trochlear* *CN 6: abducens*	Pupillary Size (mm), reactions, eyelid opening (CN 3). Eye movements (extraocular movements, EOM), CNs 3, 4, and 6
CN 5: trigeminal	Sensory (face and anterior scalp) Corneal reflexes, direct and consensual (with CN 7) Motor (mastication)
CN 7: facial	Facial expression Taste
CN 8: acoustic	Auditory acuity Air vs. bone conduction (Rinné), Weber (lateralization)
vestibular	Balance, head–eye coordination and orientation
CN 9: glossopharyngeal	Palate, pharynx, larynx (gag, phonation, swallowing, articulation)
CN 10: vagus	Visceral functions, larynx
CN 11	Shoulder shrug, head turning and flexion
CN 12	Tongue (motor)

Integration with head and neck examination

Examination of the head and neck, as described in the last chapter, obviously overlaps the cranial nerve examination. When should you test the eyes, the throat, or the tongue and where should the findings be recorded? You will probably find it convenient to include the funduscopic examination, inspection of the ears, tongue, nose, and throat in the head and neck section of the general physical examination. In contrast, specific neurologic and sensory functions (V/A, pupillary reactions, hearing, gag reflex, etc.) should, at least for now, be tested and recorded under the cranial nerve section of the neurologic examination. Testing and interpreting cranial nerve functions are best learned within the neurologic context, after which you may choose to reintegrate more of the cranial nerve examination into the head and neck examination, especially in patients who do not present with neurologic problems (see Chapter 19, section on screening examination).

SEGMENTAL VS. SUPRASEGMENTAL COMPONENTS OF CRANIAL NERVE FUNCTIONS

Problem

Why bring in the terms and concepts of "segmental" and "suprasegmental" at this point? The reason is this: confusion over the meaning and localizing value of a "cranial nerve sign" is very commonly encountered in working with students, medical residents, and even non-neurologist attendings. Thus, although you can examine cranial nerve functions without reference to the concept of segmental and suprasegmental organization, your interpretation (and proper recording) of the findings will be greatly assisted by understanding it.

Testing function

1 We test functions mediated by cranial nerves, not cranial nerves themselves, in isolation. In testing limbs, we assess strength in order to find any weakness in an arm, but we do not call this "cervical anterior root" testing. Similarly, we test strength in the face knowing that the result is a product of a chain of functions that includes CN 7 as one component. However, clinicians often say they are testing "seven" (CN 7), when they are really looking for facial weakness, whatever the localization of the lesion.

Preview of Chapter 14

2 Cranial nerve function, such as movement of the face, results from suprasegmental and segmental links (Table 5.1).

Principle of crossing

3 Cranial nerves are uncrossed (see exceptions under CN 3 and 4), which is the general rule for segmental outflow and inflow. Supraseg-

Table 5.1 Chains of function: suprasegmental and segmental links

Functional testing (examples)	Linkages in chains of motor function			Local, non-neurologic defect
	Suprasegmental: upper motor neuron (UMN)	Segmental: lower motor neuron (LMN)	Muscle/neuromuscular junction	
Facial expression – smiling, frowning, etc.	Motor cortex (face area) – corticobulbar tract	Facial nucleus in pons – facial nerve (CN 7)	Fibers of facial muscles	Example: swollen lips cause "twisted" smile
Tongue protrusion	Motor cortex (tongue area) – corticobulbar tract	Hypoglossal nucleus in medulla – hypoglossal nerve (CN 12)	Genioglossus muscles for tongue protrusion	Example: tumor of mouth deviates tongue
	Linkages in chains of sensory function			Local, non-neurologic defect
Function tested (example)	Suprasegmental	Segmental afferent nerve, roots, ganglia, (nucleus)	Segmental sensory receptors	
Pin sensation in the face	Trigeminal–thalamic tract; thalamocortical projection	Trigeminal roots, ganglion, descending tract and nucleus of CN 5	"Free endings" of trigeminal fibers in the face	Example: swelling, scar may alter pin sensitivity

mental pathways cross: the corticospinal and corticobulbar tracts typically cross, at least in part, before reaching their lower motor neurons. The anatomy of long tracts is summarized in Chapter 13 and segmental and peripheral organization in Chapters 14 and 16.

Segmental

A segmental level or unit is an embryologically derived cross-sectional component of the central nervous system (CNS) together with the associated outflow to or inflow from the peripheral structures that are anatomically and physiologically related.

Spinal segment

A spinal segment (in its simplest form) consists of the anterior and posterior horns of the spinal cord gray matter at one level (such as the 5th cervical) and all of their peripheral processes and connections at that level – the anterior roots, the dorsal root ganglion cells and posterior roots, components of the peripheral nerves, and muscles and receptors to which they are distributed. On the motor side, the smallest unit of segmental organization is the motor unit – one anterior horn cell and its peripheral axon, and the muscle fibers it innervates. Together, all these axons from one spinal level (such as C5) form the C5 anterior root. On the sensory side, the hallmark of segmental organization is the dermatome, the stripe of skin that, when stimulated, sends afferent messages to one dorsal (posterior) root ganglion (the right C5 ganglion, for example) and then on (in part) to the posterior horn gray matter of the right side of the spinal cord at C5 (see Figs 13.15 and 16.1).

Brainstem segment

Similarly, the brainstem has a basically segmental organization (which you can see manifested as an orderly emergence of cranial nerves on each side, from the midbrain to the medulla. For example, the most caudal part of the medulla contains the CN 12 nuclei which are the brainstem (bulbar) components of the segmental organization. The hypoglossal (CN 12) nerves course peripherally and innervate muscles of the tongue, analogous to the spinal organization described above for C5.

Suprasegmental

The pathways from higher CNS centers (such as cortical areas) that communicate with each segmental level of the brainstem (or spinal cord) constitute the suprasegmental (sometimes called supranuclear) control mechanism. In the example of tongue movement, the upper motor neurons of the frontal cortex – and their axons that course downward to the brainstem to synapse at the CN 12 nuclei in the medulla – represent the suprasegmental control mechanism in its simplest form. These upper motor neuron tracts controlling the brainstem motor nuclei are called corticobulbar tracts (Fig. 5.1). They are analogous to the corticospinal tracts which originate in the cortex and synapse on anterior horn cells (the spinal lower motor neurons) at the various spinal cord levels.

Construct: a two-neuron chain

Thus, for the execution of fine motor control we employ a simplified construct of neural organization – a two-neuron chain: (a) the upper motor neuron of the motor cortex which sends its axon in the corticobulbar tract or the corticospinal tract; and (b) the lower motor neuron of the brainstem or spinal cord that innervates muscle (see Table 14.2).

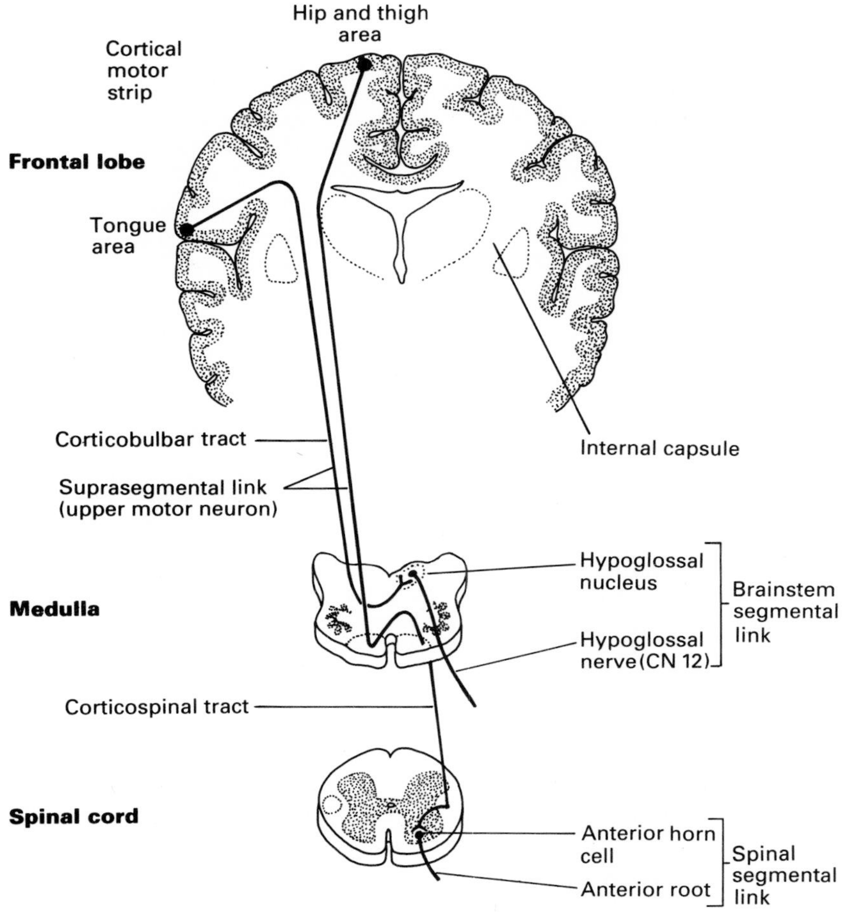

Fig. 5.1 Suprasegmental and segmental motor pathways: the two neuron chain of fine, voluntary control. At the top in a corneal section through the posterior frontal lobes, the upper motor neuron tracts – the corticospinal tract from the thigh area of the motor cortex and the corticobulbar tract from the tongue area – descend towards the brainstem. In the next section, the medulla, the corticobulbar tract crosses to synapse on the segmental lower motor neurons of the CN 12 (hypoglossal) nucleus, from which CN 12 exits. The corticospinal tract crosses in the pyramidal decussation and descends to synapse with lower motor neurons (anterior horn cells) in the lumbosacral spinal cord.

Localization of lesion

When we observe tongue deviation to one side as a result of weakness, we need to interpret whether the problem lies in the suprasegmental (upper motor neuron) link of the chain, or whether it is a segmental, neuromuscular lesion affecting the hypoglossal nucleus, CN 12 extending peripherally from the nucleus, or tongue muscles. Except in special instances, you cannot determine the answer in the acute case just by observing the weak function. You need to put this observation together

Table 5.2 Sense of smell: clinical significance

Finding	One or both sides	Both sides
Decreased or absent sense of smell	Obstruction; nasal congestion – infection or allergy; trauma; subfrontal tumor	Toxic, metabolic abnormalities (trace metal deficiences, e.g. zinc); degenerative and genetic diseases
Complaint of patient with olfactory deficit	Patient often unaware of unilateral loss of sense of smell	May emphasize loss of taste (aromatic substance) rather than smell
Positive olfactory symptoms	Foul odors or perversion of odors with purulent nasal or sinus infection; olfactory hallucinations in "temporal lobe" epilepsy (complex partial seizures)	

with other findings, as will be illustrated subsequently in this chapter and the following one. Constructs of suprasegmental/segmental control are discussed in Chapter 14. To reiterate, an abnormal finding on "cranial nerve testing" does not mean that the cranial nerve itself is necessarily the site of the lesion.

CRANIAL NERVE 1: OLFACTION (SENSE OF SMELL)

Testing

Test each nostril separately, using any aromatic, nonirritative substance (such as cloves or cinnamon kept in a test tube or small bottle). Otherwise, a soap or lotion will usually be available. Correct identification confirms perception, but is otherwise of little importance.

Indications

Test when (a) the patient complains of loss of smell or taste (since complex taste depends upon aromatic factors); or (b) when you suspect frontal pathology because of trauma, headache, personality change, or dementia – in view of the subfrontal location of the olfactory nerves and bulbs. Negative testing does not obviate the need for neuroimaging (see Table 5.2 for clinical correlations and Fig. 5.2).

CRANIAL NERVE 2: VISION AND REACTION TO LIGHT, FUNDUSCOPIC EXAMINATION

Overview

Examination of the visual system deserves particular care because of the great importance of vision to the patient and because of the localizing value of visual deficits. The visual pathways span the brain from front to back: visual symptoms and signs may point not only to problems in the eye itself, but also to lesions at the base of the brain more anteriorly (optic nerves and tracts), to the thalamic area (lateral geniculate nuclei), to the temporal, parietal, and occipital white matter (optic radiations), and to the visual cortex, most posteriorly.

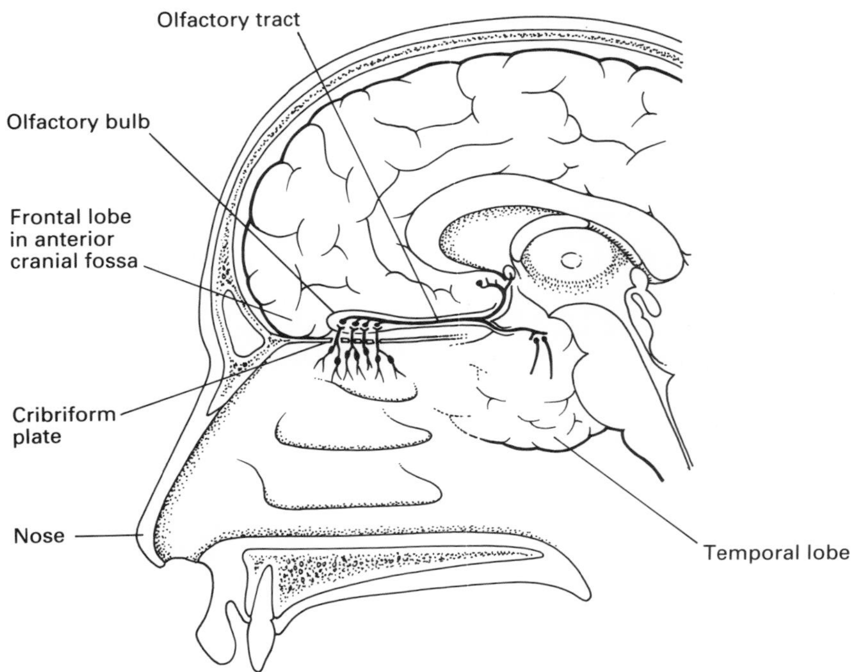

Fig. 5.2 Olfactory fibers: passage from the nasal mucosa through the cribriform plate, where they are vulnerable to disruption from frontal and nasal injury. Within the anterior cranial fossa the olfactory pathway fibers may be compressed by mass lesions at the base of the frontal lobes.

Pupillary light reflex

The afferent limb of the pupillary light reaction traverses the optic nerves, tracts, and their connections with the midbrain. The examination is usually recorded under CN 3 (efferent limb of the reflex arc, see CN 3).

CASE 5A
Left-sided loss of sight

Les Brooks, a 57-year-old left-handed man, was playing golf when he suddenly experienced "trouble seeing out of my left eye." The doctor evaluating his problem in the emergency room first ascertained that there was no foreign body in the eye and that there was no other obvious ocular abnormality that would require immediate treatment. Further clarification of the complaint was necessary: was this a difficulty seeing out of the left eye only, or was it rather a problem with seeing in the left side of space, assumed by the patient to involve only the left eye? What would be the effect of covering one eye or the other? Was there a dimness of vision, a loss of ability to see detail vs. a reduction in the scope of vision? Mr Brooks had not yet tried reading, covering one eye and then the other, or other test maneuvers, so these questions were carried over into the examination of the two main aspects of vision: V/A and visual fields (the findings will be presented subsequently).

Visual acuity

Definition

V/A is the ability to resolve small objects; testing quantifies the sharpness or strength of central vision. It is an expression of the function of the macula (for definition see Chapter 4, section on funduscopic examination) and its neural connections. In common terms, acuity expresses how well one sees directly ahead vs. peripherally.

Indications for testing

Testing should be done in the following situations:

1 complaint of altered vision;
2 other evidence of eye injury or disease (even without visual complaint);
3 baseline screening of general and neurologic health status;
4 any confusion or altered behavior that might be due to grossly impaired vision (of which a patient may or may not be aware).

Testing

Because a complaint of blurred or otherwise decreased vision has many possible causes, you should first establish whether the impairment exists in the right and/or left eye individually (Table 5.3). Cover each eye separately and inquire for clarity of vision (having assured good illumination). Then test with a visual acuity screening card ("pocket screener") if a wall chart is not readily available. Employ the patient's corrective lenses if used for reading. Test each eye separately, holding the screening card about 14 inches away, but otherwise let the patient position it to maximal advantage. In the absence of a screening card, use a newspaper or magazine to document the size of print that the patient can read (with each eye); ask the illiterate patient to point out small nearby objects or details of pictures. If the patient's corrective lenses are not available, and it is critical to obtain a best approximation of acuity immediately, test vision through a pinhole in a paper or card held close to the eye; any improvement in acuity by this method is due to elimination of refractive error.

Recording results

If you use a wall chart, record the numeric designation of the smallest number line that can be read with each eye, such as 20/30. (20 refers to the distance from the chart measured in feet; 30 indicates that this type could normally be read at 30 feet.) With the screening card, these numbers are not as accurate, but do serve to identify the smallest type that can be read.

Common errors/key points

The following are common pitfalls of testing.

1 Omission of testing (perhaps on the assumption that someone else

Table 5.3 Clinical correlation of decreased visual acuity/blurred vision

Decreased in one eye only	Decreased in both eyes, tested separately	Decreased only with both eyes tested together
Intraocular cause (retinal detachment; vascular occlusion; hemorrhage; cataract, etc.)	Bilateral intraocular disease (trauma, retinal degenerations, diabetic retinopathy, etc.)	
Optic nerve lesion (optic neuritis due to demyelination, etc.)	Bilateral optic nerve lesions	
	Certain bilateral visual cortex lesions (patient may be unaware of blindness)	
	Nystagmus (involuntary oscillating movements) affecting fixation; (turning the eyes toward the point at which nystagmus is minimized improves vision)	Incomplete double vision (binocular imbalance) – complaint of blurring, but no separation of images reported; covering either eye resolves blurring

has done it or will do it). Visual acuity testing often falls in the cracks between the general and neurologic examinations.

2 Testing both eyes together, thereby missing decreased acuity in one of them.

3 Attributing poor vision to absent glasses, but not following up with subsequent testing to be sure that the deficit is correctable.

4 Attributing poor vision to old age or disease without confirming the adequacy of or the need for corrective lenses.

Visual fields

Definitions

The scope or extent of vision of a nonmoving eye is its visual field. Moving an eye (as opposed to the head) extends its normal perimeter rather little (check this on yourself). Each eye has its own field, overlapping to a large extent the field of the other eye. The following terms will be helpful to you in describing your findings and communicating them to others.

Central field

The central field comprises the area immediately around the point of fixation (the spot you are directly looking at). The central and surrounding paracentral field extends out 15°. The central field includes the zone of maximal acuity.

Peripheral field

The peripheral field consists of the remaining extent of vision out to its anatomic limits on all sides – the extreme of vision "out of the corner of your eye." (In general, this extent is, as you can determine for yourself, approximately 60° nasally and superiorly, 70° inferiorly, and 90° temporally.)

Hemianopia

A hemianopia or hemianopsia is a defect or "cut" affecting one-half of a visual field (*hemi* = half, *a* = not or without, *opia* or *opsia* = seeing). The designation always denotes the segment of space that is visualized, not the part of the retina or visual pathways that are involved. Thus, a lesion affecting the right side of the retina of the left eye would cause a deficit in the left visual field of the left eye. A cut in the right or left field may have any configuration up to a complete hemianopia. "Hemianopia" used alone (in common neurologic parlance) implies "homonymous hemianopia" (see below and Fig. 13.17).

Quadrantanopia

Often, just one quadrant, such as the left superior quadrant, may be involved, yielding a quadrantanopia (quadrantanopsia) – in this case a left superior quadrantanopia.

Homonymous field defects

If the same sector is involved in both eyes (such as the left hemifield which is the temporal field of the left eye and the nasal field of the right eye), the hemianopia is said to be homonymous. A left superior quadrant defect in the field of each eye is a left superior homonymous quadrantanopia. (The more the defects have the same configuration within the affected field of each eye, the more congruous the homonymous hemianopia is said to be.) Nonhomonymous defects are termed heteronymous. Involvement of the temporal field of each eye is called a bitemporal, heteronymous hemianopia. An altitudinal defect affects the upper or lower field of vision.

Scotoma

A scotoma or "blind spot" is an area of impaired vision within a visual field. As noted, a central scotoma decreases visual acuity.

Physiologic blind spot

A normal scotoma, the physiologic blind spot, corresponds to the area where the optic disc is located, preventing any retinal reception in that spot. (Since the optic disc is placed on the nasal side of the macula, the blind spot will be found approximately 15° to the temporal side of the point of visual fixation.) Mapping the physiologic blind spot is not clinically worthwhile for the nonophthalmologist (but you should try it once, for interest).

Field defects and pupillary reactions

Pupillary light reflexes are not affected by hemianopias, even those caused by optic tract lesions, since the light source illuminates both halves of the retina to some degree; thus, afferent information from that eye is distributed to both optic tracts (see text and tables for CN 3).

CASE 5A
Left-sided loss of eyesight
(continued)

An evaluation of Mr Brooks' difficulty seeing on the left yielded the following findings.

1 With the right eye covered and his glasses on he could read the "20/20" line on the pocket screener. However, despite this normal corrected acuity in the left eye (OS), he stated that he could not see

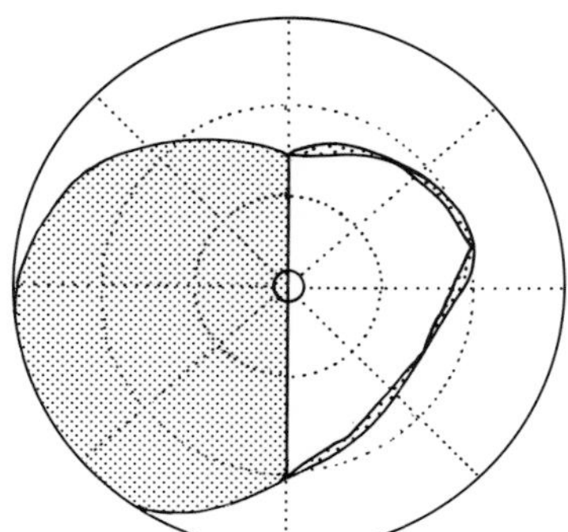

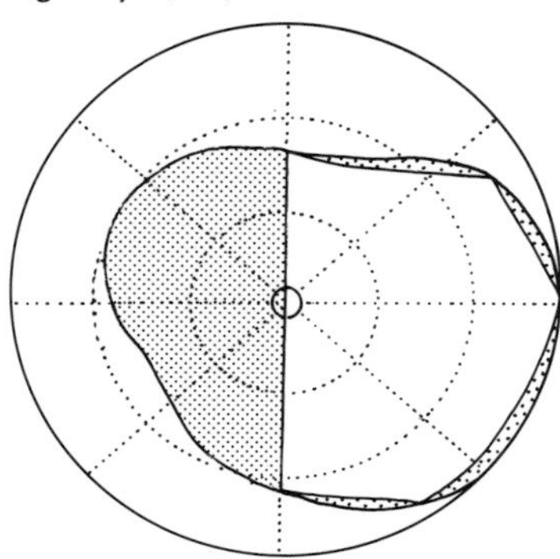

Fig. 5.3 Visual fields in Case 5A. Left homonymous hemianopia (stippled areas). Fields are plotted from the patient's point of view, i.e. as if you are the patient looking out. The large round circle for each eye represents the virtual 180° hemisphere of vision that anatomically confronts each eye, before taking into account the configuration of the orbit and nose. The irregular outline within depicts a normal field perimeter, which extends out fully temporally, but is more restricted nasally and inferiorly (because of the nose) and superiorly and inferiorly because of the orbital rims (assuming visual fixation straight ahead).

Monocular blindness vs. hemianopia

things on his left – the right side of the doctor's face was "blurred out" as he looked at her.

2 With the left eye covered, he also had normal corrected acuity in his right eye (OD), but, much to his surprise, he also could not see objects on the left side of space out of his right eye.

3 Peripheral field testing (as will be detailed in the next section) revealed a complete left homonymous hemianopia (Fig. 5.3).

In summary, Mr Brooks' difficulty with seeing "out of my left eye" was in fact a left field cut in both eyes; mistakenly attributed, as is often the case, to something wrong in the left eye itself. Work-up revealed an infarction in the right visual cortex (posterior cerebral artery territory) caused by an embolic stroke. Only partial recovery ensued, but Mr Brooks learned to compensate quite well for his left field deficit by orienting his head more toward the left and scanning frequently to the left with his gaze.

Testing visual fields

Overview

As in the above case, the three main objectives can be summarized as follows.

1 Distinguish symptoms and signs that are monocular – seen (or not seen) out of just one eye at a time – vs. those that are binocular. Cover one eye at a time, while testing the other.

2 Differentiate impaired acuity from an impaired peripheral field.
3 Compare the configuration of a field deficit in one eye with that in the other.

Testing central and paracentral fields

For screening, ask the patient to cover the other eye and look directly at you, describing any missing or blurred areas (or better still, look at a printed grid, for example graph paper). Of course, a true central field defect may have been noted already in testing of acuity. When more detailed testing is in order, use a white or other pinhead moved within the central field, against a dark background. This method depends upon steady visual fixation by the patient on a point in the background. Sometimes an early scotoma will simply take the form of relative decoloration of red or other hues.

Referral

Note that visual defects are relative and depend upon the size, color, and intensity of illumination of the test object. As a rule, any suspected central scotoma or decrease in acuity should be evaluated by an ophthalmologist.

Testing peripheral fields

Test each eye separately for maximum information, asking the patient to cover the other one. However, if you have a problem with patient cooperation (see below), start with the simpler job of testing both eyes together. While testing both eyes at once will rarely miss homonymous field cuts, a monocular defect will frequently be overlooked. As a rule, test without the patient's glasses, so that the rims do not interfere. Gross field testing, as with a wiggling finger, requires very little acuity, so beware of attributing field defects to "poor vision" (poor acuity).

Confrontation

When testing peripheral visual fields by confrontation, sit or stand facing the patient and bring the stimulus in from the periphery to gauge when the patient first perceives it (a wiggling finger or a large white or red pinhead). One traditionally prescribed approach is to compare the patient's fields with your own, but this method has the major drawback that you cannot keep the stimulus between you and the patient and still define the patient's most peripheral vision. Since an important goal of testing is to assess the actual periphery of the field, consider the following modification that many clinicians have adopted.

1 Position yourself as close to the patient as required so that your stimulus can originate outside the field of vision and move in an arc into the field of vision (Fig. 5.4). With this method you must be sure that the patient is responding specifically to the wiggling finger (or other stimulus) and not to movement of your arm.
2 Repeat this maneuver within each of the four quadrants.
3 Ask the patient to indicate verbally, or better still, by pointing to the stimulus, when it is first seen.
4 Evaluate the patient's responses by what you judge to be normal, rather than by comparison to your own fields as you face the patient. It will take some practice before you feel comfortable in estimating at what points around the periphery the patient should be able to perceive the

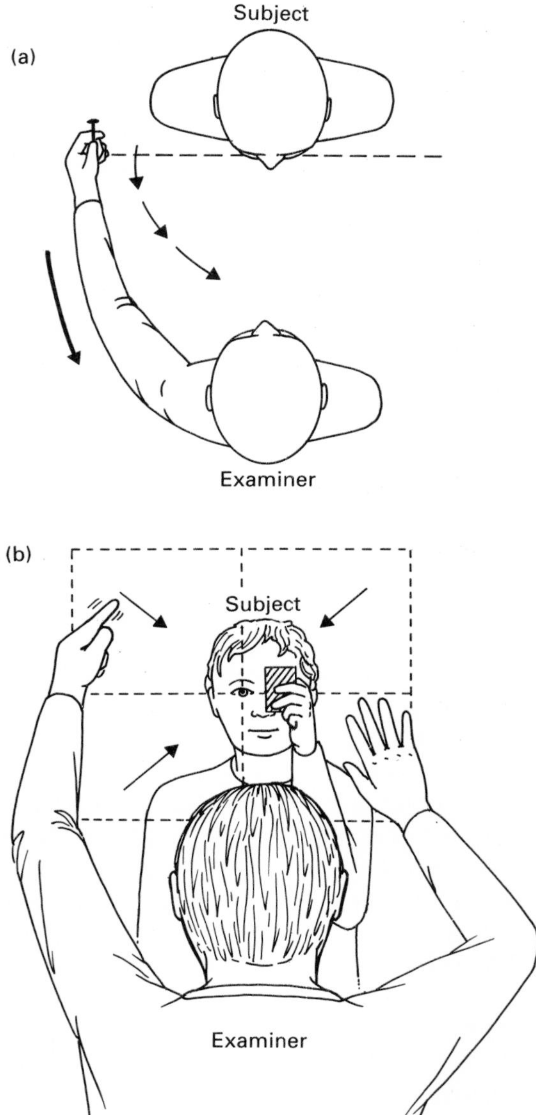

Fig. 5.4 Visual field testing. (a) Overhead view of the recommended bedside "confrontation" method, showing the stimulus originating behind the plane of the patient's vision, and then extending out in an arc, eventually to the midline. (b) The stimulus arc is repeated in each quadrant of the visual field of each eye. (Only the quadrants of the right eye, being tested, are shown; the left eye is covered.)

stimulus. (Try checking your own peripheral fields by bringing in a wiggling finger from the periphery of each quadrant.)

5 Pick a stimulus that captures the attention of the patient (pinhead, wiggling finger, waving hand). Vision within a quadrant or hemifield can also be established by flashing a certain number of fingers in that sector. (However, counting fingers requires more acuity than is necessary for perceiving a wiggling finger.) Remember that any bedside method is insensitive compared to testing with modern equipment, so if refinement is needed, arrange for "formal visual fields."

Double simultaneous stimulation

At the same time that you test visual fields, you can quickly and easily test for visual inattention to the right or left by double simultaneous stimulation: present the stimuli in the right and left fields at the same time. If the patient consistently fails to perceive the stimulus on one side (but has been able to perceive a solitary stimulus on that side), then the patient is said to show extinction, which reveals visual inattention to that side (see also Chapter 7, section on somatosensory inattention).

Testing the difficult patient

When the patient does not cooperate adequately for ordinary confrontational testing, you can still learn useful information about the visual fields.

1 Watch the patient's eyes to see whether they glance at, fix on, or follow objects in both the right and left fields.

2 Starting from behind the patient, bring your face into view from each side. A glance toward you indicates perception in that field, assuming you have emitted no sounds or other clues to your position. The human face serves as a powerful visual stimulus, as does money!

3 The stuporous patient presents special difficulties in visual field evaluation. A visual threat, such as a quick thrust of the hand toward the eye (while lightly holding the lids open, if necessary) may evoke a blink reflex when the stimulus is presented in an intact field, but not in a hemianopic field. (Be careful not to brush the eyelashes.) A lack of response on both sides does not provide reliable data on vision. Do not test by threat in the awake patient who is capable of responding to any other form of testing.

Relevant symptoms

Patients sometimes first notice visual field impairments when reading. With a left hemianopic defect (or left inferior quadrantanopia) there will be difficulty in picking up the first word of successive lines (as gaze is shifted from the end of one line at the right to the beginning of the next at the left). Conversely, with a right hemianopic defect, patients typically have trouble tracking to the right. In walking or driving there may be a tendency to bump into things on the side of the deficit. Patients often do not become aware of field defects in just one eye until the other eye happens to be covered. Slowly evolving field cuts are less likely to be noticed than acute deficits.

Clinical–anatomic correlations

Note the topographic separation of optic radiation fibers serving the upper and lower visual fields (see Fig. 13.17). A deep parietal white matter lesion may produce an inferior quadrantanopia (fibers representing the superior retina), and a temporal lesion a superior quadrantanopia (fibers representing the inferior retina). This superior–inferior separation also applies in the visual cortex. Most homonymous defects result from lesions posterior to the lateral geniculate nuclei.

Summary of visual field testing

1 You can perform good peripheral field evaluations by using a modified confrontation technique, as well as your own ingenuity. Mistakes usually involve:

(a) omission;

(b) giving up when the patient does not fully cooperate (rather than trying alternative techniques);

(c) not testing the actual periphery;

(d) failing to check all four quadrants;

(e) not testing each eye separately for monocular defects.

2 When attempting to document or rule out subtle peripheral field defects or scotomas, confirm and extend your own findings by obtaining formal visual field testing by a specialist.

3 Distinguish a field cut from deviation of conjugate gaze. The former may cause a gaze preference towards the seeing side whereas the latter stems from impaired motor control of gaze (See next section and Chapter 17.)

CRANIAL NERVES 3, 4, AND 6: PUPILS, EYE MOVEMENTS, AND EYELID ELEVATION

CASE 5B
Eye signs: emergency?

Joseph Ahearn, an emaciated, middle-aged, white male was found in a stuporous state in his boarding house room and was brought to the hospital for evaluation. Testing of pupils revealed an inequality of the pupils, the right being 5 mm, and the left 4 mm; both were reactive to light.

Which was the abnormal pupil, the smaller or the larger one, and was the difference chronic or acute? Was the larger pupil still enlarging? Might he be harboring a space-occupying lesion causing his stupor and an incipient 3rd nerve (CN 3) palsy, as part of a transtentorial herniation syndrome? (See Fig. 13.2.)

Further observation revealed no additional increase in size. Reactivity remained normal. Eventually, a prior record became available which documented the chronic pupillary inequality (anisocoria). Over the next several hours he became more alert as he sobered up. The lack of progressive pupillary enlargement, the good reactivity, and finally the access to baseline data all permitted a course of observation, rather than emergency imaging.

Table 5.4 Examining the pupils

Test	Observation	Hints
Size and shape	Estimate size in millimeters – this encourages close observation (absolute size varies with conditions)	If deep brown irises make pupils hard to see, shine light from the side – observe size before constriction
Reactivity	Observe the direct reaction of the illuminated pupil and the consensual (indirect) reaction of the contralateral pupil (observe these reactions sequentially – you cannot observe both pupils equally well at the same time)	Use a bright penlight; if there is a glare, shift the angle of illumination; if you cannot see a reaction, dim the room light, or open the lid just as you shine the light
Near reaction ("accommodation test")	Ask patient to look afar, then at end of own nose; alternatively, have patient focus on your finger 0.6 metres (2 feet) away, then follow it in towards nose; as eyes converge, pupils constrict ("near reaction")	Testing convergence of eyes accompanied by near reaction of pupils and accommodation of lenses need not be done routinely; the usual cause of absent near reaction is failure of binocular convergence (one eye loses fixation)

Testing

Careful observation of pupillary size, including measurement of diameter in millimeters (Table 5.4), is vital neurologically for the following reasons.

Marked change in size

1 In the presence of other neurologic abnormalities (such as coma), pupillary size may provide an important clue to brainstem segmental localization (e.g. a pons vs. midbrain lesion, see Table 13.2) or pharmacologic effect.

Difference in size and reactivity

2 A difference in the size of the two pupils (anisocoria), although frequently of no clinical significance, may indicate a focal neurologic process, especially if accompanied by altered reactivity (Table 5.5).

Baseline

3 Data on pupillary size, equality, and reactivity can be of great importance as a baseline observation, as you just saw in Case 5B.

Definitions

Miotic pupil: small, constricted; parasympathetic effect or sympathetic blockade.

Mydriatic pupil: large, dilated; sympathetic effect or parasympathetic blockade. (You can remember that sympathetic stimulation increases pupillary size, since the pupils "grow" large with excitement.)

The notation PERRLA (pupils equal, round, and reactive to light and accommodation), is often used (and often carelessly!) to record the pupillary examination. Since you need not test accommodation/near reaction routinely, you would note only PERRL (4 mm) (see Table 5.4).

Clinical–anatomic correlation

The pupillary light reaction helps to localize damage in the afferent visual pathways (Fig. 5.5). What would be the effect on the pupillary

Table 5.5 Comparing the right and left pupils: four examples

Example*	Observation	
	Right eye	Left eye
Anisocoria (one pupil abnormally small)	Larger right pupil is normal (note: slight asymmetry of pupillary size is not uncommon as a benign condition; sometimes genetic)	Smaller left pupil is abnormal (miotic) (consider sympathetic pathway lesion – Horner's syndrome, see Fig. 13.11 – or sympathetic antagonist drug-reactivity preserved; or, parasympathetic/cholinergic agonist drugs, e.g. eye drops)
Anisocoria (one pupil abnormally large)	Larger right pupil is abnormal; reactivity to light is decreased or absent (consider CN 3 lesion, see Fig. 5.5); parasympathetic/cholinergic antagonist; or, sympathetic agonist drug (eye drops, etc.); also, local surgical or traumatic defect (irregular shape)	Smaller left pupil is normal (note: since absolute pupillary size changes with light conditions, the essential baseline observation is the asymmetry itself)
Bilateral dilatation	Enlarged right pupil Preserved reactivity: sympathetic/adrenergic effect Diminished or absent reactivity: bilateral damage to parasympathetic supply (e.g. CN 3); pharmacologic parasympathetic antagonist/anticholinergic effect (atropine-like): systemic drug or bilateral drops	Enlarged left pupil
Bilateral constriction	Constricted right pupil Sympathetic antagonist drugs; opioids (narcotics); parasympathetic/cholinergic agonist drugs/eye drops (pilocarpine for glaucoma, etc.); bilateral sympathetic pathway lesions (see Fig. 13.11, Case 17C, and Fig. 17.4)	Constricted left pupil

* Designation of the right vs. left pupil as larger or smaller is arbitrary and for purposes of illustration only; any of the changes listed could affect either the right or left pupil (see text regarding the effect of an afferent, optic nerve lesion on pupillary size).

reaction in each eye of the following lesions? Unilateral and bilateral severance of: (a) the optic nerve; (b) the optic tract; and (c) the optic radiation (geniculocalcarine tract) or visual cortex (for answers, see Table 5.6, which also indicates the effect of a lesion in the efferent CN 3/parasympathetic pathway).

Cortical blindness

Light reception as evidenced by pupillary reaction sometimes occurs in the absence of visual perception. The fibers involved in the reflex leave the optic tract for the midbrain/pretectal area before the optic tract terminates in the lateral geniculate nucleus. Therefore, even a complete, bilateral lesion in the geniculate nuclei or more posterior parts of the visual pathways (see Fig. 13.17) will cause blindness but preserve the

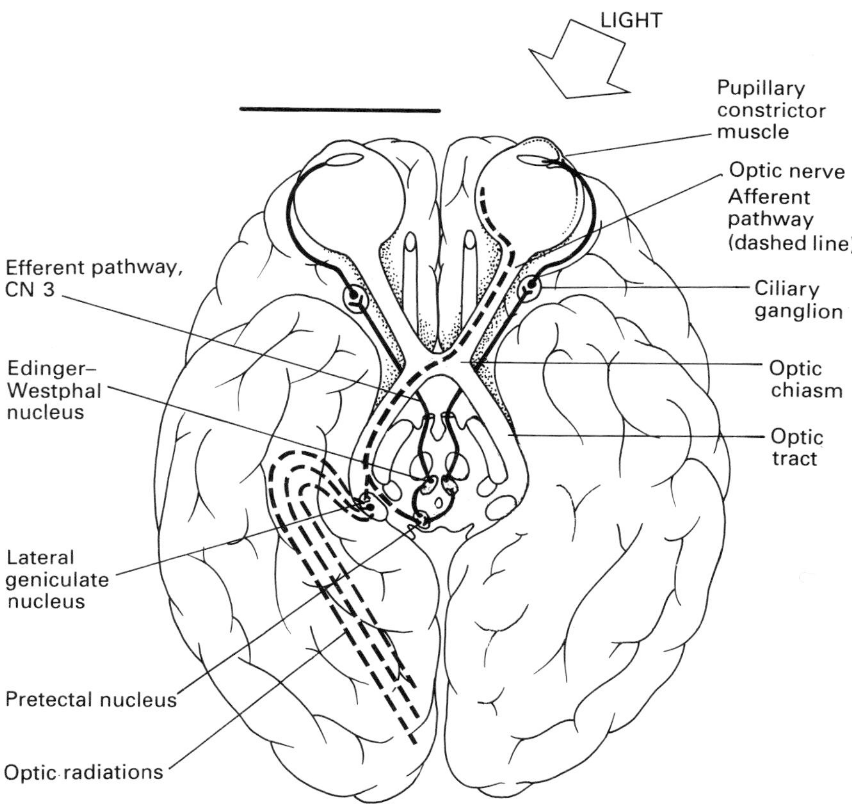

Fig. 5.5 Pupillary reflex pathways. This schematic shows the afferent pupillary pathway stimulated by light striking the retina (only the pathway from the nasal retina is shown, for clarity). The nerve impulses are transmitted through the optic nerve and cross in the chiasm to the opposite optic tract. Just before the lateral geniculate nucleus, the afferent fibers send branches to the pretectal nucleus, connecting with the Edinger–Westphal nuclei on both sides, permitting the direct and consensual light reflex. The efferent limb of the reflex arc travels from each Edinger–Westphal parasympathetic nucleus, a part of the CN 3 nuclear complex, via CN 3 to synapse in the ciliary ganglion, from which postganglionic fibers travel anteriorly to the iris of the eye. (The position of the nuclei and ganglia are rendered schematically.)

pupillary light reaction. This visual loss with pupillary reactivity is loosely called "cortical blindness," but the lesions need not actually be in the visual cortex.

Afferent defect/pupil size

What is the effect of an afferent lesion in one optic nerve on pupillary size (as opposed to reactivity)? It has been argued, and often appears to be the case, that the consensual reflex effect from ordinary light in the other eye will maintain the pupils at the same size. However, on average, the pupil ipsilateral to optic nerve lesions is slightly larger.

Table 5.6 Direct and consensual pupillary reactions: effect of complete lesions in reflex arc

Afferent limb lesion	Direct reaction (reaction in eye that is illuminated)	Consensual reaction (indirect reaction in other eye)
Prechiasmal lesion		
Optic nerve; intraocular	Absent	Absent
*Postchiasmal lesion**		
Optic tract	Present	Present
Lateral geniculate	Present	Present
Optic radiations	Present	Present
Visual cortex	Present	Present
Efferent limb (parasympathetic) lesion		
CN 3 ipsilateral to illuminated eye	Absent	Present
CN 3 contralateral to illuminated eye	Present	Absent

* Afferent pupillary reflex fibers from both optic nerves run in each optic tract which connects (via the pretectal area) with the CN 3/Edinger–Westphal nuclear complex on both sides. A lesion of one optic tract does not abolish the routine light reflex, direct or consensual, in either eye, assuming the light source illuminates the posterior pole of the retina diffusely, not just one side.

Eye movements

Definition: EOM

The movements of the eyes are produced by extraocular muscles: the medial, lateral, superior, and inferior rectus muscles and the superior and inferior oblique muscles. (The intraocular muscles change the shape of the lens and the size of the pupillary aperture in the iris.) The actions of the extraocular muscles have come to be represented by the abbreviation EOM for extraocular movements which are, simply, eye movements.

Overview

Eye movements are intimately involved with the success of visual perception: where and how well we look affects how much we see.

Analysis of eye movements often provides a key to localization, both because of neatly wired connections in the brainstem and because of the landmarks that the nerves traverse in their path to the orbits. However, most of such details need not be kept in mind by the nonspecialist. Indeed, you should concentrate on the description of your observations of what the eyes do.

You should be able to observe and document the following features of eye movements to obtain the data necessary for formulation (see also the supplementary material on horizontal and vertical gaze in Chapter 17).

1 What is the resting position of the two eyes? Are they aligned or is one eye on a different horizontal or vertical axis from the other? Are they both deviated in any particular direction?

Specific objectives of examination

2 Do they move together fully and equally in all directions? Do they move conjugately (yoked together, maintaining their alignment one to the other)?

3 Are there any adventitious or extra movements, such as jiggles, jerks, or rhythmic oscillations (for nystagmus, see below).

Adopt a systematic method such as the following.

Testing

Observe position at rest

1 Observe the eyes for their position at rest by standing or sitting directly in front of the patient. Is one eye turned outward (exotropia) or inward (esotropia), both of these being forms of strabismus (a lack of alignment of the two eyes)? Note that in the case of divergent or convergent eyes, the visually fixing eye determines which eye appears to be abnormally "out" (or "in").

When misalignment is slight, you can recognize it by shining a flashlight towards the eyes from at least 0.6 metres (2 feet) away, so as to minimize convergence.

Is there a deviation of both eyes in one direction, despite the absence of visual stimuli attracting them to that side? This is called a tonic deviation, or ongoing bias to one side, and is not dependent on whether the patient is seeing anything (see Chapter 17).

Observe spontaneous gaze

2 Observe the spontaneous movement of the eyes. Is there a tendency to look more frequently in one direction (a gaze preference)?

Test following movements

3 Ask the patient to follow a stimulus, such as your moving finger or penlight, through a full range of motion to the right, left, up, and down. (Testing oblique movements has little value for screening, but should be done if a symptom such as double vision or other findings indicate any problem with ocular motility.) To avoid the strain of convergence keep your stimulus at nearly arm's length from the patient's face. In case of very poor vision (or other difficulty with following), ask the patient simply to point the eyes fully in each direction. (For eye movement evaluation in the comatose patient, see Chapter 17, sections on Doll's Head maneuver and ice water calorics.)

4 The test for convergence of the eyes (bilateral adduction) is the same as described for the pupillary near reaction (see Table 5.4) and has little routine value.

Nystagmus

5 Look for any adventitious (extraneous) movements at rest or in any field of gaze. Nystagmus is defined as rhythmic or semirhythmic oscillation (of one or both eyes, together or separately) in any plane (horizontal, vertical, rotatory, or a combination of these). The description of your observations should be based on the following criteria.

(a) The field of gaze in which the movements occur (e.g. when looking to the right).

(b) The plane of the movements themselves (horizontal, vertical, rotatory, or a combination of these).

(c) The direction of a jerk or fast component, defined in terms of the patient's right or left. (You may see a series of fast jerk phases to the right coupled with slow return phases to the left.) Rotatory movement is documented as clockwise or counterclockwise.

(d) The amplitude of the beats (are they coarse or fine).

(e) Other characteristics (is the nystagmus episodic, does it fatigue, etc.).

An accurate description is much more valuable than a label that is subject to diverse interpretation ("right jerk nystagmus"). Incidentally, a very fine nystagmus may first be recognized on seeing the optic disc or vessels oscillate during funduscopic examination.

Endpoint nystagmus (normal)

You will find it helpful to try to distinguish between endpoint nystagmus and pre-endpoint nystagmus. The endpoint is the extreme limit of gaze in one direction, often corresponding to the point at which binocular fixation is lost. When the adducting eye loses sight of the point being followed (as when the line of vision is blocked by the nose), a fine horizontal nystagmus with the fast component towards the direction of gaze may develop. This is thought to occur because the eyes have become unyoked, due to loss of binocular fixation, or because of instability that occurs with maximum muscle contraction, or both. To help distinguish the endpoint, use a flashlight as the stimulus to be followed: as long as the patient is able to see the light with both eyes, you will be able to see its highlight reflected in the centers of the patient's corneas. When the highlight disappears from the cornea of the adducting eye (as the light source moves far laterally), the patient will no longer be seeing it with both eyes and the appearance of a few beats of horizontal nystagmus can be considered normal, as a rule.

Analyzing EOM deficits

As you see, eye movements can be tested and described without a detailed knowledge of the innervation and mechanics of individual eye movements. Yet the next step is to make anatomic correlations with specific ocular palsies for the purpose of localization, and for this a few general principles may be helpful.

1 The horizontally acting muscles for abduction (out, away) and adduction (in) are relatively simple:

(a) abduction – lateral rectus muscle (abducens nerve CN 6);

(b) adduction – medial rectus muscle (oculomotor nerve CN 3).

Effect of contraction depends upon eye position

2 Vertical movement is more complex than horizontal movement: the muscular action responsible for elevating or depressing the eye depends upon the position of the eye in the horizontal plane, that is, whether it is abducted or adducted. As evident in Fig. 5.6, the superior rectus muscle (innervated by CN 3) elevates the eye except when the eye is adducted; in that position the inferior oblique (also innervated by CN 3) is the main elevator, while the superior rectus acts to rotate it (on an anteroposterior axis of the eyeball). Similarly, the inferior rectus (CN 3) depresses the eye except when it is adducted, at which point the superior oblique (CN 4)

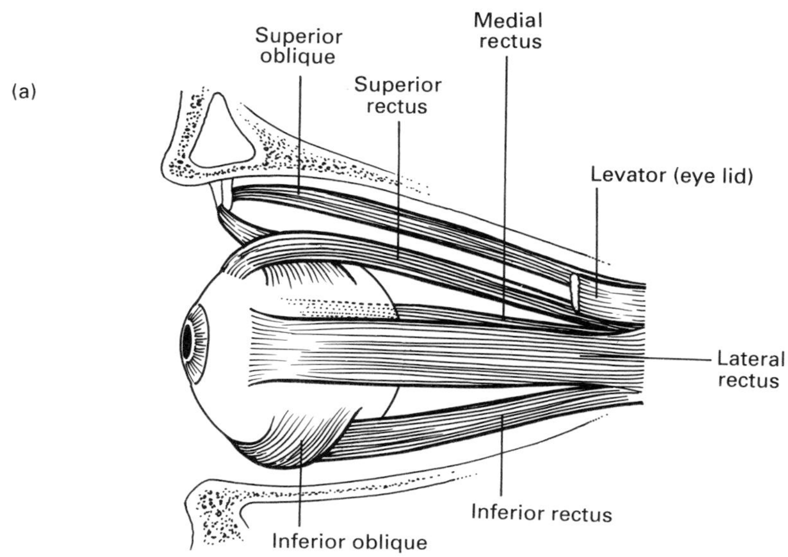

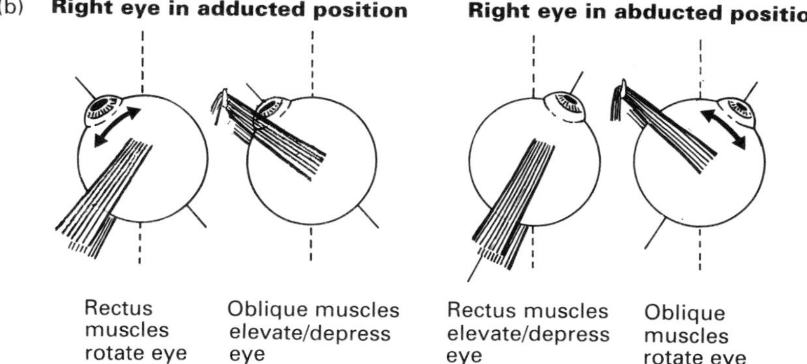

Fig. 5.6 Extraocular muscles. (a) From the origins and insertions of the muscles, the effect of contraction can be reasoned (depending upon the starting position of the eye). (b) With the right eye adducted the superior and inferior rectus muscles rotate it (intorsion and extorsion, respectively). The major elevator and depressor are the inferior and superior oblique, respectively. With the right eye abducted the rectus muscles elevate and depress the eye, and the obliques rotate (torsion). (Adapted from Cogan, D.B. *Neurology of the Ocular Muscles*. 3rd edn. C.C. Thomas, Springfield (Ill), 1956.)

turns it down while the inferior rectus rotates it. In actual function, most movements require a delicate balance of action by these muscles.

3 Note the following exceptions to the rule of uncrossed cranial nerves: CN 4 crosses dorsal to the midbrain; those fibers from CN 3 nuclei that are destined to innervate the superior rectus muscle cross in the midbrain to help form the opposite CN 3. In a similar fashion, the levator palpebrae muscle receives crossed as well as uncrossed fibers. In their peripheral courses, after leaving the midbrain region, no crossing occurs, and almost all peripheral lesions thus affect only the ipsilateral eye.

4 Remember the concept of a chain of function (Chapter 3) when analyzing any limitation of eye movement: the problem may consist of a mechanical restriction in the orbit, a primary disorder of muscle or the neuromuscular junction, a lesion in a cranial nerve peripherally, or damage in the brainstem. The lesion should not be attributed to the cranial nerve itself, just because the deficit is loosely referred to as a "6th nerve palsy." Descriptively it is a weakness of abduction. Hemispheric control is exerted on the working of the two eyes together, not on the movements of one eye or one eye muscle in isolation (see Chapter 17).

5 Do not diagnose an individual ocular palsy unless the relative positions of the two eyes change with different fields of gaze. In congenital strabismus the degree of misalignment may vary, but double vision is not experienced, since one image is suppressed. Which eye appears to be turned out (exotropia) or turned in (esotropia) depends upon which eye is fixing visually. Thus, when an eye appears "turned in," for example, do not automatically assume paralysis of abduction, as from a lesion of CN 6 (Fig. 5.7).

Double vision

Double vision (diplopia) is the cardinal symptom of an acquired misalignment between the eyes. Differentiate binocular from monocular double vision: cover each eye separately to eliminate binocular double vision and localize monocular split images to the responsible eye. Blindness or complete ptosis of one eye prevents double vision. Diplopia occurs in the plane of action (e.g. horizontal) of the two pairs (yokes) of muscles acting in that plane. The separation of images is maximal when looking in the direction of action (e.g. right) of the pair that deviates gaze to the right (e.g. right lateral rectus and left medial rectus), one of which is the paretic muscle. (A red glass over one eye identifies the source of that image, enabling identification of the paretic muscle.)

Eyelid elevation

Overview

Eye opening conveys wakefulness, just as "droopy" eyes ordinarily signify sleepiness. Closed lids may signify merely relaxation as in sleep, paralysis of lid elevation, or forced contraction.

Definitions

Palpebral fissure

Ptosis

False ptosis

The space between the eyelids – what makes an eye look big or small – is described by the width of the aperture, the palpebral fissure (Fig. 5.8). This width is estimated or measured as the vertical distance between the two lids at the middle of the eye. An abnormal droop of the upper lid is called ptosis (pronounced "toe-sis"), which can be simply a slight droop relative to the other eye or an absolute droop, evident independently, as when the lid covers part or all of the pupil. (Blepharochalasis means a sagging redundancy of the skin of the lid, which may hang down, giving an appearance of ptosis (false ptosis) even though the lid margin itself is not drooping.)

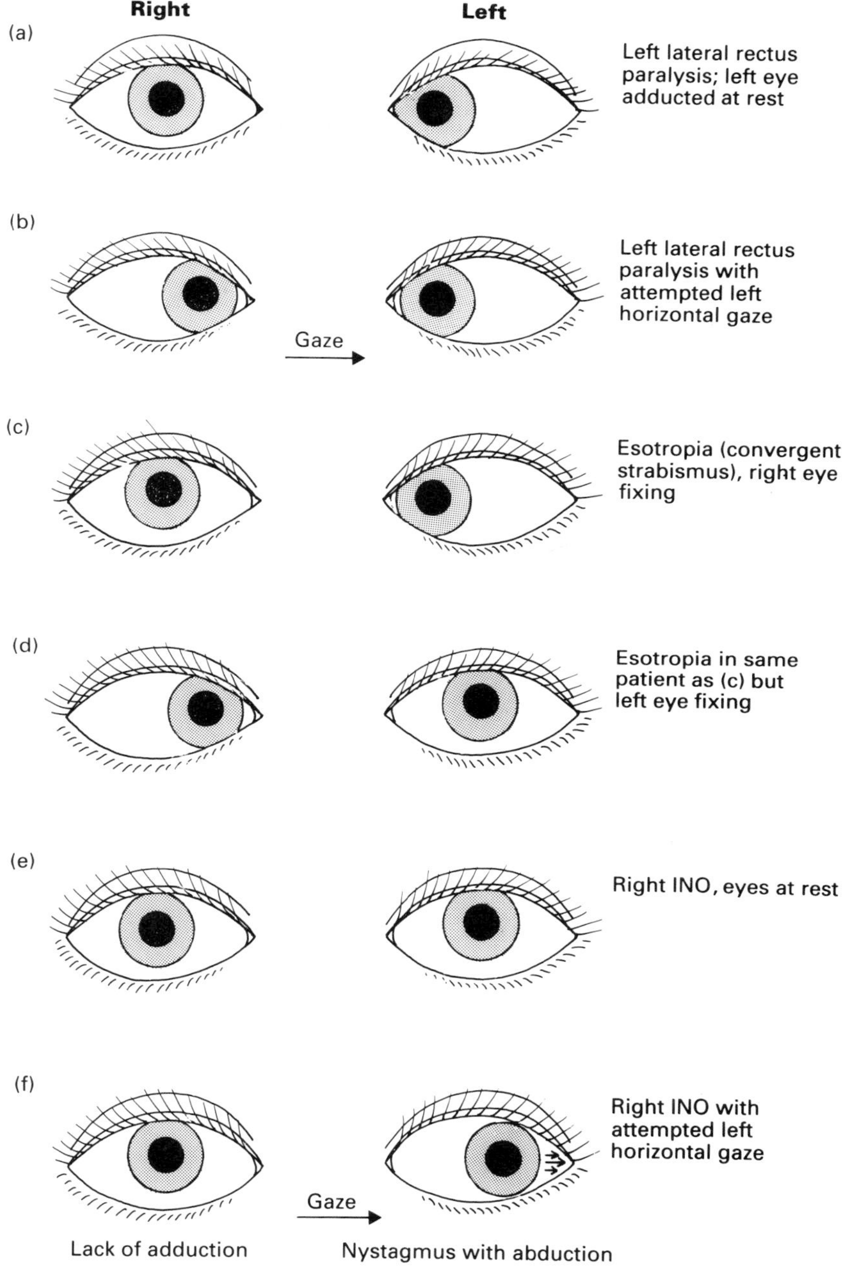

Fig. 5.7 Dysconjugate gaze (selected examples). (a) In a left lateral rectus palsy (paralysis) the left eye is adducted at rest due to the unopposed pull of the left medial rectus. (b) With attempted left horizontal gaze the right eye adducts normally, but the left eye does not abduct from its medially deviated position. (c) Strabismus (congenital, nonparalytic). With the right eye fixing, the left eye is medially deviated (esotropia). (d) In the same patient with the left eye fixing, the right eye is now medially deviated (alternating esotropia). In this case, the angle between the axes of the two eyes remains the same ("comitant" strabismus). (e) A typical right internuclear ophthalmoplegia (INO) at rest. See (g), p. 82. With no stimulus for horizontal gaze, both eyes are typically aligned in the midline. (f) With attempted left horizontal gaze in the same patient, the message to adduct never reaches the right CN 3 nucleus but the left eye abducts (with nystagmus). (*continued*)

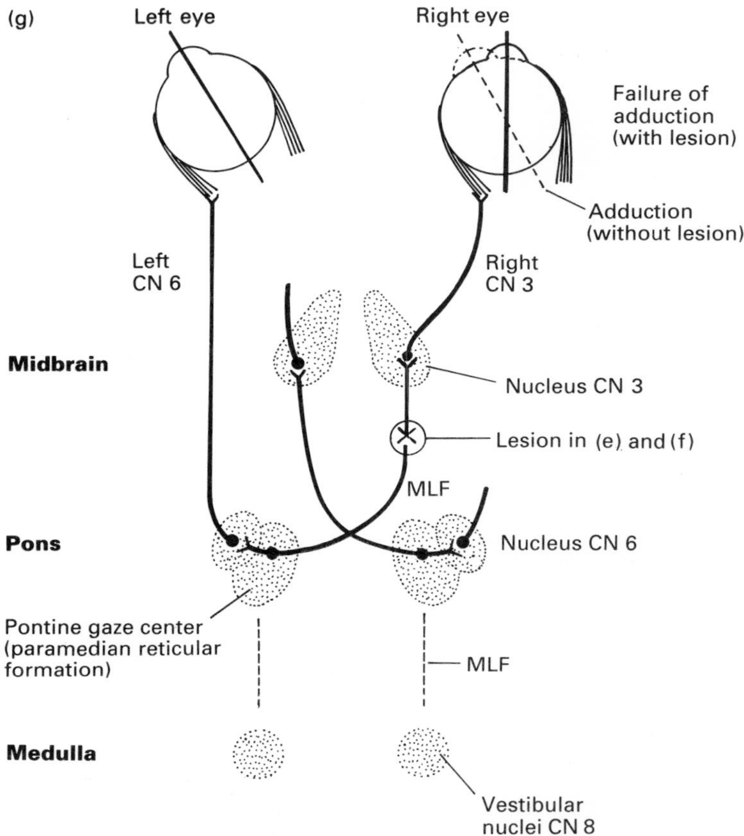

Fig. 5.7 (*continued*) (g) A schematic showing the crossed medial longitudinal fasiculi (MLF) connecting the pontine gaze centers/CN 6 nuclei with the CN 3 nuclei in the midbrain. The lesion in the right MLF causes a disconnection resulting in the abnormality shown in (f).

Testing

Both lids closed

If both lids are droopy or closed, first try arousal and then check any mechanical factor holding the lids together (like the secretions that may "glue" the eyelids in the sleepy or comatose patient). Next, is there active lid closure? Gently retract the upper lids. If the lids are just passively sagging, you will encounter virtually no resistance. With forced closure, you will feel active resistance and will be able to see the eyeballs rolling upward, a reflex called Bell's phenomenon that occurs with activation of the eye closure mechanism.

Asymmetry of fissures

More commonly, you will need to distinguish between the palpebral fissures on the right and left. Is one side too wide or the other too narrow? (See Table 5.7). Note that slight unilateral ptosis is a relatively common variant that may be familial or congenital, either in isolation or as part of a mild Horner's syndrome (see Fig. 13.11 and Table 5.7). Old photographs often reveal the chronic and static nature of the asymmetry and thus obviate the need for work-up.

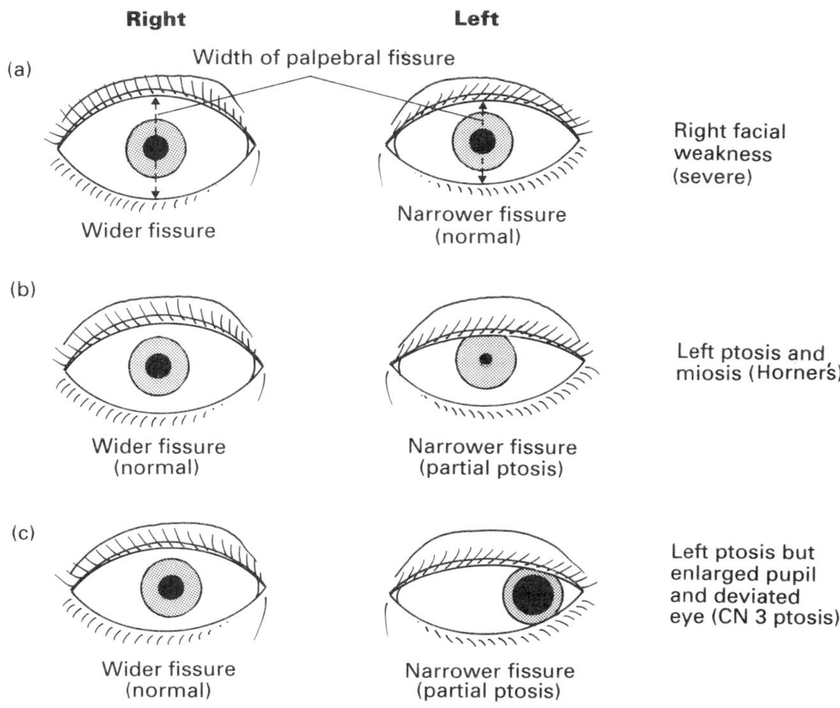

Fig. 5.8 Palpebral fissures. (a) An abnormally wide fissure on the right, due to weakness of eyelid closure (orbicularis oculi), innervated by CN 7. (The points for estimating the width of the palpebral fissures are shown by the vertical lines.) (b) A partial ptosis on the left due to a lesion of sympathetic innervation, confirmed by finding a smaller pupil on that side (Horner's syndrome). (c) A partial left ptosis associated with an enlarged pupil and laterally deviated eye, indicating a palsy of left CN 3.

Observe whether elevation of an eyelid is accomplished by raising the eyebrow, helping to retract the upper lid. Patients with ptosis will often compensate by this mechanism, and you will observe increased wrinkling above the eyebrow as a result. If ptosis is only partial, test also for fatiguing by having the patient sustain upward gaze (which is normally accompanied by elevation of the upper lid). Over time does the lid droop further (as in myasthenia gravis)? Occasionally, a patient will close one eye sufficiently to eliminate double vision, giving a false appearance of ptosis.

Innervation

Ptosis represents a failure of the lid elevating mechanism, which is partly subserved by CN 3 (fibers to the levator palpebrae superioris muscle) and partly by sympathetic innervation to smooth muscle fibers. (You can remember the latter by recalling the wide-eyed look of a person in a state of excitement or other sympathetic stimulation.) Eyelid closure is mediated via CN 7.

Table 5.7 Clinical correlation of ptosis and asymmetry of palpebral fissures

Side with narrower fissure	Side with wider fissure
Narrower side normal (other side abnormal)	Abnormally wide fissure; facial weakness on this side (decreased eyelid closure, CN 7); also, lid retraction and/or proptosis (hyperthyroidism, etc.)
This side abnormally narrow	This side normal
False ptosis: forced closure (blepharospasm); sagging upper eyelid skin (blepharochalasis); eyelid closure to block diplopia	
Ptosis: primary muscle or neuromuscular junction lesion (levator palpebrae); CN 3 dysfunction (levator palpebrae) – look for enlarged, less reactive pupil, oculomotor deficit; sympathetic lesion (smooth muscle elevator) – look for constricted (miotic) pupil and decreased sweating ipsilaterally (Horner's syndrome)	

Pitfalls

Common mistakes of interpretation include the following:
1 attributing eyelid drooping to facial weakness;
2 assuming that the side with a slightly narrower palpebral fissure is ptotic, whereas, in fact, the contralateral fissure is abnormally wide.

CRANIAL NERVE 5 (TRIGEMINAL): FACIAL SENSATION, CORNEAL REFLEXES, AND JAW MOVEMENTS

Facial sensation

Overview

The principles of testing sensation on the face are identical to those for the rest of the body (see Chapter 7). However, since the face is especially sensitive (both physically and psychologically) you should exercise special care and explain what you are doing.

Testing

Test touch before pin (as the latter can be more threatening). With pin testing, show that your pin (a new safety pin) is not too sharp by first applying it gently to the patient's hand. During testing, keep the point away from the eye. A quick temperature test for cold sensation can be done with the metal of your tuning fork, to pick up a subjective difference between sides. For a systematic survey, check each sensory modality on each side on the forehead, cheeks, and lower jaw (corresponding to the 1st, 2nd, 3rd divisions of the trigeminal nerve (CN 5) distribution). If you have received local anesthetic for dental work, you are surely aware of the innervation of the inside of the mouth by the 2nd (maxillary) and 3rd (mandibular) divisions.

Interpretation

When interpreting the boundaries of a sensory deficit on the face or scalp, recall that the area of sensation served by the trigeminal nerve (CN 5) does not include the posterior scalp or the neck (see Fig. 16.1). A deficit within the territory of one or more of the three sensory divisions of CN 5 does not necessarily mean that the lesion is in the trigeminal nerve (or division) itself: a small lesion in a CNS sensory pathway can produce a focal impairment that falls within or overlaps the territory of a trigeminal division.

Corneal reflex

Definition

The corneal reflex is a bilateral (direct and consensual) blink caused by stimulating the cornea. Despite its lack of routine importance at the bedside, this reflex will be explained because it is the source of much confusion. It is also useful to have it in your repertoire since it occasionally helps in brainstem localization.

There is an afferent limb (CN 5) and an efferent limb (CN 7, eye closure). Thus, while the reflex is discussed under CN 5 here, it could as well be listed under CN 7 or under superficial reflexes (see Chapter 9).

Issues

The main questions regarding the corneal reflex are as follows.

1 When should the corneal reflex be tested?
2 How do you test it to avoid misinterpretation?
3 Does a decreased reflex indicate a sensory (afferent) or motor (efferent) lesion? (Table 5.8.)

Table 5.8 Analysis of corneal reflex responses

Corneal stimulus	Response		Interpretation
	Right blink	Left blink	
1 Stimulate right	0	0	Right afferent lesion (patient will not feel the stimulus), or bilateral efferent lesions (severe weakness of eye closure will be evident)
2 Stimulate left	+	+	Shows left afferent and both efferents working; together with 1 above, proves a right afferent lesion
3 Stimulate right	0	+	Right efferent lesion
4 Stimulate left	0	+	Right efferent lesion

Note: an afferent or efferent lesion does not necessarily mean a lesion of CN 5 or CN 7, respectively. The corneal reflex is affected by lesions involving the cerebrum as well as the segmental inflow and outflow at the brainstem level. An acute lesion of the right or left hemisphere may depress the response when the cornea is stimulated on the contralateral side (over and above the effect that a facial weakness may have on the blink).

4 Does a decreased corneal reflex mean a brainstem or cranial nerve lesion?

Testing

To test the patient's corneal reflex adopt the procedure detailed below.

1 Explain that you will be touching the front of the eye with a wisp of cotton (show it to the patient) and that it will not hurt. Do not test patients with contact lenses in place! (Even if the lenses are out, corneal sensitivity may be affected.)

2 Touch the cornea with a wisp of cotton drawn out from the end of a throat swab. The cotton should be clean, but need not be sterile. Never use any sharp, rough, reused, or dirty material for testing.

3 Be sure to touch the cornea (over the pupil and iris), not the scleral conjunctiva (over the white of the eye), as the latter is much less sensitive. The patient experiences less visual threat if you ask him or her to look up as you approach the eye from the side.

4 Observe how brisk and complete the blink is on the same and opposite sides.

5 Now test the other eye. Sometimes the first eye tested will show a greater apparent response (startle effect) and sometimes the second eye, (anticipation effect). Before concluding that the corneal reflexes are asymmetric, go back and forth a couple of times to assure yourself of a consistent difference.

6 If the patient is stuporous or comatose and you find the corneal response hard to obtain with a very thin wisp, use a heavier strand to increase the stimulus until you get a response or can conclude that it is absent.

Clinical correlation

Analyze whether the defect seems to be in the sensory (afferent) arc and/or in the motor (efferent) arc (see Table 5.8). Remember that not just the segmental parts of the reflex ("in" CN 5, "out" CN 7) are involved, but also cerebral connections. Some supranuclear lesions, such as an acute, large, frontoparietal stroke, will cause a (transient) direct, contralateral, and consensual decrease in the corneal reflex.

Based upon your test results, if you suspect an afferent problem, test carefully for any decrease in sensation over the face, especially in the territory of the 1st trigeminal (CN 5) division to detect a segmental lesion. If you suspect an efferent problem, check voluntary eye closure and other muscles of facial expression.

Corneal reflex data are more useful in localizing intrinsic pontomedullary lesions and mass lesions of the posterior fossa that may compress the brainstem, such as cerebellar hemorrhage and acoustic neuromas (tumors of CN 8). Like other superficial (cephalic) reflexes, the presence of a corneal reflex is inconsistent with complete brain death.

There is a great deal of individual variation in normal response to corneal stimulation. A bilateral decrease, even an apparent absence of the corneal reflexes, is rarely of neurologic significance in an otherwise alert, intact patient. While corneal and other superficial reflexes may not be detectable in hysteric conversion states, the former should not be used as evidence for the latter. Local corneal changes, especially those induced by contact lenses, are the most common causes of reproducible deficits in reflex activity.

Key points on corneal reflex

Key points of corneal reflex testing are listed below.

1 I do not recommend routine testing because of the wide range of individual responses and the many non-neurologic causes of apparent abnormalities.

2 Testing is especially indicated in cases of suspected brainstem lesions, cerebellar lesions (impinging on brainstem), and CN 5, CN 7, and CN 8 lesions.

3 The corneal reflex is often decreased acutely contralateral to a major cerebral lesion.

Jaw movements

When testing jaw movements including mastication, follow the procedure described below.

Testing of jaw movements

1 Palpate the masseter and temporalis muscles on both sides during clenching of the teeth.

2 As you test the power of jaw closing and of opening (pterygoid muscles) against resistance, watch for deviation of the jaw to one side, which suggests asymmetric strength.

Clinical correlation

The muscles of mastication are innervated by the motor branch of CN 5 (3rd division, mandibular). Jaw weakness occurs rarely in primary disorders of muscle or the neuromuscular junction. (Inquire about difficulty or fatigue in chewing meat or other foods.) Unilateral hemispheric, upper motor neuron (UMN) lesions usually do not produce appreciable lateralized jaw weakness, because of the bilateral suprasegmental UMN innervation of the CN 5 motor nuclei in the brainstem.

The more common jaw problems involve aching of the masseter and temporalis muscles due to unconscious tensing, grinding of the teeth (bruxism), or pain and stiffness at the temporomandibular joints. Difficulty opening or closing the jaw suggests dislocation at these joints, a dystonic reaction to an antipsychotic drug, or muscle pain or spasm due to tetanus, parotitis, or temporal arteritis.

CRANIAL NERVE 7: FACIAL EXPRESSION AND TASTE

Overview

Facial expression provides insight into feeling and personality (allowing somewhat for cultural differences) as well as displaying a prominent aspect of motor function. There are many small muscles of facial expression and little reason for you to remember their individual names. Instead, you should concentrate on close observation of facial expression during the general encounter as well as during specific testing. In many instances you will pick up a slight asymmetry or an overall lack of mobility of facial features only in the course of watching the patient's spontaneous activity and reactions.

Testing

1 Observe both emotional facial expression, such as the appearance during laughter, and so-called volitional (planned) expression, such as a grimace that is requested during testing (see discussion below).

Nasolabial folds

2 Look specifically for symmetry of the nasolabial folds, the more or less prominent creases that run from the sides of the nose, down towards the corners of the mouth.

Eye closure

3 Specifically test forced eye closure by noting how fully the eyelashes are buried on each side. In the alert, cooperative patient, do not force the eyelids open, as these tissues are delicate and easily bruised. However, in the stuporous or comatose patient it is helpful to retract gently the upper lids in order to compare the tone of the eye closure muscles.

4 As you observe forced eye closure, also note the symmetry of the frown or grimace that often accompanies it. Or ask the patient to smile or grimace ("show your teeth"). Further testing of the muscles around the mouth could include pursing the lips and puffing out the cheeks.

5 Pay special attention to the forehead muscles, especially the ability to raise the eyebrows and wrinkle up the forehead. The involvement or lack of involvement of the upper face is valuable for analysis of facial weakness in terms of a segmental vs. supranuclear mechanism (see below).

Clinical correlation

Lower motor neuron (LMN)-type weakness

As noted in the introductory section of this chapter, the distinction between a segmental, lower motor neuron (LMN) type, and a suprasegmental, UMN, or supranuclear type of facial weakness is of fundamental localizing importance (Fig. 5.9 and Table 5.9). The LMN, or

Table 5.9 Analysis of facial weakness pattern

	Lesion of right cerebral hemisphere (upper motor neuron, UMN), corticobulbar, suprasegmental type)	Lesion of right brainstem/ CN 7 (lower motor neuron, LMN), segmental type)
Upper part of the face (forehead)	Not affected (because of bilateral UMN/corticobulbar innervation of the portion of the left facial nucleus (in pons) from which LMN fibers of CN 7 go to upper face)	Right (ipsilateral) forehead weakness, together with impaired eye closure
Lower part of the face	Weakness of left lower face (contralateral); the part of the left facial nucleus which sends fibers to the lower face receives UMN innervation "only" from contralateral (right) hemisphere	Weakness of right lower face; (together with the upper face involvement noted above) this is the pattern of weakness in the total facial distribution characteristic of a lesion of the final common pathway (LMN)

Note: eyelid closure is considered between upper and lower face; it is affected in the UMN pattern but more severely in the LMN pattern.

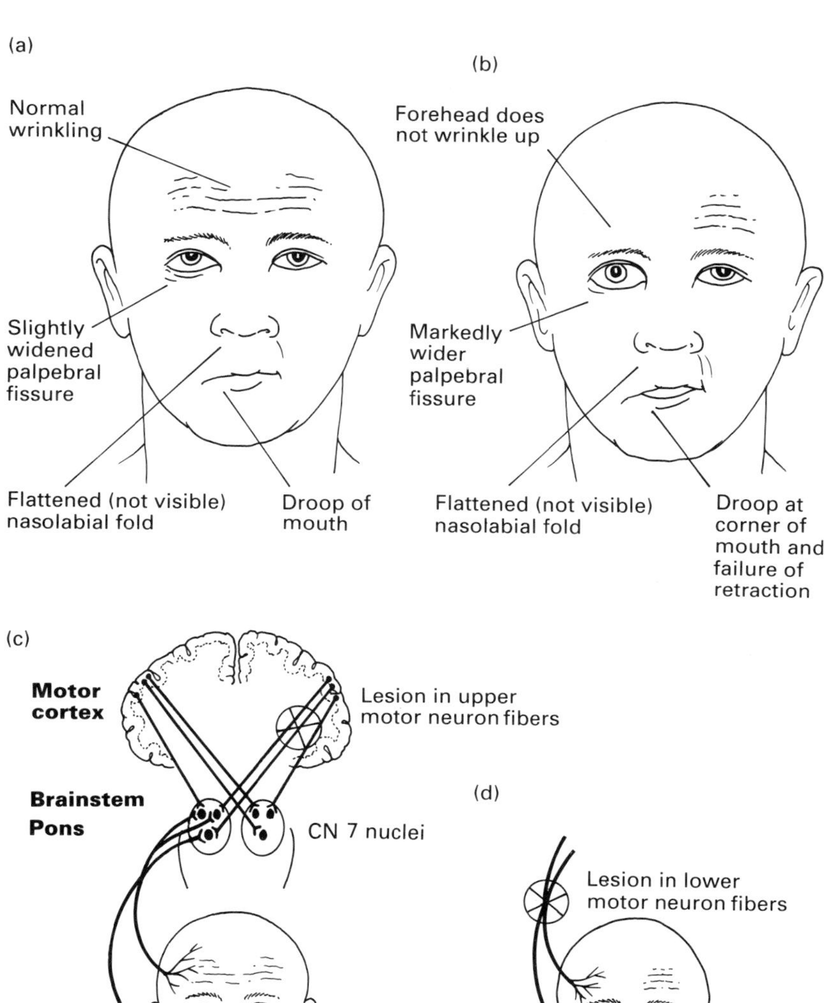

Fig. 5.9 Facial weakness: patterns and lesions. (a) Upper motor neuron (UMN) pattern of weakness with slight widening of the right palpebral fissure, a droop of the right side of the mouth, and flattening of the right nasolabial fold, but with preservation of wrinkling up of the forehead (the upper part of the face is largely or completely spared). (b) Lower motor neuron (LMN) pattern of facial weakness in which the entire right side of the face is weak. (c) Schematic showing a lesion of the UMN, corticobulbar tracts from the left motor cortex to the CN 7 (facial) nuclei in the pons. There is bilateral UMN innervation from the motor cortices to those LMNs of the right facial nucleus that will send out CN 7 fibers to the upper part of the right face, thus sparing the forehead. (d) Lesion of the LMN system, in this case affecting the right CN 7 peripherally, which is the final common pathway to the entire right side of the face.

peripheral, form is most clearly exemplified by the effect of cutting CN 7. Since this is the final common pathway, all innervated facial muscles on that side would be entirely paralyzed. In contrast, if the UMN fibers from the contralateral cortex – the fibers that descend and cross in the brainstem before synapsing on the CN 7 nucleus – were disconnected, this would result in a different appearance: the movements of the upper part of the face (mainly the forehead) would typically be preserved. In contrast, the movements of the lower part of the face, such as spreading the lips, would be diminished. Evidently, there is bilateral supranuclear innervation to the part of CN 7 nucleus that innervates the upper part of the face. This part of the nucleus receives uncrossed as well as crossed corticobulbar fibers – fibers from both hemispheres. Therefore, even a major supranuclear lesion on one side produces little or no weakness of the forehead. However, a second supranuclear lesion, this time on the other side, might then cause weakness of the entire face on both sides.

UMN-type weakness

This quirk of circuitry thus helps with the particular example of segmental vs. suprasegmental localization posed by facial weakness: the distribution of weakness within the facial nerve territory points to the source of the weakness, namely the UMN or the LMN link. Beware, however, of confusion caused by the words we use: distinguish between the upper part of the face and UMN and between a "peripheral type" of facial weakness and a lesion in the peripheral portion of CN 7. A lesion in the nucleus of CN 7 is obviously within the CNS, but produces a peripheral type of facial weakness, the segmental, LMN type which involves the upper as well as the lower part of the face! Thus, first describe the observed function of the various parts of the face and then draw your inference regarding the pattern of involvement – the entire side of the face (LMN) or just the lower part (UMN).

Eyelid closure

Is the eye considered part of the upper face or the lower? In practice, eyelid closure is impaired by most lesions causing weakness of only the lower part of the face, the UMN pattern. However, LMN lesions can produce a much more profound deficit in eye closure, sometimes causing gaping of the lids and preventing adequate blinking, which is essential for corneal protection.

Bilateral weakness

Bilateral facial weakness may be quite difficult to recognize, especially if it is very symmetric and relatively mild. The patient exhibits a sagging, "down in the mouth" facial expression and the flattened, inert mouth with slightly gaping lips can suggest a fishmouth appearance, as seen in certain muscular dystrophies.

Volitional vs. emotional expression

You may notice at times a dissociation between planned, volitional movements, such as showing teeth, and emotionally activated movements such as spontaneous smile. The latter are thought to be mediated, at a supranuclear level, by limbic and subcortical motor pathways. (Diseases may affect the direct corticobulbar pathway and alternative subcortical motor pathways differentially.)

In their subjective account of symptoms of weakness, patients will sometimes seem to be directing you to the wrong side. They may feel the mouth "pulling to the right" (and thus focus on the right) whereas the pulling occurs because of weakness on the left. Patients may also experience heaviness, swollen, or "dead" feelings in the paralyzed side of the face. This usually does not mean an actual sensory deficit.

Relevant symptoms

Sense of taste

For practical purposes, evaluation of the sense of taste is limited to testing the anterior two-thirds of the tongue. First, emphasize that the test substance will not be disagreeable or harmful. If one side of the tongue is suspected of having a possible deficit, test that side of the tongue first so that there will be no foreknowledge of the flavor. Make up a thick slurry of salt or sugar in water and paint it heavily on the side of the protruded tongue, using a clean throat swab as an applicator. The tongue and jaw should remain as immobile as possible during testing to avoid diffusion of the test flavor.

Testing

There are two principal reasons for testing taste: first, the patient complains of loss of taste, which may represent loss of smell (see CN 1). Total loss of taste is very unusual. Patients are often unaware of unilateral loss of taste. Second, and much more common, is the occurrence of a LMN type of facial weakness. Taste on the anterior two-thirds of the tongue is subserved by afferent fibers that travel in the petrous bone with the trunk of CN 7. A lesion in this portion of CN 7 (Fig. 5.10) causes not only a LMN type of facial weakness, but also a decrease or loss of taste on that side of the tongue (anterior two-thirds). Thus, testing taste in this situation contributes to localization. Routine taste testing is not indicated.

Clinical correlation

Example: Bell's palsy (an inflammatory CN 7 syndrome)

CRANIAL NERVE 8: HEARING (ACOUSTIC) AND VESTIBULAR FUNCTION

Hearing

The most important thing about testing hearing is simply to do it! Determine specifically how well the patient can hear in each ear. The embellishments of the examination are of minor importance by comparison. A mild bilateral or more severe unilateral hearing loss is often inapparent in conversation.

Overview

Having inspected the ear canals and tympanic membranes with an otoscope, you should test auditory acuity in each ear separately, preferably using a high-frequency stimulus, such as a 512 Hz tuning fork, a ticking watch, or rubbing fingers together. (High frequencies are usually lost first, thus justifying the use of a high-pitch stimulus for screening.) Try to document the threshold for hearing by determining the

Testing acuity

High-frequency threshold

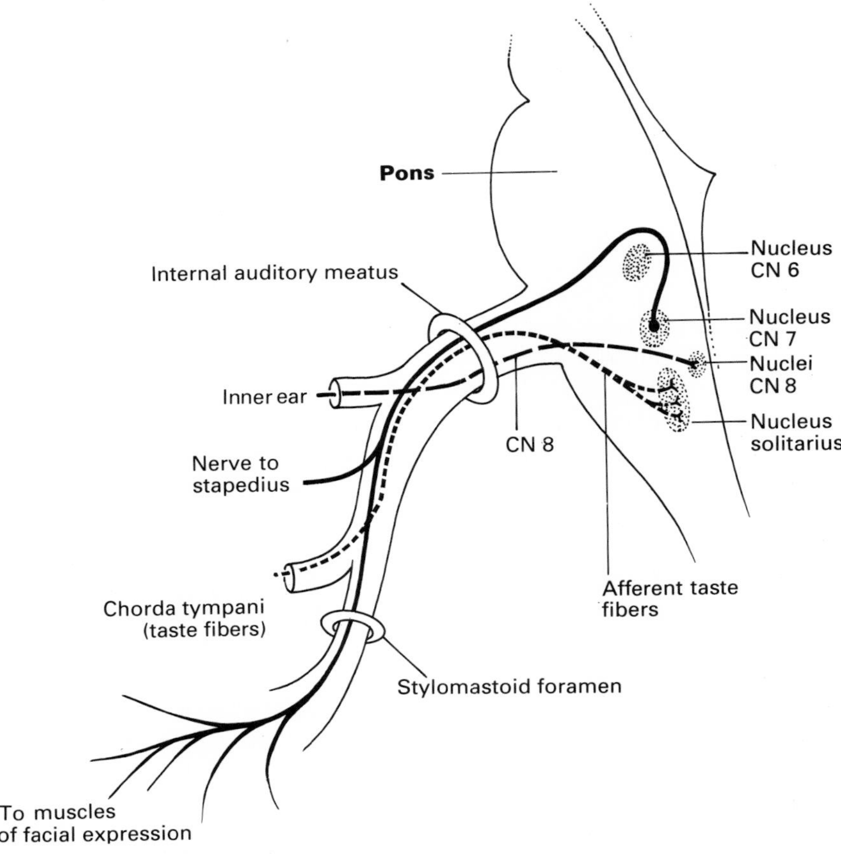

Fig. 5.10 Facial nerve (CN 7) with taste fibers. Highly simplified schematic view of the relationship of CN 7 with taste fibers. Lesions of the facial nerve, depending on location, may affect not only the innervation of the muscles of facial expression, but also the taste fibers in the chorda tympani and the nerve supply to the stapedius muscle. (Afferent and secretory fibers are not shown.)

softest perceptible stimulus: how far from the ear can a given stimulus be heard? If you have normal hearing, determine whether you can still hear the stimulus after the patient can no longer hear it. (To save time, start with a very soft sound so that you will not need to wait through the whole decay curve.)

Discrimination

If the patient demonstrates particular difficulty catching your words, even when you seem to be speaking loudly enough, you should assess speech discrimination by whispering in each ear, while masking the other. After assuring yourself that the problem is one of discriminating sounds (and not an aphasia or deficit in language comprehension which can be tested in writing), seek an audiologic consultation.

Air vs. bone conduction (Rinné)

Compare air conduction with bone conduction by asking the patient which sound is louder – when the foot of the tuning fork is placed on the skull near the ear (mastoid process) or when the vibrating tuning fork is then held in the air close to the ear (air conduction)? (This is the Rinné test which, together with the Weber test, I perform only when air conduction is impaired.)

Lateralization (Weber)

The sound of a tuning fork placed in the middle of the forehead should not normally lateralize: the sound should be heard in the middle, throughout the head, or in both ears, not primarily from one ear. As you test for this, be sure that the patient is not localizing the feeling of vibration, which would naturally be to one side if the fork were placed off-center. Because of the excellent conduction through bone, the sound of a laterally placed tuning fork will be well heard in both ears. In the Weber test, the sound lateralizes to the side of decreased air conduction. To understand the experience of bone conduction, note the effect of plugging one of your ears as you do the lateralization test with a 512 Hz tuning fork placed both laterally and in the middle of your own forehead (alternatively use a 256 or 128 Hz tuning fork). (See Further reading section for explanation of the Weber lateralization, which involves complex physics.)

Sequence of testing

First, test acuity in each ear. If acuity appears normal and conversational speech is easily heard and understood, you can dispense with further testing in the patient without other auditory symptoms. In case of impaired auditory acuity check whether bone conduction surpasses air conduction and whether the Weber test lateralizes. If air conduction is diminished but better than bone conduction, the problem lies either in a minor defect in air conduction or in the sensorineural mechanism involving the inner ear, CN 8, or cochlear nuclei. Any hearing impairment should receive formal audiologic evaluation unless due to a transient or remediable problem in the middle ear or external ear canal.

Relevant symptoms

Patients are often unaware of, or ignore, hearing impairment, especially if in the "nontelephone" ear. In older patients always assess hearing, whether or not there is a complaint. Also inquire for local symptoms (such as pain, fullness in the ear) and for the associated auditory symptoms of buzzing or ringing (tinnitus). Symptoms arising from nearby vestibular and coordination centers include dizziness, poor balance, and clumsiness. Background factors include medications, allergies, recent airplane travel, swimming, probing of the ear canal, respiratory infections, noise exposure, and a family history of deafness.

Clinical implications

Most hearing problems involve the ear, and do not point to a neurologic lesion. However, benign tumors of the posterior fossa, especially "acoustic neuromas" of the CN 8 Schwann cell sheath, represent "don't miss" diagnoses: they are curable if excised before damage to adjacent structures occurs.

Balance and other vestibular functions

Definition and overview

The vestibular system comprises the labyrinths of the inner ears and their connections via the vestibular division of CN 8 to the vestibular nuclei of the medulla, and their brainstem, cerebellar, and other connections. Vestibular function plays an important role in balance, sense of orientation in space, and coordination. However, because motor, cerebellar, proprioceptive, and visual capacities also contribute to a patient's balance, it is difficult to evaluate the vestibular system in isolation. Aside from trying to reproduce vertigo (an illusion of movement) and associated nystagmus, there are no clinical tests specifically for vestibular function that are both simple and generally useful.

Relevant symptoms

Find out what the patient means by dizziness. Referral for sophisticated vestibular testing is not ordinarily indicated for nonvertiginous dizziness. Instead, you should pursue history and examination relevant to postural blood pressure changes, other causes of syncope (fainting) or presyncope, visual problems, anxiety, etc. Note that a change in body position from supine to upright may induce two different reactions: first, a postural (orthostatic) blood pressure drop, causing a presyncopal form of dizziness; second, a positional vertigo due to movement of the head, but entirely unrelated to blood pressure.

In addition to relating dizziness to vertical changes in head or body position, ask about the effect of rapid turning, including rolling over in bed in one direction or the other. Is the vertigo worse when eyes are open or closed? Does visual fixation help? Ask about hearing impairment, ringing, or buzzing in the ears (tinnitus), and background factors as listed in the preceding section on hearing.

Inquire about headache or other pain at or near the onset of the dizziness. Since the more common inner ear causes of vertigo are painless, (except for abdominal discomfort and headache after retching), headache and neck pain are "red flag" warnings of possible posterior fossa hemorrhage or other serious neurologic events. (Patients with migraine headaches often complain of vague dizziness, but only rarely of true vertigo.)

Positional testing

Positional testing is a provocative tactic for eliciting vertigo and nystagmus. First, ask the patient to position or move his or her head in any way that has caused dizziness before. (Be prepared to hold the patient in case such a maneuver causes severe vertigo.) If vertigo and nystagmus are not produced, then do systematic positional testing, performed as follows (Fig. 5.11).

Starting from a sitting position, lay the patient back with the body flat and the head hanging straight back, 30–45° over the edge of the examination table. Subsequently, repeat this with the right ear down—head rotated to the right—and then the left ear down (the order is not important). Maintain each change of position for at least 15–30 seconds, watching for nystagmus as you test full eye movements and noting

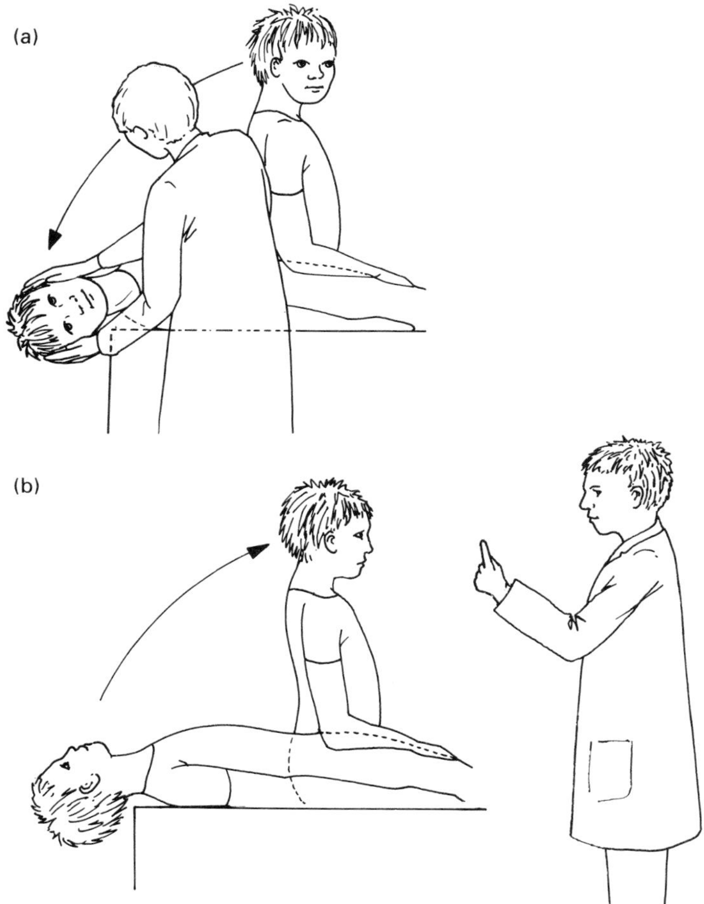

Fig. 5.11 Positional testing for vertigo and nystagmus. This test is employed in patients with complaints of vertigo, especially occurring with change in head position. (a) The patient is tested with the head hanging and turned to the right. The eyes are observed for nystagmus (as they follow through a full range of motion) for at least 30 seconds (nystagmus may appear after a latency), and then the patient is restored to the erect sitting position and again observed for nystagmus or complaint of vertigo. The procedure is repeated with the head hanging and turned to the left. In (b) the patient is shown after arising from the head-straight-back position and is being tested for nystagmus in the erect position.

any complaint of dizziness or nausea. Restore the patient to the sitting position, again checking for nystagmus, etc. Then try the next reclining position, etc. The reason for the prolonged observation after each change of position is that vertigo and nystagmus may appear only after a short latent period. Describe any nystagmus as suggested earlier (in the section on cranial nerves 3, 4, and 6). Note that simply spinning the patient around in an uncontrolled fashion is not a useful bedside or office test. Also, you should not perform ice water calorics (see Chapter 17) to assess dizziness. Caloric testing for dizziness should only be done in a controlled laboratory setting in order to obtain reliable information that justifies the discomfort to the patient.

Past-pointing (an often misused term)

Past-pointing refers to a tendency to miss a target or deviate from a line of intended movement in a systematic way, because of a bias or drift to one side (especially evident with eyes closed). This bias can be demonstrated, usually in a vertiginous patient, by finger–nose testing with eyes closed, or by asking the patient with eyes closed to raise one arm (or both) vertically and then return to the horizontal. In the presence of vestibular dysfunction (including brainstem and cerebellar components of the vestibular system) a deviation may occur towards the side of the lesion. As will be indicated in Chapter 8 (coordination), past-pointing is not synonymous with dysmetria, but is a particular form of it.

Ataxia with and without vertigo

If possible, test limb coordination and gait at a time when the patient does not feel dizzy in the head. When vertiginous, the patient is almost sure to be ataxic. But if the patient exhibits incoordination when not dizzy, then you should look for a neurologic explanation outside of the peripheral vestibular system.

CRANIAL NERVES 9 AND 10: PHARYNGEAL AND LARYNGEAL FUNCTIONS

Overview

Functions mediated by CN 9 (glossopharyngeal) and CN 10 (vagus), such as swallowing, phonation, articulation, and palatal action, are usually grouped together. You can accomplish most of your evaluation by eliciting a good history and by careful observation during the history and the head and neck part of the general physical examination. For neurologic screening in the asymptomatic patient you may dispense with the formal examination, but the testing skills should be in your repertoire.

In addition to motor and sensory functions of the palate, pharynx, and larynx, CNs 9 and 10 also carry important autonomic fibers: parasympathetic fibers that travel with CN 9 innervate the parotid glands; parasympathetic nerves from the dorsal motor nucleus of the vagus innervate smooth muscle of the pharynx, larynx, upper gastrointestinal tract and its glands, as well as the heart and the vascular smooth muscle of the heart and lungs. While not ordinarily testing these parasympathetic pathways in a neurologic examination, we do make observations that bear upon the functions they serve. Symptoms of nausea and faintness, are characteristic of vagal discharge. Every pulse and blood pressure measurement reflects, in part, this parasympathetic activity (as well as sympathetic activity mediated through the thoracolumbar spinal cord).

Testing

For swallowing, note any pooling of secretions in the mouth, coughing or gagging after swallowing, and, in particular, difficulty with liquids, which, because they go down faster, stress the neuromuscular mechanism of swallowing more than solids do. To test further, have the patient drink sips of water. If these are swallowed without any problems, increase carefully to larger draughts. Should the patient be unable to handle a clear liquid, try a bland, thick liquid or soft solid, such as a milk shake or pudding, which may be easier to swallow but carries more risk than water, in case aspiration should occur.

Phonation

Listen to the quality of phonation or sound production, especially an exaggerated nasal quality that might suggest insufficiency in closing off the nasopharynx. Persistent hoarseness or any other difficulty with sound production requires laryngeal visualization by an expert.

Articulation

Listen for the ability to enunciate specific letters, syllables, and words. Differentiate thickness or slurring of speech (dysarthria) from an abnormal rhythm of speech or difficulty with word finding. Ask the patient to repeat guttural sounds, such as "go" which particularly involve the pharyngeal musculature, as opposed to labial (lip) sounds such as "me" and palatal/lingual sounds such as "kay," "tee," or "la." Dysarthria may result from cerebral (and especially bilateral cerebral) lesions, upper and/or lower motor neuron lesions in the brainstem, or (less often) peripheral cranial nerve or muscle problems. Lack of teeth (edentulous state) may affect articulation.

Palatal function

You can test motor, sensory, and reflex function of the palate and the pharynx directly. Initially, try not using a tongue blade, since in some patients you will be able to inspect palatal movement without it. (A more complete view of the pharynx usually requires use of a tongue blade.) Ask the patient to say "ah" to observe the soft palate rising on both sides, and with it the uvula. (Deviation of the uvula by itself is not likely to be significant: look for decreased elevation of one side of the palate that may deviate the uvula.)

Gag reflex

Sensation of the soft palate or posterior pharyngeal wall is usually tested in the course of eliciting the gag reflex. Whenever tested, be sure to stimulate each side, and observe for elevation of the palate on both sides (as with the pupillary light or corneal reflexes). There is a wide range of normal gag responses. A bilaterally decreased or absent gag is not necessarily abnormal unless there is difficulty with phonation, speaking, or swallowing. While a good gag reflex suggests a capacity for safe swallowing (protection against aspiration), the ability to swallow and protect one's airway is more complex. The proof is in the eating and drinking.

Localization

As with other cranial nerve-mediated functions, any observed abnormality results from dysfunction somewhere in the chain of function—cerebral, brainstem, or peripheral—but not necessarily in CNs 9 and 10 themselves. Abnormal phonation, for example, occurs with lesions at many different sites—from the basal ganglia to the neuromuscular junction, not to mention the vocal cords themselves.

Pseudobulbar palsy

Swallowing, phonation, articulation, and certain other brainstem/

cranial nerve-mediated functions are under at least partial bilateral UMN (corticobulbar) control. It is not surprising, therefore, that bilateral UMN lesions would be likely to cause dysphagia, dysphonia, and dysarthria, as well as increased jaw jerk and snout reflex (see Fig. 9.3). Lability of affect (expression of emotion) is also commonly associated. This constellation of signs constitutes the core of the pseudobulbar palsy syndrome. In fact, it is not really pseudo – it is just the bilateral dysfunction of corticobulbar innervation of brainstem nuclei (bulbar, especially medullary), analogous to corticospinal lesions affecting anterior horn cells. (We do not say that a stroke, for example, causes a pseudospinal palsy.)

CRANIAL NERVE 11 (ACCESSORY): SHOULDER SHRUG, HEAD TURNING, AND FLEXION

Overview

The trapezius muscles enable us to display our indifference or displeasure by shrugging. They also participate synergistically in many other functions of the shoulder girdle. The right and left sternocleidomastoid muscles (especially the medial or sternomastoid portions) together flex the neck. The lateral part of the muscle that arises from the clavicle bends the head laterally toward the same side, but turns the head away: as you can observe and palpate, the muscle inserts into the mastoid process of the skull, which is behind the axis of rotation of the head (Fig. 5.12). Contraction causes the posterior half of the head to rotate forward and the face to turn to the opposite side. Since this contralateral action is at least superficially counterintuitive, it can be useful in assessing a patient's suggestibility or malingering (see Chapter 18).

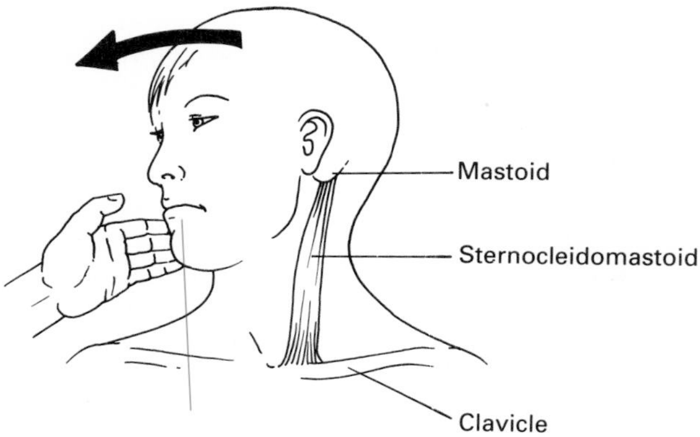

Fig. 5.12 Sternocleidomastoid muscle (CN 11). Since the insertion in the mastoid process is behind the axis of rotation of the head, and the origin from the sternum and clavicle anterior to it, contraction of the left-sided muscle pulls the mastoid forward rotating the head to the right.

Testing

Shoulder shrug

To test shoulder shrug (trapezius function) watch the symmetry and speed with which the patient elevates the shoulders toward the ears; also, gauge the power of this elevation against your active resistance. Observe for atrophy and asymmetry, but note that many normal people have uneven right and left shoulders.

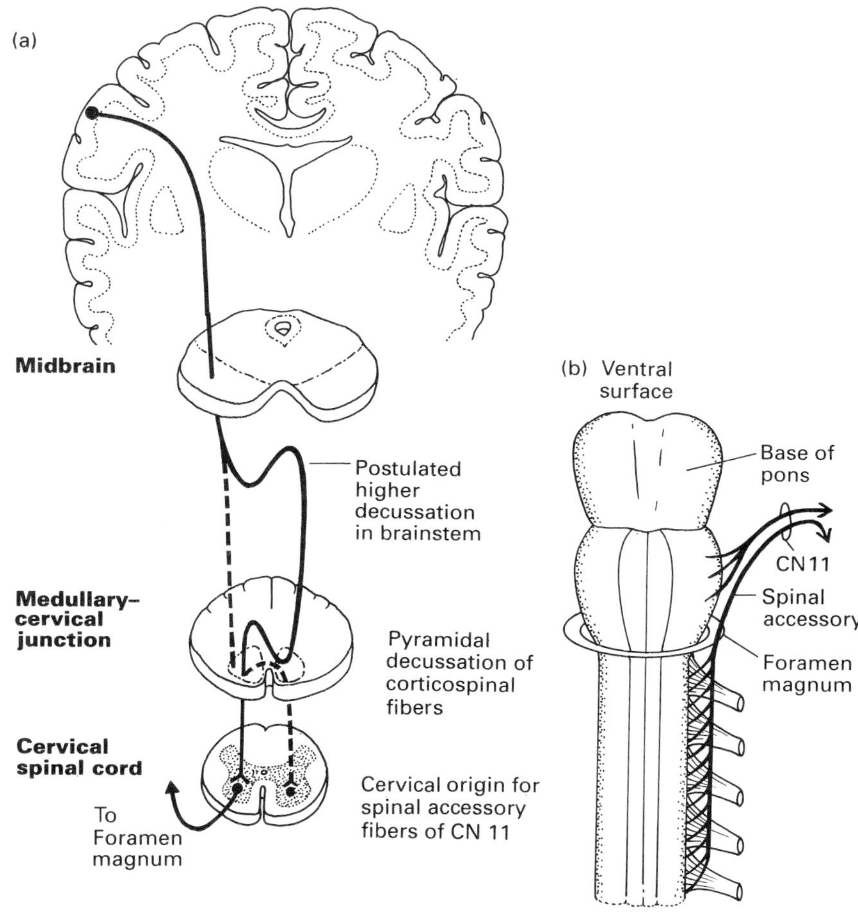

Fig. 5.13 CN 11 (accessory nerve). (a) Suprasegmental fibers to neurons in the CN 11 nucleus are both crossed and uncrossed. (The motor tract from the cortex is shown on just one side.) A double decussation of upper motor neuron fibers controlling sternocleidomastoid function has been postulated to account for cortical stimulation causing head deviation to the opposite side. Control of trapezius function is mainly crossed. (b) Spinal origin of CN 11 (accessory nerve). Fibers from the upper cervical motor roots (C1–C5, but mainly C2–C4) are seen to join together and ascend upward through the foramen magnum. (They then descend through the jugular foramen, joining with direct cervical fibers to innervate the sternocleidomastoid and trapezius muscles. The cranial fibers that briefly join with CN 11 are really part of CN 10, the vagus.)

Head turning

Assess the power of head turning (rotation) as you resist with your hand against the patient's cheek or jaw. At the same time, observe and palpate the contracting muscle – which is on the opposite side from the direction of head turning. (If you have trouble remembering whether the right or left muscle turns the head toward a particular side, just test it on yourself or on the patient.)

Head flexion

Test head flexion against resistance by pushing with your hand against the patient's forehead. (Extension of the head may be tested at the same time, but this function is served mainly by part of the trapezius and paraspinal muscles.)

Anatomic note

Of the two parts of CN 11, the first or bulbar part is functionally a component of the vagus nerve and will not be further considered here (see CNs 9 and 10). The second part, or spinal accessory nerve, should be thought of as cervical: these roots (mainly from C2 to C4) happen to course upward through the foramen magnum into the posterior fossa and then down through the jugular foramen to the ipsilateral sternocleidomastoid and trapezius muscles (Fig. 5.13). These muscles are also directly innervated by upper cervical motor roots.

The suprasegmental control of head turning is also peculiar: for the left motor cortex to turn the head to the right, the *left* sternocleidomastoid muscle must be activated. But descending corticospinal fibers to the C2–C4 segments would cross from left to right, at least partially, in the pyramidal decussation. Anatomists have postulated an earlier left to right cross higher in the brainstem, which takes the fibers from left to right; these fibers then cross back to the left in the pyramidal decussation.

Clinical correlation

The inclusion of a decreased shoulder shrug with weakness of the limbs on that side helps to establish a motor level (in the same way that the upper border of pin or touch impairment establishes a sensory level, as will be seen in Chapter 7). In either case the pathologic lesions must be at least as high as the clinical level. A neural lesion causing weakness of shoulder shrug must be at the C4 level or higher (since the roots arise from segments C2–C4). Bilateral trapezius and sternocleidomastoid weakness might also be due to primary muscular pathology involving the shoulder girdle (as in certain dystrophies). Damage to the accessory nerves can occur in the upper neck or in the course of their peculiar loop into and out of the posterior fossa.

CRANIAL NERVE 12 (HYPOGLOSSAL): MOTOR FUNCTIONS OF THE TONGUE

Testing

Observe the appearance and bulk of the tongue as part of the general examination of the oral cavity. In particular, note any atrophy. This is often first apparent as a thinning and shrivelling along one or both edges of the tongue. Are there adventitious (extraneous, involuntary) movements evident with the tongue at rest or protruded?

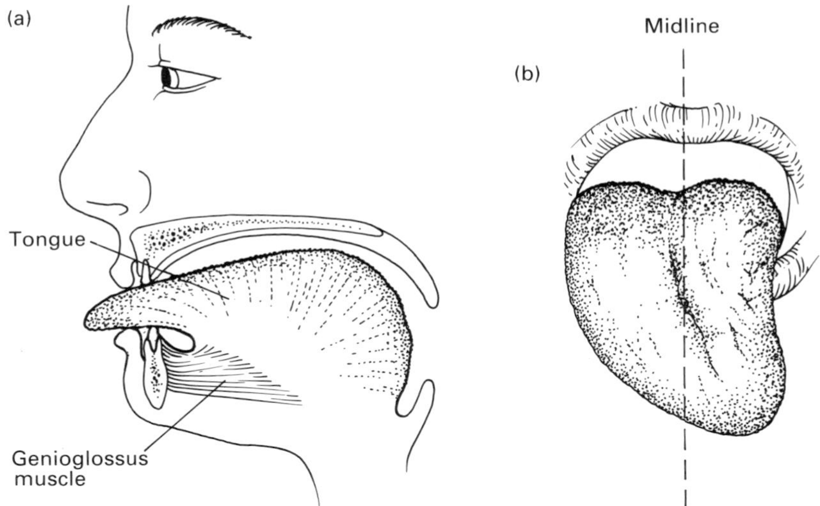

Fig. 5.14 Tongue protrusion and deviation. (a) The position of the genioglossus muscle (shown on one side only) demonstrates how (bilateral) contraction pulls the base of the tongue forward in order to protrude it. (b) In a left CN 12 lower motor neuron lesion, the tongue protrudes towards the side of the lesion, because of the unopposed action of the right genioglossus muscle which, in pulling the tongue forward, deviates it to the left. Atrophy and fasciculations also occur on the affected side.

Table 5.10 Analysis of tongue deviation and related signs (tongue deviating to left)

Types of nervous system lesion	Segmental, lower motor neuron (LMN)	Suprasegmental, upper motor neuron (UMN)
	Left CN 12/hypoglossal nucleus or nerve lesion prevents the forward pull of the left genioglossus muscle; the unopposed protruding action on the right causes left deviation	Right corticobulbar lesion (of fibers that will cross to synapse on left CN 12 nucleus). Unopposed right genioglossus muscle deviates tongue to left (actual occurrence is variable)
Associated acute signs	Weakness in out-pouching tongue into right cheek; possible dysarthria for lingual sounds	Weakness in out-pouching tongue into right cheek; possible dysarthria for lingual sounds
Associated subacute to chronic signs	Neurogenic atrophy (left side); fasciculations (left side, see Tables 6.1 and 6.2)	The acute signs of a unilateral UMN weakness, including deviation, tend to resolve

Observe for deviation of the tongue to one side or the other as it is protruded (Fig. 5.14). You can also assess the power of the tongue by asking the patient to outpouch the cheek with it; you can then feel it and resist by pressing against it from the outside of the cheek.

Clinical correlations

The protruded tongue may normally exhibit undulating or rippling movements that may be mistaken for fasciculations. (See Chapter 6). Most of these nonfasciculatory movements will subside when the tongue is rested for a few moments in the floor of the mouth. Significant fasciculations persist at rest and indicate a nonacute, LMN lesion (Table 5.10). Beware of diagnosing fasciculations in the absence of atrophy. Dyskinetic twisting or protruding movements of the tongue suggest "tardive dyskinesia," a disorder of nonvoluntary "extrapyramidal" aspects of motor function, induced by disease or by drugs (such as antipsychotic medications).

Interpreting a deviation of the protruded tongue is often a source of confusion (see Table 5.10). A minimal deviation of the tip – less than 1 cm – is often not clinically significant.

SUMMARY

Priorities

1 Visual fields: peripheral and central fields (including acuity) require testing, not simply inference from symptoms. Monocular defects localize to the retina or optic nerve; bitemporal, binasal, or altitudinal field cuts usually implicate the chiasm/pituitary area; homonymous field deficits indicate a postchiasmal lesion, usually of the temporal, parietal, or occipital lobes.
2 Pupils: baseline information on symmetry and reactivity can be crucial, especially in neurologic emergencies. Changes in reactivity and/or size reflect alteration of function in one of the following: the afferent, receptive limb of the reflex arc (especially the optic nerve); the efferent limb (parasympathetic fibers associated with CN 3); the sympathetic pathway (c.f. Horner's syndrome).
3 EOM: acute or progressive weakness of individual eye movements is usually signaled by double vision, which differentiates an ocular palsy from congenital strabismus. Abolishing double vision by covering either eye confirms that the diplopia is truly binocular. If you learn the direction of pull of each of the eye muscles, you will then be able to recreate the effect of contraction with the eye in different resting positions. Gaze palsies (see Chapter 17) provide the key to localization of many strokes and seizures.
4 Facial weakness: distinguish the suprasegmental, UMN type that affects just the lower part of the face from the segmental, LMN type that affects the whole side of the face. The difference stems from the bilateral (crossed and uncrossed) UMN (corticobulbar) innervation of the part of the CN 7 nucleus that controls the forehead. Remember that the LMN output is the final common pathway: a complete lesion must involve the entire side of the face.

5 Auditory and visual acuity: measuring these capacities is important in the assessment of the overall function of the patient, above and beyond specific neurodiagnostic clues.
6 Swallowing: difficulty handing secretions and swallowing liquids, especially, can result from the full range of neurologic and neuromuscular dysfunction, particularly if bilateral. Deficits often result in aspiration pneumonia, and thus present in "non-neurologic" guises. Testing of actual swallowing is more definitive than merely testing the gag reflex.

Pitfalls

1 Not establishing the actual periphery in visual field testing.
2 Not covering each eye separately to assess visual fields and double vision.
3 Not really looking carefully at pupillary size (especially comparative size) and reactivity: if a baseline record is vague or inaccurate, it is worse than useless.
4 Mistaking a nonparalytic, congenital strabismus for an acute ocular palsy (especially mistaking a congenital esotropia, or in-turned eye, for an acute "6th nerve palsy").
5 Assuming that the narrower of the two palpebral fissures signifies ptosis: often it is the other, wider one that is abnormal, due to facial weakness.
6 Misidentifying normal, undulating, or "restless" movements of the tongue as fasciculations.

PROBLEMS FOR SELF-STUDY

Problems

1 A patient presents with acute onset of weakness on the right side of the face. What additional cranial nerve examination data would you especially wish to have?
2 A patient is noted to have an enlarged left pupil that does not react when a flashlight is shone in. What further data on cranial nerve functions do you need to obtain in order to interpret this?
3 A patient complains of sudden onset of difficulty reading, specifically reading more slowly and losing her place. Her spoken language seems normal, and reading and understanding single words and short phrases present no problem. What would you emphasize in the patient's visual examination?

Comments

1 In addition to testing sensation on the face, the pattern of weakness would be the key. Does it affect the forehead as well as the lower parts of the face? If so, this is the LMN (segmental) type which could result from a lesion of the CN 7 nucleus or the cranial nerve itself. CN 6 function should be checked because of close anatomic proximity in the brainstem. Taste should be tested on each half of the tongue, since taste fibers run with CN 7 in part of its peripheral course. Confirm

that no other weakness (i.e. parts of a hemiparesis) exists on the right side, especially if the facial weakness appears to be of the UMN type.

2 First determine whether the afferent or efferent limb of the pupillary reflex arc is not working. If the eye were blind, the consensual pupillary reaction in the other (right) eye would also be absent. However, light stimulus to the right eye would cause consensual response in the left eye, assuming the parasympathetic/CN 3 efferent mechanism were intact. An afferent lesion alone would not cause great pupillary enlargement, since the consensual mechanism would result in constriction. If CN 3 were affected on the left, you would probably also find ptosis and weakness of eye movements mediated by CN 3.

3 The symptoms suggest difficulty with scanning ahead across a line of print and/or a decrease in the length of line seen in a given visual fixation. You should check for a right homonymous hemianopia or a right inferior quadrantanopia. (If the field cut were on the left, finding the beginning of the next line on the left would be difficult.) The available information indicates that acuity is sufficient and that this is probably not a dyslexia (a language problem).

FURTHER READING

Baloh, R.W., Honrubia, V. *Clinical Neurophysiology of the Vestibular System*. 2nd edn. F.A. Davis, Philadelphia (PA), 1990. A comprehensive source for delving deeply into this complex system.

Brazis, P.W., Masdeu, J.C., Biller, J. *Localization in Clinical Neurology*. 2nd edn. Little, Brown, and Company, Boston (MA), 1990, pp. 93–285. Detailed localization of cranial nerve and brainstem functions and dysfunction.

Duus, P. *Topical Diagnosis in Neurology*. 2nd edn. Thieme Medical Publishers, New York (NY), 1989. Highly illustrated clinical–anatomic correlations of deficits in cranial nerve functions (Chapter 3).

Mayo Clinic. *Clinical Examinations in Neurology*. 6th edn. Mosby, St. Louis (MO), 1991. Further details of basic neuroophthalmology (Chapter 6), understandably presented.

Tonndorf, J. Bone conduction. In: Keidel, W.D., Neff, W.D. (eds) *Auditory System. Clinical and Special Topics, Handbook of Sensory Physiology*. Vol. V/3. Springer-Verlag, New York (NY), 1976. The physics of the Weber test in its normal and pathologic contexts. Recommended for those who are truly curious about the basis of Weber lateralization (a matter of much disinformation in teaching).

Troost, B.T., Patton, J.M. Exercise therapy for positional vertigo. *Neurology* 1992; 42:1441–4. Vertigo is one of the most vexing of the common neurologic problems; positional vertigo is reviewed, and helpful treatment reported for the benign, paroxysmal variety.

chapter 6

Motor Examination

All behavior is expressed by some form of motor activity. The bedside or office examination condenses the many dimensions of basic motor function into four components, each of which has a specific objective (Table 6.1).

A more complex aspect of motor activity, coordination, which depends to an even greater degree upon integration with other neural systems, will be discussed in Chapter 8, after the motor and sensory examinations have been introduced.

Relevance of examination

Once engaged in the details of the examination, it is easy to lose sight of the totality of motor function in the patient's frame of reference. Your assessment of the motor system begins with the patient's attempt to convey a practical difficulty with activity. You then test the patient and express certain findings in terms of the medical model of neuromuscular status. But when the formal examination is over and done with, do not forget to question whether you have captured the patient's problem: do the findings relate to the trouble the patient is having? For example, does normal strength tested at noon adequately address the fatigue of holding the head erect at the end of the day?

Table 6.1 Motor examination: main components of evaluation

Objective	Test/observation
To document normal power	Strength (active resistance to opposing force)
To show normal relaxation of joints/ muscles	Tone (resistance to passive movement)
To recognize unintended or extraneous movements (and postures)	Adventitious ("involuntary") movements noted by observation
To disclose wasting or other changes in the appearance of muscle	Muscle bulk and consistency recognized by observation and palpation

The integration of symptoms and signs in a diagnostic formulation will be discussed in Part 3, but even at this point the relevance of testing to symptoms needs to be kept in mind. Otherwise, you may find that you have completed your data gathering in a way that is technically competent, but not diagnostically pertinent. Table 6.2 summarizes: (a) the vocabulary of the patient's symptoms due to motor deficits; (b) common signs of motor abnormalities; and (c) examples of motor disabilities.

Chain of motor function

In preceding chapters I have referred to the basic suprasegmental and segmental organization of the nervous system and the schema of upper motor neuron (UMN) and lower motor neuron (LMN) components of the motor control system. Oversimplified as this simple linear chain of function is, it remains the cornerstone of analysis of many motor deficits that you will encounter (see Chapter 14).

Upper and lower motor neurons

The UMN or suprasegmental part of the motor chain (Fig. 6.1) refers to the cortical motor neuron and its axon which travels down through the

Table 6.2 Motor deficits – basic symptoms, signs, and disabilities

Deficit	Symptoms	Signs	Disabilities (examples)
Decreased strength	"Weak; slow; tired; numb; heavy; etc."	Impaired power and spontaneous movement; clumsiness; premature fatigue of sustained contraction	Impaired walking, climbing, rising from chair, lifting; impaired ability to sustain use of arms above head; dropping things
Increased tone (rigidity; spasticity)	(Often no direct symptoms) "stiffness; tightness; aching"	Lead-pipe or cogwheel rigidity; spasticity (clasp-knife effect)	Little disability in routine activities from mild rigidity, *per se*; greater degrees may affect fluidity of gait and limb movement
Adventitious movements	"Twitching; flailing; jumpy; uncontrolled"	Tremor; chorea; myoclonus; tics; flexor spasms; dyskinesias; etc.	Psychosocial stigma and reactions; dropping things; difficulty feeding and writing
Atrophy of muscle	"Losing muscle; wasting away"	Neurogenic atrophy; disuse atrophy	Disability results from associated weakness

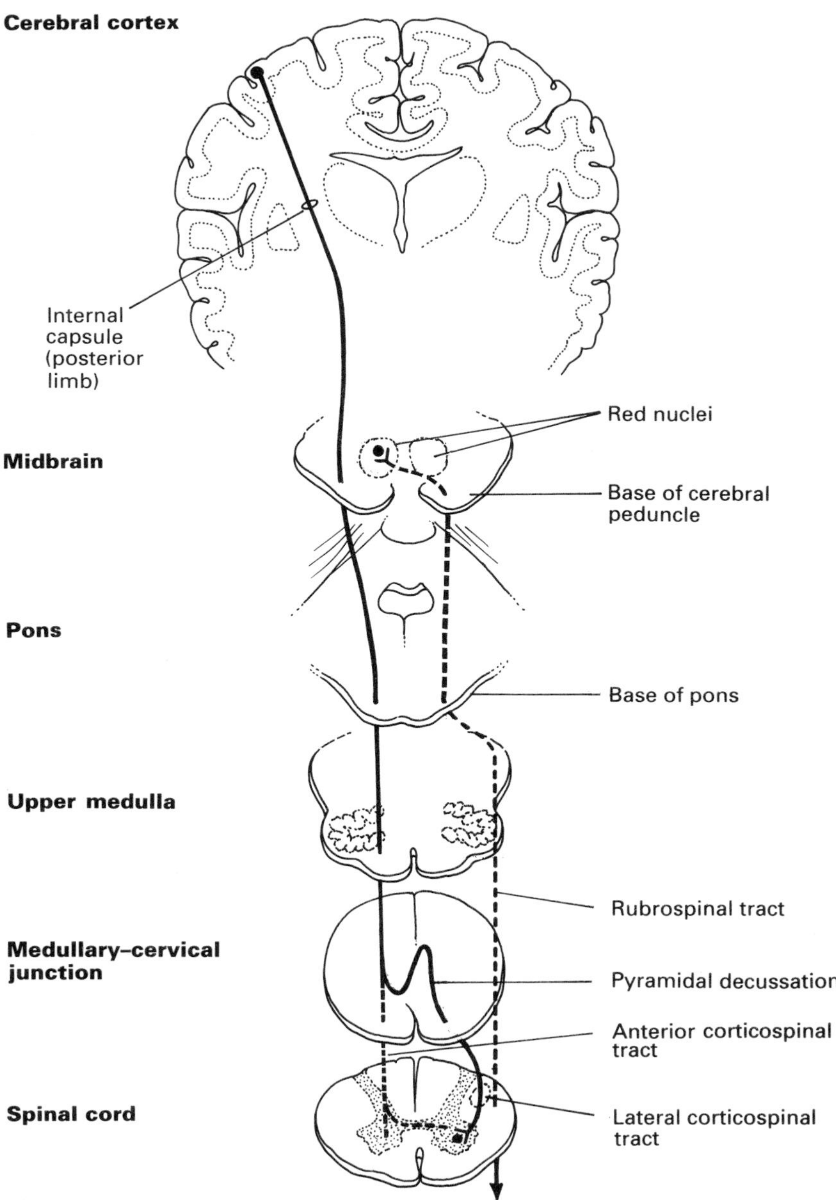

Fig. 6.1 Corticospinal (pyramidal) tract. Schematic showing the course of an upper motor neuron fiber from the cortex through the corona radiata of cerebral white matter, through the internal capsule, the base of the cerebral peduncle in the midbrain, the base of the pons, the medullary pyramid, the pyramidal decussation at the medullary–cervical junction, and into the lateral column of the spinal cord to its synapse in the anterior horn. Also shown, to represent the multiple other descending motor tracts, are the rubrospinal tract and the anterior corticospinal tract (which terminates in the thoracic region).

Table 6.3 Motor signs: upper motor neuron vs. lower motor neuron patterns

	Upper motor neuron (UMN) lesion	Lower motor neuron (LMN) lesion
Strength	Weakness of muscle group or groups (see text); extent depends on size of cortical lesion or degree of motor tract involvement (see Chapter 14)	Weakness of one or more individual muscles (often those innervated by a particular anterior root or peripheral nerve)
Tone	Increased tone because of UMN dysfunction – spasticity; (tone may be normal or decreased); also, extrapyramidal rigidity	Decreased (or normal); LMN lesions never directly increase tone, but resistance may be secondarily increased by contracture, etc.
Adventitious movements	Myoclonus; tremor; dyskinesias; dystonias (cortical, basal ganglionic, cerebellar, etc.); convulsive movements (usually cortical in origin)	Fasciculations (twitching of small groups of muscle fibers, see text); usually insufficient to move a body part, but can move a small digit; cramps (some neurogenic) are involuntary, painful muscle contractions
Muscle bulk	Diminished by disuse (disuse atrophy)	Neurogenic atrophy (loss of trophic function); disuse atrophy

cerebral hemisphere and brainstem to synapse with the LMN – the anterior horn cell in the spinal cord (or cells of the motor nucleus of a cranial nerve in the brainstem). LMNs send their axons out into the motor roots and peripheral nerves. (Although not part of the neuronal chain, the muscle, as end organ, is part of this segmental motor organization.) Basic clinical correlations between motor findings and UMN vs. LMN lesions are presented in Table 6.3.

Individual muscle testing

Comprehensive instruction in testing of specific muscles will not be presented here, as the goal is now to achieve competence in a general approach to motor evaluation. In Chapter 16 certain key muscle tests for peripheral nerve and root disorders are shown (see Figs 16.7–16.10 and Further reading section).

STRENGTH

Definitions

1 Paresis describes a partial degree of weakness, as in hemiparesis;
2 -plegia implies complete paralysis, as in hemiplegia (one side of the body); quadriplegia (all four limbs); paraplegia (both legs, lower half of the body); and monoplegia (one limb).

Relevant symptoms

Weakness is expressed by patients not only as failure to generate specific muscular output and accomplish tasks of muscular exertion, but also as low energy, fatigue, or slowness. Although pain is not a primary symptom of weakness, patients may focus on the pain that arises when weakened muscles are overstressed or when unaccustomed, compensatory postures are adopted.

There are multiple dimensions to motor output that you can test.

Motor parameters

1 Resistive strength: graded at peak power (a weight lifter requires great peak strength which does not need to be sustained).
2 Sustained exertion or endurance: the time–strength curve is more critical than peak strength alone (a gymnast needs to be able to sustain a high level of output, but rarely uses maximum strength).
3 Ability to accelerate: a sprinter depends more on this capacity than on overall strength and endurance.

For specific bedside testing, resistive strength should be emphasized and the following points observed.

Testing

1 Position: resistive testing is usually conducted with the patient lying or sitting. (Some actions, such as flexion of the thighs, may be harder to evaluate in some patients in the sitting position, in which case the test should be repeated supine.)
2 In limb testing, use one of your hands for active resistance and the other to stabilize the limb proximally to the joint being tested. Test action across just one joint at a time.
3 Instruct the patient to push or pull streadily against you, or alternatively, to resist you. Frequently, much encouragement is needed to elicit maximum performance. Test in midposition of the range of motion, not in full flexion or in a fully extended, "locked" position.
4 Inquire initially and as exertion mounts for any pain (see below) or other interference with the patient's best effort.
5 Push resistive testing to maximum capacity, allowing for the patient's comfort and safety, general medical condition (e.g. cardiac), fractures, healing wounds, etc.
6 Practice testing exertion in all planes at each major joint (for example, at the shoulder test abduction, adduction, flexion, extension, internal and external rotation) although you will not routinely test all of these in practice.
7 Test for ability to maintain the arms and hands outstretched (eyes closed). Look for downward drift and also for pronation (when the forearms initially are supinated). These signs of weakness may only appear with the occurrence of fatigue after 20–30 seconds or more. For greater efficiency, you may wish to test for drift during the Romberg test (see Fig. 8.1). With arms pronated and the hands dorsiflexed, asterixis or "flap" (occurring most commonly in hepatic or other metabolic/toxic dysfunctions) may be observed.
8 Dorsiflexion and plantar flexion of the feet can also be assessed by asking the patient to walk on heels and toes, respectively. (Do not confuse these tests with heel-to-toe walking or tandem gait. See Chapter

Table 6.4 Grading systems for resistive motor testing: definition and comparison of two widely used scales

Observation	"Absent to excellent"	"0–5"
No contraction	Absent	0
Flicker or trace contraction	Trace	1
Active movement with gravity eliminated	Poor	2
Active movement against gravity	Fair	3
Active movement against resistance	(G−) Good (G+)	(4−) 4 (4+)
Full strength	Excellent	5

8.) Overall, direct resistive testing of foot strength is more likely to detect subtle deficits.

Grading of resistive motor testing

For resistive motor testing several grading systems are in use. The choice of system is not important, only that the scale is specified, and that it discriminates among significant differences in power exerted. Two widely used scales are defined and compared in Table 6.4.

The grade recorded for each test should be the patient's best performance, or peak strength. If you find substantial inconsistencies, make a side comment to that effect. Note that "4" or "good" is too broad a category, without (+) or (−) interpolations (see Chapter 11).

Use of a grading scale not only inspires the confidence of others who read the medical record that you have done a careful examination, but will prompt you to do a better examination. Even more importantly, grading serves much better than general recollection to identify and document changes found on serial examinations.

Standards of normal

Factors that may affect "normal" strength include: (a) age; (b) size/gender; and (c) state of muscular development. Over time you will develop a sense of what level of strength can be expected from different individuals, according to their build, background, or walk of life. However, even your best estimate will serve only as a rough guide.

Comparing sides

In general, we rely quite heavily on comparison of strength between corresponding parts of the right and left sides, especially if no gross weakness is apparent. Aside from the risk of missing bilateral weakness, emphasis on lateralized differences must take handedness into account.

Handedness

Handedness, or cerebral motor dominance (see Chapter 14), results in a discernible difference in strength, especially in the upper extremities. How much effect handedness has – and therefore how much the examiner should allow for it in setting a standard of normal – depends on the patient's habitual pattern of use of the limbs. (Inquire about handedness for various purposes, not just writing. In some patients the pattern of usage can be evaluated by comparing calluses, the size of a particular muscle (such as the biceps), and overall development of a body part, such as breadth of the palm or diameter of the forearm.)

CASE 6A
Losing his grip

Eddie Hodges, a 63-year-old right-handed man, was brought to his health plan center by his wife because he had had an episode of loss of power in the right hand. He was using a screwdriver and suddenly felt that he was "losing his grip." He experienced no numbness or impairment of feeling when he touched his right hand with his left.

General and neurologic examinations revealed no abnormalities except for the following: strength in the right arm, tested first, seemed very good and was initially assumed to be normal. However, on testing the left side, strength was even better – it was "rock hard," compared to a slight "give" in certain right-sided groups.

The following results were recorded:

(3 pm)	Right	Left
Finger spreading	4++/5	5/5
Wrist dorsiflexion	4++/5	5/5
Wrist volar flexion	5/5	5/5
Forearm (elbow) extension,	4++/5	5/5
flexion (supinated and pronated)	5/5	5/5
Arm (shoulder) abduction	5/5	5/5

It was also noted that Hodges was a very powerfully built man, that the minimal weakness on the right was only noticeable by comparison with the left, and that at the time of testing he was no longer aware of any deficit himself.

His carotid pulses were normal (2+) and no bruits were appreciated. He was hospitalized for observation with a diagnosis of a possible transient ischemic attack (TIA). After a negative cranial computerized tomography (CT) scan (to rule out bleeding or a mass), he was started on antiplatelet therapy with aspirin. Over the next week a complete recovery of strength ensued, confirming that the slight relative weakness of the right hand had indeed represented a real deficit. A repeat CT scan was negative. The presumptive diagnosis was a mild left frontal, ischemic stroke of embolic type, source unknown.

Problems of interpretation

Erratic or hesitant performance

Some patients require considerable encouragement to produce their best exertion or to sustain their maximal effort until you signal for release. Nonetheless, you will encounter resistive output that is hesitant, quickly collapsing, or otherwise erratic. Such performance is often assumed to be hysteric or otherwise psychologically determined (see Chapter 18). While this could be the case, some patients who are genuinely weak can muster fairly good strength momentarily, but not sustain it, thus leaving an impression of erratic effort. On the other hand, the patient's degree of exertion should not parallel the resistance of the examiner: physiologically, a patient should not exhibit moderate arm power against the resistance of your whole arm and then weak arm power against your one or two fingers.

Fatiguability

Progressive loss of strength with continued testing suggests the possibility of a myasthenic condition (decremental strength or "fatigue" due to disease at the neuromuscular junction). However, more often the failure is one of effort or systemic exhaustion.

Effort

Factors determining effort include pain, fatigue, depression, distraction, malaise, and systemic effects of illness or injury. When assessing effort, try to establish any variation among different parts of the body. If any part can respond with good strength – whether this be a hand, a thigh, the neck, or the jaw – then impaired strength-testing performance elsewhere should not be attributed to a general motivational problem or diffuse physical factors; that is, the patient is not just overly fatigued, "washed-out," or uncooperative.

Pain

A willing patient can be tested even in the presence of some pain. If resistance falters, ask whether the pain became too severe or whether the limb just gave way. Even when pain or guarding do influence testing, you can make some inferences about strength that are worth documenting: peak strength is at least as good as the best exertion noted. This does not enable estimation of true neuromuscular capacity, but performance and recording of the strength examination provides a kind of "floor" upon which to base subsequent comparisons.

Pitfalls in assessing strength

Common pitfalls in evaluating strength include:

1 lack of sufficient intensity of testing (is strength really excellent or only quite good?);
2 absent or inadequate grading of strength;
3 omission of proximal strength testing;

4 presumption that the obvious weakness is the only weakness, for example, in a case of foot drop (weak dorsiflexion), be sure to test the strength of plantar flexion, inversion, eversion, and more proximal movements to define the complete pattern of weakness;
5 excessive discounting of expected strength in women, in people of slight build, and in the elderly;
6 overreliance on right–left comparisons, which risks missing mild, bilateral weakness;
7 failure to test functional capacities; to reproduce the symptomatic situation: observe the patient getting up from a chair or bed, climbing stairs, etc., as indicated.

TONE

Definition

Tone is defined operationally as resistance to passive movement of the limbs, parts of limbs, or spine (Fig. 6.2). (Passive movement means that the examiner manipulates the patient's body part through a range of motion, the patient offering no voluntary resistance.)

Determinants of tone

Resistance to movement is produced by the elasticity of the muscle plus the neural "set" – the level of impulse activity in the segmental control mechanism as influenced by its suprasegmental (UMN) input.

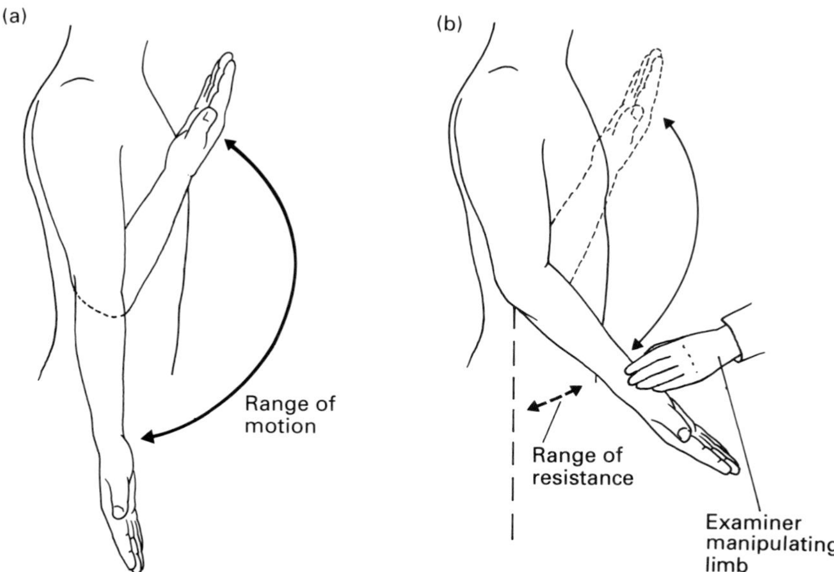

Fig. 6.2 Testing range of motion and tone. The range of flexion and extension at the elbow joint is defined by the anatomy of the joint. Within this range of motion, an examiner may find increased resistance to passive motion at any point, shown here as increased flexor tone occurring during extension, at about 45° short of full extension.

Increased resistance can also be referred to as rigidity or hypertonia, and decreased resistance as hypotonia (flaccidity being a state of no discernible tone). Spasticity is a kind of hypertonia associated with hyperreflexia and other corticospinal (pyramidal) signs (see Table 6.5). Extrapyramidal rigidity is most definitively characterized by a cogwheel (ratchet-like) quality.

The so-called extrapyramidal system is part of the suprasegmental motor control system of which the basal ganglia are important components (see Fig. 14.2).

Tone (as defined neurologically) should be distinguished from the lay meaning of tone which refers to firmness or flabbiness, or the state of conditioning. You will probably see reference to extensor tone and flexor tone, terms which frequently cause confusion. Excessive contraction of extensor muscles causes increased extensor tone which is elicited by passive flexion. For example, passively flexing the forearm at the elbow elicits the tone of the forearm extensors, primarily the triceps. Thus, extensor tone is not tested by extending.

Tone vs. range of motion

Resistance to passive movement should be differentiated from range of motion of a joint. A full range of motion is that allowed by normal anatomy of the joint and its supporting structures. This range can be

Table 6.5 Increased and decreased tone

Site of lesion	Increased tone	Decreased tone
Suprasegmental/upper motor neuron Brain and spinal cord tracts	Hypertonia – may be of "spastic" type (clasp-knife) and associated with hyperreflexia, Babinski sign, clonus	Hypotonia may be present acutely (later hypertonia); rarely chronic hypotonia
Basal ganglia/ extrapyramidal disorders (Chapter 14)	Rigidity (lead-pipe or cogwheel)	Rarely hypotonia in a few basal ganglia diseases
Cerebellum	None	Decreased tone may be hard to detect (see text)
Segmental/lower motor neuron; nerve roots and peripheral nerves	None (except secondary contractures and cramps)	Focal hypotonia if most or all of the innervation of relevant muscle groups is damaged (e.g. flaccid ankle in case of sciatic nerve palsy)
Neuromuscular junction and muscles	None (except contracture, myotonia, and cramps)	Hypotonia hard to assess and rarely important in adults, but a significant issue in infants ("floppy babies")

restricted by disease or injury involving the joint or periarticular tissues. Tone is tested within the available range of motion (see Fig. 6.2), but in case of marked resistance you may have difficulty separating extreme hypertonia from other causes that inhibit motion.

CASE 6B
Tripping

A 50-year-old man complained of a progressive tendency to trip while walking. Neurologic examination was completely normal with the exception of increased tone in the legs. A repeat examination shortly thereafter showed a further bilateral increase in tone, as well as Babinski signs, but no weakness, as yet. Radiologic work-up demonstrated thoracic spinal cord compression, due to a treatable tumor. In this case, a mild spastic hypertonia provided the earliest clue to a UMN type of dysfunction caused by pressure on the descending motor tracts. (For cord compression, see Fig. 14.8; for another type of increased tone and for an additional relevant example, see Cases 8A and 14A respectively).

Always test tone

Assessment of tone is frequently neglected, partly because patients rarely complain of it directly (i.e. stiffness). Moreover, observation will not necessarily detect mild to moderate hypertonia. Therefore, you must test for it specifically. In doing so you will discover cases of early Parkinson's disease and other treatable conditions.

There are several steps in evaluating tone.

Steps in evaluation

1 Ask whether the patient is aware of any joint that hurts when it is moved.

2 Ask the patient to let the limb (or neck) go loose and floppy so that you can move it. (This may also be expressed as "relaxing"; "let me do all the work – don't help me at all"; "let go like a rag doll"; "let me feel the weight of your arm.") You should support the limb fully so that the patient does not feel the need to do so.

3 Put each limb to be tested through a full range of motion, one joint at a time. Move it in all directions – extension, flexion, abduction, adduction, internal rotation, external rotation – any movement of the joint that anatomy permits. While any joint can be tested in this way, tone is most commonly tested at the wrists, elbows, knees, ankles, and neck. Vary the speed of manipulation.

4 Even if there is an inability to achieve a full range of motion (such as restriction of the last 30° of extension at the elbow) you can still assess tone within the available range of motion.

5 If the patient is lying down, a good way to evaluate extensor tone at the knee (tone in the extensors of the leg) is to place a hand under the knee, then lift quickly so as to buckle the knee (Fig. 6.3). Normally, the heel will slide up the bed towards the thigh. If tone is increased, the heel

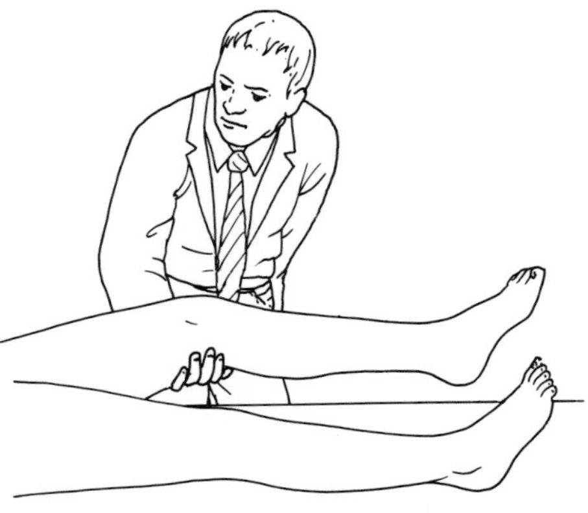

Fig. 6.3 Testing extensor tone at the knee. The knee is buckled by means of a quick lift so as to test tone in the knee extensors (quadriceps). Normally the heel will slide along the bed or table surface. In hypertonia, the heel lifts off the bed because of the poor quadriceps relaxation.

may lift off the bed because of the failure of the leg extensors (quadriceps femoris) to relax quickly when passively stretched.

6 A technique sometimes called "activation" enhances rigidity of an extrapyramidal type (described below). Ask the patient to draw circles or write in the air with a contralateral limb to augment abnormal resistance to passive motion in the limb being tested. (The passive manipulation should be asynchronous with the patient's active motion on the other side.) A momentary increase in tone may occur normally.

Standards of normal

Ordinarily you should be able to move a limb through its range of motion with almost no sense of resistance from the muscles being stretched out. In adults a pathologic decrease in tone is difficult to detect and to distinguish from normal, complete relaxation. Some normal people have relatively tight hamstring muscles of the posterior thigh, as evident in routine athletic stretching. You will also note some differences in how far you can dorsiflex the feet ("stretching the heel cords"). It should be possible to dorsiflex the feet at least slightly past neutral (90° angle of the foot with the leg) with minimal resistance. (A "tight heel cord" really reflects shortening of the gastrocnemius–soleus calf muscle group rather than a primary shortening of the tendon itself.)

Description of increased tone

The type of resistance encountered upon passively moving the limbs may be difficult to describe, but the following terms are often used.

Plastic or leadpipe rigidity: a more or less continuous, steady resistance through much or all of the range of motion.

Clasp-knife rigidity: a "spastic" resistance associated with UMN lesions. With increasing stretch, resistance mounts until there is a sudden release. UMN hypertonia often exists without this phenomenon being evident, however.

Cogwheel rigidity: a ratchet-like or catching quality. This may be felt intermittently and in only part of the range of motion. Wrists and elbows are especially good for testing. Cogwheel rigidity is characteristic of parkinsonism, the most important extrapyramidal disorder (see Chapter 14).

Paratonia or Gegenhalten: a resistance that increases the more quickly the examiner moves the limb and diminishes or disappears with slower manipulation. (This response might simulate wilful resistance.)

Recording findings

Describe the results of testing in the following ways:

1 which body parts or joints have normal or abnormal tone;
2 the character of the resistance (such as cogwheel) and the degree (mild, moderate, severe);
3 any asymmetry or disproportion between upper and lower extremities, axial structures (spine) vs. appendicular structures (limbs), distal vs. proximal, right vs. left;
4 effects of "activation," if tested;
5 effects of posture (such as standing vs. lying), especially if neck or trunk tone is at issue.

Other factors affecting resistance

Psychophysiologic factors that decrease relaxation, as well as disorders of muscles, joints, and periarticular structures, also influence resistance and should be identified before ascribing hypertonia to specific lesions of the motor system. Some of the more common causes affecting resistance are described below.

Guarding?

The most common cause of increased resistance is pain or guarding against anticipated pain.

Tension?

Difficulty relaxing due to tension is a problematic issue. Is the patient tense physically, mentally, or both? Anxious patients often find it difficult to relax, but the state of voluntary relaxation is notoriously difficult to judge. Beware of overattributing "poor relaxation" (increased tone) to psychologic tension. If you are unsure about your findings because of this factor, repeat this part of the examination at a later time.

Arthritis?

Acute or chronic inflammation or damage to the joint or periarticular tissues should be revealed by a thorough joint examination.

Chronic contracture?

Contracture is a shortening of muscle not due to active contraction. (Example: the calf muscles may shorten, producing a tight heel cord in a case of prolonged, uncorrected foot drop in which the weak dorsiflexors failed to counteract the strong plantar flexors.)

Rigidity in old age

With far advanced age, increased tone may be manifest for physiologic reasons that are poorly understood.

Key points

The key points to remember when assessing tone are as follows.

1 Remember to test tone. Omission is by far the most common error. You may well miss diagnosing early Parkinson's disease or early UMN lesions by not testing tone (see Cases 6B and 8A).
2 Test through a full range of motion, not in just one part of it.
3 In adults, establishing the absence of increased tone is more important than guessing whether tone is decreased.
4 The distinction between psychologic difficulty relaxing and patho-

logically increased tone can be difficult. Do not form snap judgments. Follow-up to see whether your findings are reproducible. Ask for help.
5 True hypertonia means a suprasegmental disorder – extrapyramidal or pyramidal (corticospinal). Neurologic increased tone rules out a LMN abnormality as the sole problem.

ADVENTITIOUS ("INVOLUNTARY") MOVEMENTS

Definition

Adventitious movements are extraneous or apparently unintended, occurring either spontaneously or in response to external stimuli. In fact, it is not always easy to judge whether a movement is truly involuntary (another term that is often used).

Overview

If you study a person's motor activity, you will observe some movements that are clearly volitional (like reaching for a glass of water) and others that occur automatically like breathing or swallowing. Some movements are not purposely initiated, but are within the patient's control to some degree. Fidgeting with the hands is rather easily controlled. Tics – intermittent contractions of specific muscles – appear to be wholly involuntary, but can be temporarily suppressed by an act of will. Certain pathologic movement disorders represent severe exaggerations of normal reactions (for example, recurrent, severe startling in response to mild sound or touch stimuli). Other adventitious movements, such as tremor, may bear a superficial resemblance to normal reactions (the trembling of severe fright) but actually have a different physiologic basis, as in "essential" (action) tremor.

Voluntary or involuntary

How does the observer decide whether movements are voluntary or involuntary, purposeful or intrusive? Our decision is based on the following: (a) the patient's own description, (which is subject to lack of insight or self-deception); (b) the degree of control the patient is able to exert over them; and (c) whether it is possible to duplicate the movement voluntarily. (This last is fraught with hazard because of the wide variation in what different people can control: some people can even produce a kind of nystagmus at will.) With certain triggered movements, like startle, the reaction time may be less than a person could volitionally reproduce.

Patients sometimes incorporate apparently involuntary movements into purposeful actions: an arm movement may start out as a quick involuntary fling and end up with scratching an ear. Thus, in observing and evaluating movements, you should describe carefully the characteristics of the movement, but avoid hasty presumptions as to what extent it is volitional. Videotape analysis helps greatly.

Common types

Some adventitious movements, like tremor, are oscillating. Others are nonrhythmic, such as a single quick jerk (myoclonus), the relatively quick twitches or "dancing" movements of chorea (Case 2C), or the complex, sinuous changes of posture that characterize athetosis. A fasciculation (twitch of a muscle fascicle) ordinarily does not move a body part, as would contraction of a whole muscle, but is nonetheless visible as a twitch or ripple beneath the skin. Involuntary movements may occur spontaneously or be elicited by stimulation or activity.

Testing

Testing for adventitious movements depends primarily upon close inspection of spontaneous activity, but also upon observing the effect of triggering stimuli.

Describe these movements in terms of:

1 parts of the body involved;
2 orientation in space (flexion–extension, rotational, chaotic, etc.);
3 frequency (estimate of movements per second);
4 amplitude (amount of displacement – often loosely called "coarse" or "fine");
5 pattern: single, multiple, clustered, synchronous, stereotyped.

Assess the effect of stimuli or changes in the internal or external environment, such as:

1 sudden noise, tap, pain;
2 application of psychologic stress; effect of sleep;
3 maintaining or changing postures;
4 directed motor activity, e.g. reaching.

Clinical correlations

Many pathophysiologic mechanisms, some fairly well understood and some as yet totally baffling, underlie adventitious movements. Customarily, the term "movement disorder" refers to dysfunction of the motor control system including the basal ganglia, thalamus, and cerebellum. However, the following groupings offer a broader view of involuntary movements, since you may not find the nature of the motor activity obvious from observation.

1 *Epileptic seizures*: tonic–clonic convulsive movements caused by cortical electrical discharges.
2 *Extrapyramidal disorders*: involving the basal ganglia and their connections, including such phenomena as dystonia, chorea, athetosis, dyskinesias, tremor, etc. (see Chapter 14).
3 *Cerebellar system disorders*: such as intention tremor (see Chapter 8).
4 *Segmental neuromuscular disorders*: including *fasciculations*. A fasciculation is a twitch of a group of muscle fibers (of one motor unit, i.e. innervated by one α motor neuron); this occurs when the nerve cell body or its axon is injured or diseased, but still in synaptic contact with the muscle. Fasciculations are not considered to be a movement disorder, since they are usually insufficient to move a body part. However, a small part like a little finger can be moved, which sometimes creates confusion with focal tremor, myoclonus, or seizure activity. Not all twitching or rippling within a muscle indicates pathologic fasciculations. The rapid trains of twitching felt in muscles, especially in the eyelids, are almost always benign and are frequently triggered by stress and fatigue.

5 *Miscellaneous*: tics, certain spasms and complex cramps, and numerous other troublesome movements do not fit into neat categories.

In summary, your main resources in assessing movement disorders will be a sharp eye, an open mind, and access to experienced help. Describe the characteristics of the movements, but also try to obtain a videotape and the opinion of a more experienced person, since movement abnormalities are hard to capture in words, and labels should not be prematurely applied. Beware of uncritical assumptions as to whether an observed movement is voluntary or not.

MUSCLE BULK AND THE DIRECT EXAMINATION OF MUSCLES AND NERVES

Overview

Examination of the muscles themselves (as opposed to their function) reveals information about certain primary diseases, but also reflects the status of the connecting motor neurons. The two most important questions are: (a) is there atrophy (wasting) due to denervation, disuse, or primary myopathy? and (b) are there fasciculations? In addition, the consistency and local reactivity of muscle (which may provide clues to primary muscular or systemic diseases) can be assessed, as well as the size or tenderness of palpable peripheral nerves.

Testing

Muscle bulk is first assessed by inspection. This requires adequate lighting and the patient needs to be sufficiently undressed. In a patient without a complaint of weakness or other neuromuscular symptom, thorough observation of the musculature is not necessary. In the course of a general physical examination, you can quickly "size up" the musculature (but your inspection will yield greater dividends in the detection of skin lesions!).

Observation

In observing the musculature generally, look for disproportions between:

1 upper and lower limbs;
2 proximal and distal groups;
3 the right side of the body vs. the left.

Palpation

Palpate any muscles or muscle groups (both at rest and in contraction) that are weak, atrophied, or exhibit fasciculations. Also, carefully feel any muscle identified by the patient as a site of pain, swelling, or stiffness. Some muscles are better assessed routinely by palpation than observation: feeling the masseters with the jaw clenched is the best way to assess their bulk, and similarly for the sternocleidomastoids, the 1st dorsal interosseus muscle (in the web space between the thumb and 1st finger), and others.

Measurement

The girth of the individual muscles cannot be measured, but the circumference of limbs can be quantitated with a tape measure. Since more than one muscle group is included, the result reveals only the sum of bone, muscle, and other tissues at that level. Nonetheless, comparisons between sides, as well as changes over time, are useful in following the course of atrophy. For purposes of comparison, the site of measurement needs to be specified, for example:

Calf circumference right: 37 cm
(10 cm below knee) left: 34 cm

Clinical correlations

Normal muscle development varies greatly: small muscles are not necessarily atrophic muscles. Rarely an apparent increase in bulk results not from muscle tissue, but from deposition of other tissues (such as fat).

Common causes of greater muscle bulk in one limb are:

1 handedness;
2 occupational utilization;
3 compensation for impaired use of other muscle groups.

Decreased bulk

Decreased muscle bulk can usually be attributed to one of the following.

1 *Disuse atrophy*: muscle size diminishes with lack of use, as when a leg is casted. This involves all groups that are not active and becomes apparent gradually over weeks and months. Muscles do not vanish as they may in neurogenic atrophy or end stages of primary myopathies. With exercise, the disused muscles will enlarge and regain normal consistency and strength. Systemic catabolism also wastes muscles.

2 *Neurogenic atrophy*: with interruption of the LMN (anterior horn cells, anterior roots, and peripheral motor or mixed nerves), only the denervated muscles show progressively severe atrophy, due to loss of trophic function of the nerve, as well as disuse. Shrinkage of muscle bulk is evident clinically in 2–3 weeks and progresses to a near-maximum in several months. Therefore, keep in mind the time scale when interpreting atrophy or the lack of it: absence of atrophy does not exclude a LMN lesion in the acute stage. Neurogenic atrophy follows the distribution of the denervation, and thus may affect part of one or more muscles, a whole muscle, or groups of muscles. Since most muscles are innervated by fibers from more than one nerve root, a lesion at a single segmental level will cause only partial atrophy. Reversal of neurogenic atrophy may occur through reinnervation.

3 *Primary myopathic disease*: in late stages, affected muscles may virtually vanish, as in some advanced dystrophies.

CONSISTENCY, TENDERNESS, AND REACTIVITY OF MUSCLE

Consistency

Consistency is the palpable quality of the muscle tissue as felt by the examiner when the muscle is at rest (which should not be confused with tone – the resistance to passive movement at a joint). A person with normal muscles (not "muscle bound") will exhibit no increase in limb tone. In cramping of a muscle, all or part of it feels knotted due to extreme contraction. Infiltration with fibrous fatty or other abnormal tissue may produce a woody, doughy, or mushy feeling. Flabbiness results from disuse, denervation, or primary wasting disease of muscle.

Tenderness

Tenderness over a muscle may occur with disorders (such as inflammation or traumatic injury) not only of the muscle itself, but also of skin, bone, tendons, and other tissues. Try gently pinching a skin fold to distinguish tenderness of skin or subcutaneous tissues. Muscle tenderness is absent in most myopathies; even in polymyositis, an inflammatory myopathy, true muscle tenderness is often lacking.

Reactivity

You can assess the reactivity of muscle by direct percussion with a reflex hammer. A local contraction (idiomuscular response) should be distinguished from a reflex. (This is especially pertinent to the brachioradialis or supinator jerk, which is elicited by tapping the lower third of the radius, not the forearm muscles.) In myotonic disorders, percussion of a muscle group (such as the thenar eminence of the palm) produces a sustained contraction, often with dimpling of the overlying skin. (This myotonic phenomenon occurs also in voluntary contraction, such as a handshake that does not release as quickly or fully as intended.)

PALPATION AND PERCUSSION OF PERIPHERAL NERVES

Indications

Palpation of specific peripheral nerves is indicated when symptoms of weakness, numbness, or autonomic disorder suggest the possibility of either a diffuse polyneuropathy or a lesion of a particular nerve trunk. The two major nerves that are normally accessible to palpation are the ulnar nerve at the elbow and the common peroneal nerve at the head of the fibula. In most patients you can feel each of these and roll them under your fingers, assessing for enlargement or tenderness (see Chapter 16).

In certain conditions of increased neural reactivity, tapping over the nerve will elicit a muscular twitch. For example, tapping over the facial nerve and its branches may elicit contraction of facial muscles (the Chvostek sign – see Chapter 9). A similar type of reaction is seen with percussing the common peroneal nerve over the fibula.

Tinel's sign

In an injured or regenerating nerve, percussion over the nerve may yield tingling in the nerve distribution, when the stimulus occurs at the site of injury or the leading edge of regeneration. Thus, one can follow the progress of regrowth of a superficial nerve. Percussion of normal nerve may also produce tingling or an electric shock feeling (e.g. ulnar nerve at the "funny bone").

To summarize the direct examination of muscle and nerve:

1 In routine examination, integrate inspection of musculature into the motor or general physical examinations. Palpation and percussion of muscle and nerve palpation need not be included in your examination in the absence of relevant symptoms or signs.

2 In the case of muscular complaints, carefully inspect, palpate (and, when indicated, percuss) the muscle groups of that part of the body—look especially for atrophy and fasciculations.

FUNCTIONAL ASSESSMENT OF THE MOTOR SYSTEM

By way of completing this chapter as a whole, let us return to a question asked earlier: has the examination fully addressed the patient's problem? Has determination of tone, resistive strength, muscle bulk, and presence or absence of "involuntary" movements related adequately to the patient's difficulty—for example, progressive slowness in physical activities of daily living? If not, you will penetrate the problem better by reproducing the situation that gave rise to the complaint. Observe the patient's inability to reach up to a high shelf or difficulty in climbing stairs. By witnessing the patient's actual experience you may be able to appreciate dimensions of motor difficulty reflected in symptoms but missed in the routine format of examination.

SUMMARY

Key points in the testing and observation of strength, tone, muscle bulk, and involuntary movements, as well as the direct examination of muscle and nerve, have been listed at the end of each of these sections.

Priorities

1 Tone: testing tone carries special importance because the patient's complaints may not direct you to this part of the examination. A spastic increase in tone may be one of the first signs of UMN dysfunction. Cogwheel rigidity often provides the key to insidiously developing Parkinson's disease.
2 Strength testing: go beyond right–left comparisons to evaluate strength (both distally and proximally) against a normal standard. In myopathies and neuromuscular junction disorders (as well as some cases of spinal cord or other CNS disease), mild weakness will be missed because of its symmetry. When strength testing does not reveal the weakness that might have been expected from the patient's complaints, try to reproduce the symptomatic situation by functional testing, e.g. climbing stairs.

Pitfalls

1 Attributing increased resistance upon passive movement to psychologic tenseness / "poor relaxation" rather than a neurologic cause of increased tone.
2 Not testing tone through a full range of motion, especially full extension at elbows and knees.
3 Attributing weakness, especially if symmetric, to thin musculature or old age, rather than to a neurologic disorder.

PROBLEMS FOR SELF-STUDY

Problems

1 A 41-year-old woman complains of unsteadiness when standing and walking. She is found to have symmetric weakness of the hip girdle muscles bilaterally. What other aspects of the examination would you most like to test?

2 A 64-year-old man presents with acute weakness of the left arm and leg; tone is not increased. Deep tendon reflexes (DTRs) are decreased relative to the right side. Would you expect to see fasciculations and neurogenic atrophy in the left arm and leg?

Comments

1 First, determine whether there is also bilaterally symmetric weakness in the shoulder girdle and neck flexors. If so, and distal muscles are strong, with no sensory or major reflex changes, then the probable diagnosis would be a myopathy, which could be further tested by electromyography (EMG), etc. If, on the other hand, there are UMN signs of increased tone, hyperreflexia, and Babinski signs – and/or concomitant sensory loss – then the CNS would be implicated (see Chapter 14).

2 Weakness in the arm and leg on the same side usually indicates a UMN lesion at a cervical level or higher. Although normal to decreased tone and reflexes are most often associated with LMN and other segmental disorders, this pattern can occur with an acute UMN problem, such as a stroke. Usually, tone and reflexes will subsequently increase. You would not expect the LMN signs of fasciculations and neurogenic atrophy at any time in this case, assuming that the responsible lesion is limited to the corticospinal tract and does not involve any LMNs. A lesion within the cervical spinal canal on the left might produce LMN signs of weakness, fasciculations, and eventually neurogenic atrophy in the involved cervical segment (implying damage to anterior horn cells or anterior roots). Ipsilateral UMN signs would appear caudally (including the leg), if the left corticospinal tract were affected (see Chapters 13 and 14).

FURTHER READING

Brooke, M.H. *A Clinician's View of Neuromuscular Disease*. 2nd edn. Williams and Wilkins, Baltimore (MA), 1986. A practical and accessible approach to primary and secondary disorders of muscle.

Dalakas, M.C. Polymyositis, dermatomyositis, and inclusion body myositis. *N Engl J Med* 1991; 325:1487–98. Polymyositis and dermatomyositis are treatable conditions with which every clinician should be familiar.

Davidoff, R.A. The pyramidal tract. *Neurology* 1990; 40:332–9. Scholarly review of the anatomy of the pyramidal and other descending motor tracts; discusses modern revisions of classic concepts of UMN control.

Davidoff, R.A. Skeletal muscle tone and the misunderstood stretch reflex. *Neurology* 1992; 42:951–63. Muscle tone is reviewed and misconceptions exposed.

Griggs, R.C., Mendell, J.R., Miller, R.G. *Evaluation and Treatment of Myopathies*. F.A. Davis, Philadelphia (PA), 1993. An up-to-date clinical text on muscle diseases.

Joseph, A.B., Young, R.R. (eds) *Movement Disorders in Neurology and Neuropsychiatry*. Blackwell Scientific Publications, Boston (MA), 1992. A multiauthored reference source for the myriad disorders of movement – mainly too much, but sometimes too little.

Kandel, E.R., Schwartz, J.H., Jessell, T.M. *Principles of Neural Science*. 3rd edn. Elsevier, New York (NY), 1991. The neuroanatomy and physiology of the motor system (Chapters 38–40).

Love, L.A., Leff, R.L., Fraser, D.D., *et al*. A new approach to the classification of idiopathic inflammatory myopathy: myositis-specific autoantibodies define useful homogeneous myopathy patient groups. *Medicine* 1991; 70:360–74. An attempt to categorize polymyositis and related inflammatory myopathies neurobiologically – an essential step in advancing research and specific therapy.

Medical Research Council of the UK. Aids to the examination of the peripheral nervous system. Memorandum 45. Pendragon House in North America, Palo Alto (CA). Reprinted by permission, Her Majesty's Stationery Office, 1976. An illustrated pamphlet on muscle and nerve testing, widely used for learning and for ready reference (see also Chapter 16, Further reading section).

Phillips, C.G., Landau, W.M. Upper and lower motor neuron: the little old synecdoche that works. Clinical neuromythology VIII. *Neurology* 1990; 40:884–6. Brief review of Gowers' still-useful concepts.

Sacks, O. A neurologist's notebook: a surgeon's life. *The New Yorker*. March 16, 1992, pp. 85–94. Captivating account of a successful surgeon with a movement disorder: the "tic" syndrome of Gilles de la Tourette.

chapter 7

Sensory Examinations

Most sensory data are familiar

As with other aspects of neurologic testing, you could easily invent most of the sensory examination (Table 7.1): you merely need to think of the kinds of sensations you experience – the various modes of perception of environmental or bodily stimuli. In addition to the special senses of sight, hearing, taste, and smell, you perceive the outside world by touching or being touched, lightly or with pressure, with a dimension of colder or warmer temperature, and by the experience of sharpness or pain. More complex perceptions are, among others, texture, shape, weight, and position or movement of a body part in space. Even changes in ticklishness can be significant!

"Inner" and "outer" symptoms

Sensory symptoms result both from what patients feel "within" (spontaneous or unstimulated sensations) and what they experience from "without" (the result of cutaneous stimuli). Many of these cutaneous stimuli come from the patients themselves. People do a great deal of tactile exploration, purposeful or inadvertent. Some sensory deficits are discovered by patients themselves in this way, in the course of rubbing, scratching, and washing.

Self-examination

Thus, patients often come to you not only with symptoms, but with

Table 7.1 Sensory testing: what to test, where and how

Sensory modality	What is the stimulus?	How slight a stimulus can you feel? How normal is it?	Where is it abnormal?		
			Right–left difference?	Nerve or root pattern?	Distal–proximal gradient?
Pain: Test with disposable safety pin, etc.	Compare point vs. dull end	Find mildest pinprick felt as pointed	Subjective comparison of sharpness	Map abnormal area	March pin proximally to normal
Temperature: Test coldness with metal tuning fork	Identify cool vs. warmer object	Not routinely assessed	Subjective comparison of coldness	Not usually mapped	Compare regions, e.g. foot vs. leg vs. thigh
Vibration: Test with 128 Hz (or 256 Hz) tuning fork	Vibration of fork vs. pressure only (sham vibration)	Allow decay until vibration no longer felt	Stimulus felt on one side after extinction on the other	Not usually assessed	Compare toes, ankles, knees, pelvis, spine, hands, etc.
Joint position sense	Upward vs. downward motion of body part	Define least excursion consistently and correctly identified	Compare least movement correctly perceived	Not usually assessed	Distal to proximal joints
Touch: (Test with cotton wisp)	Touch vs. no touch	Lightest touch felt (threshold); normal quality?	Compare threshold and quality	Map abnormal area	March stimulus proximally

the results of self-examination (see Table 1.2). In your assessment you can capitalize upon this by making the patient a partner in the ongoing assessment. Ask the patient to map out for you where stroking the skin does not feel normal. Similarly, he or she may be able to help you to decide whether pinprick is slightly decreased in one area vs. another by self-application of the pin to both regions. Since the patient's brain is in communication not only with the stimulus received but with the application of the stimulus, the patient has an advantage in discounting variations in stimulus strength (see Table 7.2).

These are but a few examples of the ways in which patients can participate meaningfully in a sensory evaluation beyond simply responding "sharp" or "dull" to a pinprick. To participate effectively the patient must be alert, attentive, able to understand instructions, and not overly suggestible. The sensory evaluation is, therefore, also a form of mental status test. If mental function is impaired, not only will the patient be a difficult partner and subject, but interpretation of results will be particularly troublesome.

Hyperawareness

On the other hand, the very sensitivity of perception may cause problems: the nervous system is flooded with stimuli, making it difficult to distinguish trivial variations from significant alterations. Symptoms

Table 7.2 Subjective and objective elements of sensory examination

Modality	Bedside rating	Recording result
Pain	Subjective: your estimate of strength of stimulus; patient's threshold for "pointedness." Objective: sharp point vs. dull	Example: "mild pin stimulus not felt as pointed on toes, but first felt at ankles, shading to normal at midshin bilaterally"
Temperature	Subjective: patient's estimate comparing sides or regions	Example: "stimulus felt as much colder on left than right – over entire left side up to sternal notch"
Vibration	Subjective: how long vibration is felt on one side after loss on other side; also, total duration in seconds. Objective: vibration vs. pressure (sham vibration)	Example: "stimulus felt for 5 s on left ankle after extinction on right; total 20 s right, 25 s left"
Joint position sense	Objective: degree of least excursion reliably identified	Example: "estimated 1 cm (or 30°) movements of thumb reliably perceived bilaterally"
Touch	Subjective: your estimate of strength of least stimulus felt; normal in quality? Objective: touch vs. nontouch	Example: "slight touch with wisp perceived on dorsum of toes, right and left, but touch triggered prickly feelings on right"

may arise from normal phenomena that would go unnoticed if the patient were not overly "tuned in" to sensory feelings. Therefore, we need to enable the patient to let the body "speak for itself" – to send signals of altered perception, but not to exaggerate self-awareness.

Standards of normal

We credit people's minds and muscles with natural differences, but sometimes find it hard to accept that patients differ in their thresholds of perception. Being "thick-skinned" or "thin-skinned" refers figuratively not only to emotional sensibilities, but also to pin sensitivity: certain areas of the body are "tougher" (that is, have a higher sensory threshold) than others. Some differences are intrinsic to the nervous system, while others are extrinsic, for example, the tough callused skin caused by hard use. Thus, the standard of normal requires continual adjustment. In testing, beware of comparing areas that are not similarly coarsened or judging threshold by stimulating just one arbitrary area. If the response to pin is "dull" in one place, such as the dorsum of the great toe, test other toes and surfaces before concluding that there is more than just a local pin deficit.

Frustrations of sensory testing

Frustrations arise from the subjectivity of sensory responses and from disparities between the patient's symptoms and formal test results. People possess remarkably sensitive perceptual systems, but our bedside testing tends to be crude by comparison. Detailed testing entails a significant commitment of time and energy. The deterrants to good sensory testing are similar in many ways to the barriers that confront a good history (see Table 1.3). To make sensory testing more manageable, you will need to learn to be selective.

Selective testing

You may wonder whether you need to test sensation everywhere on the body to do an adequate examination. Definitely not! To map the entire body surface is neither practical nor necessary. The following clues will help to guide your selective survey.

1 In order to gain the most useful data with maximum economy of time and effort, capitalize upon the topographic clues provided by the patient's symptoms. (For example, the "sciatic" symptoms of low back pain radiating down the posterior thigh would indicate the need for careful testing in the lumbosacral dermatomes.) Sensory symptoms are of great localizing value, whether or not "confirmatory" signs are delineated. (Normal findings never invalidate or nullify honest sensory symptoms.)

2 Reproduce the patient's reported self-examination (such as the discovery that hard scratching does not hurt in an area on the lateral thigh). Test pin there.

3 Correlate with other neurologic deficits (such as weakness) that focus your attention on a particular area.

4 Look for vascular, dermatologic, or other abnormalities (like signs of repetitive trauma) that raise a question of altered sensory function.

5 In addition, document certain key sensory tests (such as pin and vibration in the toes) that are important as baseline screening observations (see Chapter 19).

6 Finally, when you detect a sensory abnormality, pursue it: test other modalities carefully; look for a wider extent on the same side of the body or in the opposite limb; retest for subtle motor or reflex signs in the same area (see Chapter 16).

The basic clinical method of sensory testing will be less intimidating if you clearly establish the goals of the examination:

Modality

1 Can the patient distinguish one modality of sensation from another – the sharpness of a pin stimulus from the dullness of a soft touch or blunt end of the pin?

Threshold

2 Is the threshold of each sensory modality normal? What is the lightest stimulus perceived?

Topographic pattern

3 Are there significant topographic differences, comparing right with left, distal with proximal, upper extremities with lower, trunk with head and neck – or differences among parts of these? Do the boundaries suggest a dermatomal or peripheral nerve distribution? (See Figs 16.1–16.4.)

Technology

The implements of testing (see Table 7.1) such as safety pin and tuning fork serve well for ordinary bedside and office practice. Calibrated pins and hairs have long been available but are rarely used, even by neurologists. More advanced technology has now enabled much better quantitative testing, as in the case of calibrated vibrators. Helpful as these may be for clinical research and other specialized purposes, they have not yet supplanted the clinician's traditional tools (see Chapter 11, Further reading section).

PAIN

Overview

From the standpoint of sensory evaluation, pain is most important for its decrease or absence as tested by pin sensation. An isolated impairment of pain sensation typically is unaccompanied by any persistent, positive symptoms. ("Pins and needles" are not typical of loss of pin sensitivity.) Physical injury may announce a deficit in sensitivity, since the usual painful warnings of impending tissue damage are missing.

Two main types of altered pain sensitivity are recognized.

Definitions

1 *Analgesia (hypalgesia)*: the absence (decrease) of pain sensitivity.

2 *Hyperpathia*: an abnormally increased or exaggerated reaction to a painful stimulus (not a decreased threshold to the perception of painful stimuli). The hyperpathic sensation is often experienced with a slight delay (the term *hyperalgesia* is also used).

Pin testing and painful testing

Pain testing is usually done with a pin, but you should not use it to inflict pain. Paradoxic as this sounds, the perception of "pain" sensation can be evaluated by testing sharpness or pointedness. This should not ordinarily be carried to the point of discomfort, because by hurting the patient you have not only exceeded the usual requirements of testing, but you have risked alienating the patient from maximum cooperation.

Tools

Safety pins serve well for most testing: they are not too sharp, they are inexpensive, and should be discarded after each patient (avoid drawing blood which is upsetting and risks transmission of infection). Indicate to the patient that the pin has not previously been used. In addition, the act of discarding the safety pin into the designated container for "sharps" shows your sensitivity to concerns about the human immunodeficiency virus (HIV) and other infections. Use of a sharp broken end of a throat stick or tongue blade has also been advocated as a disposable testing device.

CASE 7A
A spinal stroke

George Pardee, a 54-year-old financier, was sitting in church when he suddenly doubled over from excruciating midback pain. As the pain wore off over the next 20–30 minutes he became aware that he could not move his legs or feel any pain when he pinched them. When first evaluated at the hospital shortly thereafter he was no longer in any pain whatsoever, but his legs were paralyzed and insensitive to pin stimulus. A neurologic consultation was immediately obtained.

Techniques of testing

The following discussion of pin and temperature testing will exemplify the methods used to evaluate a sensory deficit as in the above case (see

Tables 7.1 and 7.2). This is followed by a presentation of the findings.

Distinguishing sharp from dull

1 For recognition of the pointedness or sharpness of the pin, you may wish first to test the patient's hand gently to show that testing will not be painful (unlike the dreaded needle stick! Let squeamish patients try out the pin themselves). Then, with the patient's eyes closed or averted, determine whether the patient can distinguish the point of the pin from a dull stimulus, such as the opposite, blunt end (this can be done on the toes of each foot or any other areas). Correct responses establish that pain sensation in that area is present, but not necessarily intact, since the threshold has not yet been determined.

Threshold

2 To test for threshold of pain perception, determine the very least stimulus that is recognized as sharp, as opposed to mere touch or pressure. An overreaction to the stimulus or complaint of a burning sensation or other hyperpathia suggests a sensory abnormality, but not an increased sensitivity (in the sense of a lowered threshold of perception).

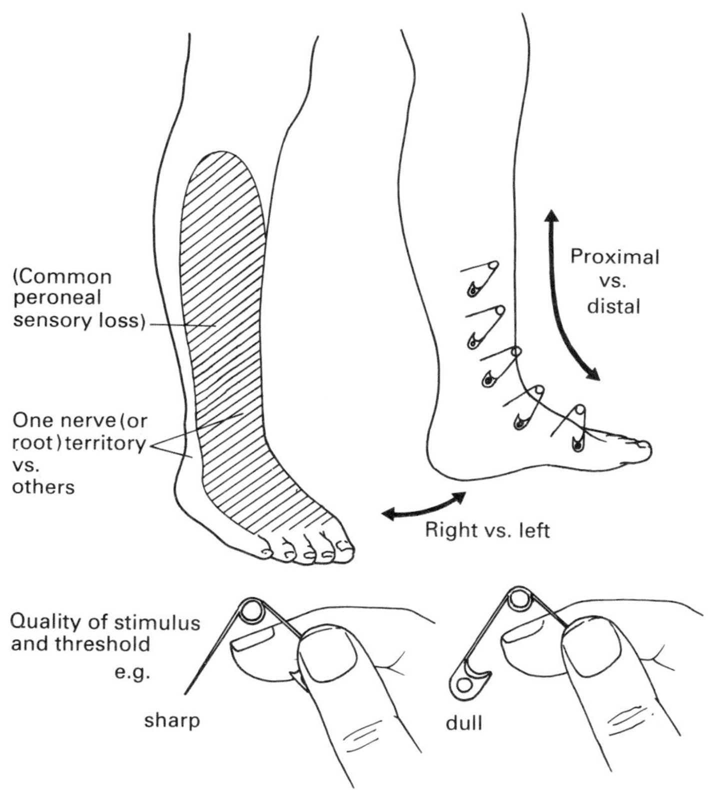

Fig. 7.1 Sensory comparisons. Using pin testing as an example, the pin stimulus is compared with dull touch; the pin is marched from distal to proximal, and compared between the right and left foot; an area of sensory loss (shaded) in the superficial peroneal sensory distribution is distinguished from an adjacent unaffected.

Topography

3 To complete pin testing, compare the threshold (as well as the character of the response) in different areas (Fig. 7.1). Testing the toes on each foot measures the threshold at the ends of the longest nerves (which are more likely to be affected in the common diffuse diseases of nerves, the axonal polyneuropathies). Marching the stimulus up the foot and leg enables detection of a shading from a more distal blunting of sensation to a more proximal sharpness (as occurs in the so-called stocking–glove distribution that is characteristic of most polyneuropathies (see Fig. 16.11). When applying successive pin stimuli, do not repeat them too rapidly or too close to one another: the phenomena of temporal and spatial summation increase perception. Delivery of about one stimulus per second at distances of 1–2 cm from one another is usually satisfactory when moving the stimulus along the skin.

The most important topographic feature to uncover is a sensory level. A sensory level is any segmental level below which one or more modalities are impaired and above which sensation is normal. Most often (as will be elaborated subsequently) a sensory level indicates a spinal cord lesion and therefore deserves immediate further evaluation (see Fig. 14.6).

CASE 7A
A spinal stroke (*continued*)

As earlier noted, Mr Pardee's intolerable back pain had subsided, leaving him unable to feel a pinprick to the legs. More detailed sensory evaluation then disclosed a complete absence of ability to recognize sharpness, up to the level of the T7 dermatome on the trunk on both right and left sides. Nor could he tell warm from cold. Both pin and temperature sensation were normal above this level. Below that approximate level he perceived touch normally or nearly so; vibration and position sense were completely intact throughout. He was also paraplegic, but evidenced no lower extremity hypertonia, tendon reflexes, or Babinski signs. (These upper motor neuron (UMN) findings appeared in later weeks after the state of spinal shock subsided.) Voluntary bladder and bowel function were lost.

The diagnosis of an anterior spinal artery syndrome was made – a spinal cord infarction of the anterolateral two-thirds of the spinal cord (supplied by the anterior spinal artery) – involving, in this case, the midthoracic cord. The posterior columns (vibration, joint position sense (JPS), and some touch) were spared. The pathogenesis of the arterial occlusion was never elucidated (see Chapter 14, section on sensory levels, and Fig. 14.3 for the anatomy of this case).

This tragic event dramatically illustrated the occurrence – below a defined anatomic level – of a dissociated sensory loss: the absence of pain and temperature sensation with preservation of vibration, position, and some touch. He experienced no positive sensory symptoms in the legs. In fact, he was aware only of the paralysis until specific testing revealed to his amazement that he could not feel the sharpness of the pin or distinguish hot and cold (see Chapter 14, section on dissociated sensory loss).

Deep pain

Deep pain results from noxious stimulation of viscera or other noncutaneous structures. Historically, impaired deep pain sensation has been a factor (along with decreased JPS) in the joint trauma and deformity known as Charcot joints, a classic sign of spinal tabetic neurosyphilis. Many physicians were taught to elicit deep, visceral pain by applying pressure to a testicle or firmly squeezing the Achilles tendon between two knuckles. Certainly, squeezing a testicle, nipple, or other sensitive organ has no place in routine neurologic testing.

TEMPERATURE

Screening tests

While formal evaluation of temperature sensation need not be a part of the ordinary neurologic examination, simple testing serves as an adjunct to pain evaluation. For the quickest screening, you can simply touch both arms, legs, or sides of the face with the broad surface of a tuning fork. Request the patient's subjective impression as to whether one side or the other is consistently different – the abnormal side feeling less cool. The coldness of the tuning fork can also be compared with the rubber of your reflex hammer.

Correlation with symptoms

Patients often complain of feeling cold in some region (for either primary vascular or neurologic reasons), but perceive cold or warm stimuli well. Conversely, as with pain, patients may be unaware of loss of temperature sense, and hence burn themselves accidentally (for syringomyelia see Fig. 14.4).

VIBRATION

Unlike pain, temperature, or touch, the sense of vibration does not seem like a natural or obvious candidate for testing. Yet vibratory testing has achieved an important place in the sensory examination because it provides a rather sensitive measure of the ability of large, heavily myelinated nerve fibers to conduct the rapid trains of impulses that the vibratory oscillations trigger.

Testing

From the standpoint of bedside or office practice, testing vibration is fairly quick and reproducible in the alert patient and can be semiquantitated (see Table 7.2). Be sure that the patient reports the vibratory sensation ("buzzing feeling") itself and not just the pressure of the tuning fork. You can confirm this understanding by trying a sham stimulus (fork not vibrating) or by extinguishing the vibration with the fork remaining in place. To save time, start with a low-intensity stimulus, so that you will not need to wait through a long vibratory decay period each time you place the tuning fork.

As with other modalities of sensation, establish the threshhold of perception (see Table 7.1). If you simply place a strongly vibrating fork on a bone and the patient feels it, you will not have learned very much – and you certainly cannot record vibratory sense as "intact."

Clinical correlation

No symptoms are specifically attached to loss of vibratory sense, although tight, encased, band-like, or constricted feelings may provide a clue to posterior column dysfunction more generally. Vibratory sense impairment tends to be prominent in peripheral neuropathies, as well as in spinal cord syndromes involving the posterior columns (Case 7B).

Anatomic note

(Recall that the same dorsal root ganglion neuron that sends a peripheral process out into a peripheral nerve also sends a central process into the central nervous system (CNS), and many of these ascend in the posterior columns.) Of course, vibratory sense impairment, like other sensory modalities, may result from lesions more rostrally, namely in the brainstem, the thalamus, the thalamocortical projections, and in the sensory cortex. At the level of the thalamus and above, lesions tend to diminish the primary sensory modalities as a group rather than selectively (see Figs 13.13 and 13.14).

PROPRIOCEPTION

Overview

The most common measure of conscious proprioception is JPS, also sometimes referred to as kinesthetic sense. However, this is not the only way to evaluate the sense of relative position, or change of position of the body or its parts in space. The Romberg test (which will be described in the next chapter) assesses proprioception in the trunk and legs by comparing balance with and without the aid of visual orientation (see Fig. 8.1). Unconscious proprioceptive capacities are almost continuously utilized in providing feedback for control of our every posture and motion.

Testing

To test JPS (or direction of movement) at the great toe, stabilize the proximal phalanx and hold the distal phalanx at the sides. The patient (with eyes closed) should report whether the direction of movement of the toe is in an up or down direction. Determine what is the smallest discrete movement up or down that the patient can correctly and reproducibly identify on both right and left sides (see Tables 7.1 and 7.2). If JPS is not normal on the first toe tried, test other digits. (A deficit limited to one toe, usually due to local damage from trauma, is rarely of larger neurologic significance.) If digit JPS is abnormal, try it at successive proximal joints until normal function is demonstrated.

Another way of assessing proprioception is by static JPS testing (as opposed to the dynamic or kinesthetic testing of the direction of joint movement described above). Move the patient's arm (or leg) to some position in space and then, maintained in a fixed position, ask the patient (eyes closed throughout) to point to the exact location of the thumb (or great toe). This clearly requires not only a sense of where the specified part is, but good proprioception in the pointing limb as well. Alternatively, ask the patient to extend the arms fully out to the side and then bring them together, so that the index fingers touch end to end.

Interpretation

Correct naming of the direction of a large movement does not establish that JPS is normal. In order to document intact JPS, the degree of movement must be the least that which a normal person can perceive. Occasional errors are of little importance. Obviously, a 50% correct answer rate is no better than chance alone. Try to make the pattern of movement random. JPS testing is more objective than vibratory testing in that you can validate every answer: it is up or down, right or wrong.

Pathologic interference with JPS can occur in the peripheral and central pathways leading to the thalamus and cortex. As a discriminative or so-called "cortical" modality, JPS (or other proprioception tests) may be affected by parietal lobe lesions that spare the perception of vibration or ordinary touch.

TOUCH

Overview

A sense of touch not only registers contact with the environment, but enables you to manipulate objects: "getting the feel" of a keyboard, for example, depends on a subtle interplay of mechanics and sensory feedback; displaying a "fine touch" involves exquisite tactile sensation as well as position sense and well-tuned motor output.

Fine touch

Fine touch is clinically associated with other modalities served by the so-called posterior column (medial lemniscal) pathways (see Chapter 13). Lesions of the posterior and posterolateral columns of the spinal cord that affect vibratory and conscious position sense are typically accompanied by deficits in touch (often mild). While anatomy books cite the role of the ventral (anterior) spinothalamic pathways in subserving touch, the posterior pathways appear to be important for fine, tactile sensation with high spatial discrimination. (Note that in Case 7A, severe infarction in the ventral cord territory of the anterior spinal artery left the patient with nearly normal touch sensation.)

Anatomic note

CASE 7B
"Swollen" feet

Alice Burgess, a 34-year-old physical therapist, noticed slight tingling on the sole of her right foot upon arising from the dinner table one evening. She passed it off, thinking that she had been sitting on a hard chair too long. However, the next morning when she got out of bed her feet felt swollen and her soles did not seem to be making close contact with the floor. However, her feet did not look swollen.

She went to her health center for an examination, but her nurse clinician found no significant past history and noted no swelling or circulatory abnormalities. Neurologic examination was initially normal, but on the following day certain abnormalities were detected—diminished light touch, as well as JPS and vibratory sense. Her findings will be described in more detail after the examination for touch sensation is introduced.

Testing

Qualitative changes

The patient's subjective impression as to qualitative and quantitative alterations in touch is often revealing. Not only will the patient's symptoms often guide you to an area of abnormality, but the patient may already have done some mapping by exploratory touching. If not, a good way to start the examination is to ask the patient to ascertain, by light stroking, whether there are any "feelings of difference"—any areas that just do not feel entirely normal. Alternatively, run your hand lightly over the patient's skin. This may induce paresthesias or feel leathery, distant, or just less sensitive. Unless the quality of the sensation is normal do not conclude that sensation is intact.

Threshold

In testing light touch (see Tables 7.1 and 7.2), note that a moving stimulus creates temporal and spatial summation of impulses, increasing the chance of perception. Thus, if a single touch is not felt, augment the stimulus by using a stroking motion (or a heavier strand). It is hard to establish by tactile testing that the sense of touch is truly intact, but it is possible to demonstrate that it is very good.

Relevant symptoms

In contrast to the spinothalamic system, lesions that produce light touch deficits commonly announce themselves with a variety of positive sensory symptoms. These include a constricted or swollen feeling, an illusion of being encased in some material, and numb or novocaine-like feelings and paresthesias ("pins and needles").

CASE 7B
"Swollen" feet (*continued*)

Having come with a complaint of her feet feeling swollen, Ms Burgess found that when she stroked the skin of her feet and lower legs, the touch felt strangely distant, as if she were touching a callus on her toe. She could map this out to include not only most of both feet, but her right leg and lower thigh as well, although no sharp boundary could be defined. Light cotton wisp stimuli were not as consistently felt on the right leg as on the left above the ankle. In addition, vibratory and position sense were decreased in both lower extremities, worse on the right.

Over the next 3 days these abnormalities ascended to her abdomen, almost to the level of the umbilicus. Subsequently the symptoms and signs stabilized and eventually resolved entirely. She was diagnosed as having transverse myelopathy – a pathologic derangement affecting all or part of a cross-section (transverse section) of the spinal cord. The pathology was presumed to be demyelination, in the posterior columns, at or above T10. Had magnetic resonance imaging (MRI) been available, it might have been possible to localize the exact level of the lesion. Later episodes led to the diagnosis of multiple sclerosis. Fig. 7.2 shows the spinal cord plaques in a patient with multiple sclerosis.

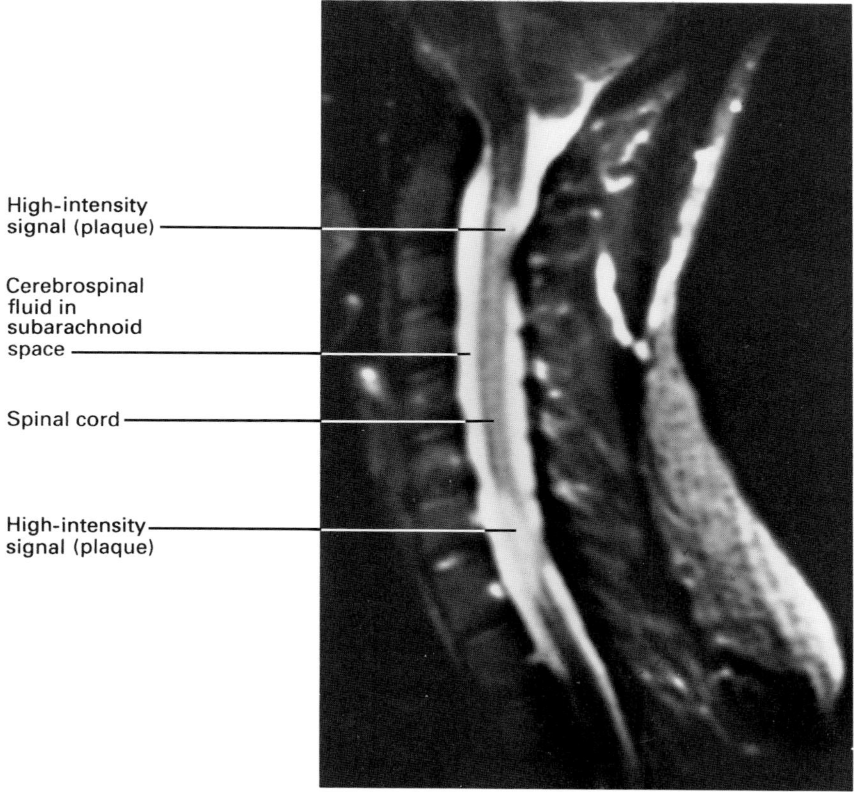

Fig. 7.2 Spinal cord demyelination (case similar to Case 7B). This spinal magnetic resonance image (T2-weighted image) shows two high-intensity (bright) lesions in the cervical cord of a patient known to have multiple sclerosis. (Courtesy of Jonathan Kleefield MD.)

SENSORY LEVELS

As you have seen in this case (and in Case 7A in which the patient lost pain and temperature sensation below the midthoracic region) lesions in certain ascending sensory tracts in the spinal cord create sensory levels. A sensory level is not necessarily crisply defined at one static level on the body. Most disease processes are partial and changing, which results not only in a changing degree of sensory loss, but also in a changing sensory level. With a partial lesion there may be some ascending fibers that are totally affected, yielding a zone (up to the groin – marked by L1 dermatome – for example) of severe loss of vibration and altered touch, etc., then a zone of progressively milder sensory loss up to the lower chest at approximately T7, and then an upper level above which sensation is entirely normal (such as T2 and above). This gradation is due to the topographic lamination of fibers in CNS tracts (see Fig. 14.6).

Clinical level vs. anatomic (cord) level

The best demarcation of the clinical sensory level is that level separating normal sensation above from any objective or subjective alteration below. A single cord lesion responsible for a clinical sensory level can never lie below that level, but may be above it.

Brown–Séquard syndrome

The extreme example of a hemitransection of the cord illustrates another facet of sensory levels. Touch and other posterior column sensory modalities (and motor functions) are affected ipsilateral to the lesion, whereas pain and temperature are affected contralaterally. This is because the pain and temperature pathways cross within several segments of the cord level at which the root fibers enter and synapse. This "dissociation" of pain–temperature sensation from "posterior column" modalities (and UMN motor loss) is characteristic of an intrinsic spinal lesion (see Fig. 13.16 and Chapter 14, section on dissociated sensory loss).

Remember that a sensory level is not necessarily "level." As you can see from a dermatome chart (see Fig. 16.1) the upper thoracic dermatomes are quite circumferential, whereas the lower ones descend anteriorly, as do the ribs. Once the lumbar dermatomes move off the trunk and onto the lower limbs, the boundary (between L3 and L4, for example), becomes nearly vertical. But a sensory demarcation at L4 (sensation preserved in higher dermatomes and impaired in lower ones) is nonetheless a sensory level.

Vertebral level

This brings up a third kind of level – the vertebral level. Because the cord itself ends at about T12–L1, the lumbosacral cord segments are more rostral than their respective vertebral bodies (for example, cord segment L5 is in the region of T12 vertebral body, well separated from the more caudal L5 vertebral body. Therefore, a protruding intervertebral disc at the L4–L5 vertebral interspace could not be responsible for compressing the L5 cord segment. This disc could compress the L5 roots after they have descended in the spinal canal as part of the cauda equina and before their exit at the L5–S1 interspace). Neuroimaging focused on the L4–L5 and L5–S1 vertebral levels would miss a lesion at T12 vertebral level responsible for an L5 cord segment compression (see Figs 13.9 and 14.6).

DISCRIMINATIVE SENSORY TESTS

Definition

At a practical level, the discriminative sensory tests are those that require not only the recognition of a simple stimulus (such as touch), but appreciation of more complex qualities (such as texture). Dynamic JPS testing requires a spatial decision as to direction of movement, in addition to recognition of movement; JPS therefore includes a discriminative aspect. Clearly, some tests are more discriminative than others, but the ones described below fit this label and are commonly employed for this purpose. (As will be seen, they are also referred to as cortical sensory tests, because lesions in the sensory cortex of the parietal lobes may produce deficits that predominantly affect these discriminations.)

Overview

Several general points are worth remembering about discriminative tests.

1 The primary modality of sensation must be sufficiently intact to permit meaningful discriminative testing. If there is a major deficit in touch sensation, a test that depends on tactile perception (like graphesthesia) will not produce meaningful results.

2 Do not choose a test that depends upon some other function, such as an ability to palpate or to point (as in the tests of stereognosis and touch localization) if the patient cannot carry these out adequately from a motor standpoint.

3 While most discriminative tests are usually done on the palms of the hands or the fingertips, be prepared to choose another site if the hands are unavailable or if the major neurologic deficits are elsewhere. For example, if the only other abnormality found thus far is a weakness in the right leg and foot, do not limit your discriminative sensory tests to the hand, but compare these functions on the feet as well.

4 Since the range of normal in the bedside mode of testing is quite broad, comparison between sides takes on particular importance.

Testing graphesthesia (writing on skin)

An ability to recognize numbers or other figures drawn on the skin tests tactile and spatial capacities. Most simply, you can write with your finger on the patient's palm (eyes closed). The task is easiest for the patient if you hold the palm in front of the patient, like a blackboard, and write from the perspective of the patient. (To face the patient and write from your own perspective results in a figure that is reversed for the patient and therefore must be mentally transposed.) If there is a mild deficit in light touch, be sure to apply a sufficiently strong stimulus for the patient to perceive, otherwise the discriminative aspect cannot be judged. While comparison of number writing on the right and left palms is the usual format of this test, you can also do it on the face, arms, legs, and soles, or use a finer stimulus (like a pencil point) on the finger tips.

Stereognosis

Stereognosis, or the ability to recognize shapes by feeling, is often tested with coins, keys, safety pins, or other readily available small objects. The patient must be able to palpate the item. Instruct the patient to "move the (coin) around and feel it really well" (with the test hand only and eyes shut). In fact, your observation of how well the patient manipulates the object may provide a bonus in terms of data on motor, proprioceptive, or other components of dexterity. If the patient has difficulty with specific identification, try to ascertain what qualities can be perceived: is it round? Is the material hard, soft, light, or heavy? What does the edge feel like? If the denomination of the coin (penny) cannot be stated, is it more like a dime or a quarter? Or, can the patient match it to a known sample? Clearly, the ability to "feel" the shape of an object (as a group of sensations) depends upon "feeling" the object well in the sense of motor manipulation.

Two-point discrimination

This test assesses the patient's ability to distinguish two simultaneous stimuli applied at varying distances from one another: as the touch stimuli are applied more and more closely to one another, eventually the patient will perceive only one. "Two-point" does not mean two sharp points (as the purpose is not to elicit pain) but simply two discrete stimuli. The most precise tool is a caliper or compass with points sufficiently dull that they will not prick. A practical bedside alternative consists of the bare ends of two throat swab sticks. Hold these in one hand, at equal length, so that both ends touch the patient's skin at the same time. In testing the palm, start with a 2–3 cm separation and reduce the distance until the patient (with eyes closed) reports only one point felt, which normally occurs at 1 cm or slightly less. Finer points can be distinguished at a few millimeters separation on the finger tips. At more proximal limb and trunk locations the minimum separation needed to discriminate two points will be greater. In addition to its use as a "cortical" test, in which case right–left comparisons are especially important, two-point discrimination is also used to test fine tactile function in cases of peripheral nerve injury and dorsal column dysfunction.

Touch localization

In this test, the patient is asked to localize exactly where a touch stimulus is applied, which requires not only perception, but a kind of spatial discrimination. Since accuracy of localization varies over different parts of the body, you should compare performance at the same location on the right and left sides. One way for the patient to indicate the location of the stimulus is to touch exactly that point with a finger of the other hand. If the patient is unable to execute this, a verbal description of the site can be substituted, but is less accurate.

You can conveniently add an additional test for extinction at this time (as is done in visual field testing). By applying double simultaneous stimuli to the right and left, you can assess whether the patient fails to report the touch on one side. (If reproducible, and not due to primary blunting of sensation, extinction suggests a relative neglect of that side, usually associated with a deficit in contralateral parietal function.)

Clinical correlation

A lateralized (but nonfocal) deficit in sensory discrimination implies dysfunction of the contralateral parietal lobe. Before arriving at this conclusion, however, you should ordinarily be able to demonstrate impaired discrimination by more than one test. Also, beware of confusing local factors, such as calluses on the palm or fingers: try other areas nearby and more distant. If performance is poor bilaterally, be sure that the patient understands the test, and that no disorder of communication is responsible for the errors.

SUMMARY

Priorities

1 Thresholds: when testing pin, touch, vibration, and JPS, try to establish the least stimulus that can be perceived correctly.
2 Comparisons: after checking that one stimulus can be differentiated from another (sharp vs. dull, vibration vs. pressure, etc.), compare right vs. left and distal vs. proximal gradients. Also, seek differences in one aspect of a limb (e.g. anterior vs. lateral) to expose a peripheral nerve or dermatomal pattern to any deficits found.
3 Screening: be sure to test at least vibration and pin (pain) sense on the toes of the right and left feet. This samples the two main sensory systems and will pick up most polyneuropathies.

Pitfalls

1 Not sufficiently crediting purely subjective alterations in sensation – and therefore not enlisting the patient in mapping them.
2 Performing a perfunctory, rather than problem-oriented examination. Do not test pin and touch in a scattered fashion over the body, while neglecting to check proprioception in a clumsy hand.
3 Interpreting and recording a sensory modality that is merely present (e.g. strong vibration felt at the ankle) as "intact" or "normal."
4 Not following distal deficits (in any modality) proximally to establish an upper limit – and possibly detect a sensory level.
5 Calling sensation normal when only one modality, such as pin, has been tested, thus leaving the possibility of a major deficit in vibratory sense, for example.

PROBLEMS FOR SELF-STUDY

Problems

1 A 23-year-old man is found to have absent pin sensation in the toes bilaterally. Sharpness is felt at the ankles and knees. What additional testing would be most helpful?
2 A 55-year-old woman with diabetes is found to have decreased JPS in the right foot, which is attributed to diabetic neuropathy. How would you go about assessing this diagnosis from the standpoint of the neurologic examination?

Comment

1 In addition to testing other sensory modalities, continue the pin test-

ing on the thighs, hips, and trunk to ascertain a sensory level. Some ability to perceive pain should not be equated with normal. Although it might appear that the pin loss has followed a distal–proximal gradient in the lower extremities consistent with a polyneuropathy, the deficit must be mapped to the point or level of normality. If the transition to normal is found on the trunk, the lesion is almost surely in the cord rather than the peripheral nervous system. Motor and reflex testing would also help with localization (see Chapters 13 and 14, and Figs 14.6 and 14.7).

2 The examination and its documentation must include not only the extent of the JPS deficit, but the distribution of impairments in other modalities. If the JPS loss in the right foot were part of a pattern of JPS loss on the right side of the body, then a left parietal lesion should be considered; other discriminative ("cortical") modalities of sensation should be evaluated. A pattern of some loss of all modalities in the right foot should be mapped to ascertain a particular peripheral nerve distribution, such as the common peroneal. If present, this could be a diabetic mononeuropathy. It would not represent the more common polyneuropathy, in which vibratory sense is usually affected more than JPS, but, most importantly, all deficits are symmetric and worse distally than proximally. Reflex and motor testing would also help define the localization (see Chapter 16).

FURTHER READING

Davidoff, R.A. The dorsal columns. *Neurology* 1989; 39:1377–85. Another of this author's scholarly reviews of key neural systems – the present one explaining revisions in concepts of the spinal transmission of vibration, fine touch, and JPS.

Kandel, E.R., Schwartz, J.H., Jessell, T.M. *Principles of Neural Science*. 3d edn. Elsevier, New York (NY), 1991. Anatomic and physiologic basis of somatosensory perception (presented in Part V, Sensory systems of the brain).

Matthews, W.B., Compston, A., Allen, I.V., Martyn, C.N. *McAlpine's Multiple Sclerosis*. 2nd edn. Churchill Livingstone, Edinburgh, 1991. Multiple sclerosis often presents with sensory symptoms; this book covers the entire subject, and is the place to look after general medical and neurologic texts.

Sacks, O. *The Man Who Mistook His Wife for a Hat*. Summit Books, New York (NY), 1985. The case of "the disembodied lady" illustrates the problem of proprioceptive deafferentation: what it is like to lose a sense of one's position.

Sandson, T.A., Friedman, J.H. Spinal cord infarction. Report of 8 cases and review of the literature. *Medicine* 1989; 68:282–92. Varieties of the anterior spinal artery syndrome were seen eight times in less than 5 years in a community hospital; this article presents the cases and reviews the subject.

Simon, R.P., Aminoff, M.J., Greenberg, D.A. *Clinical Neurology*. Appleton and Lange, Norwalk (CT), 1989. Sensory disorders (Chapter 7) may be among the hardest to diagnose, but with careful attention to symptoms and signs may also be the most precisely localizable.

chapter 8

Coordination and Balance

Overview

Coordination denotes the harmonious integration of all elements of movement into an efficient whole. Coordination includes the following characteristics (which overlap):

1 accuracy of a targetted movement (as in reaching for a door handle or threading a needle);

2 fluidity, synergy, and economy of movement (as in drawing or throwing a ball);

3 rhythmicity, smooth alternation, and controlled modulations (as in typing or playing a musical instrument);

4 balance and steadiness of posture and movement (as in dancing or skating).

We all have some experience with incoordination; clinicians and patients can communicate well on this point! Even if one's system of coordination is not disordered, it may need to compensate for the environment: on shipboard in a rough sea one reels and staggers, but learns to adapt (by such means as spreading the legs – a wider "base" to maintain better equilibrium). In testing, we use the reverse of this mechanism (standing with feet together or walking a line heel-to-toe) to "stress" a patient's balance and coordination.

Coordination testing and cerebellar function

From the standpoint of testing and interpretation, coordination is often too narrowly identified with cerebellar function. What we test is coordinated movement – not cerebellar function in isolation. We cannot directly test the cerebellum and its connections apart from the other anatomic systems that contribute to the integration of movement. Smooth, steady, balanced, well-targetted motor performance requires a sufficient degree of strength, relaxation of tone, and proprioceptive feedback, as well as vestibular and visual orientation in many instances. Integration of other systems is at least part of what the cerebellum seems to do. For this reason the term "coordination testing" is preferable to "cerebellar testing," so as not to prejudge which of the component anatomic and physiologic mechanisms may be at fault in producing an observed deficit. (The distinction is not just semantic; as a concept it has real, practical importance. See Case 14A and the Further reading section at the end of this chapter).

Role of history and functional testing

Assessment of coordination offers a prime example of the limitations of routine testing. The maneuvers that you will learn to use at the bedside are pale reflections of the demands of real life on balance and coordination. Therefore, if the patient imparts a history of difficulty, but performs your bedside tests quite well, assume that there is more of a problem than meets your eye as a neurologic examiner. In addition, try to reproduce the functional situation in which the patient has experienced difficulty. This might be as simple as lifting a coffee cup to the lips or as complex as typing.

In general, feel free to devise your own tests of coordination that will help to capture the patient's problem. At times, the need for such innovation is imposed by constraints such as a cast on an arm or a shoulder in pain from bursitis. As long as you can bear in mind the goals of your testing, you can usually invent some substitute test that will produce useful, if only partial, data.

STANCE AND GAIT

Definitions

Stance obviously refers to the attitude of standing (such as an erect, military posture, a slouch, a precarious stance, or a particular batting stance). (*Station*, as used in the phrase "station and gait," is a bit of jargon conveying the same meaning.)

Ataxia denotes incoordination – an irregularity or lack of order – in movement. Ataxia can be applied not only to gait (locomotor or gait ataxia) but also to limb activity, the components of speech, and even to eye movements.

Relevant history

Patients describe disequilibrium of stance and gait in a variety of ways, often using the terms dizzy, weak, off-balance, staggering, "walking like I'm drunk," veering to one side, falling or "afraid of falling," etc. For clarification, try to establish whether the patient feels off-balance in the absence of faintness, a sense of impending collapse, or dizzy sensations (spinning, rocking, or other movement) in the head. Are the symptoms spontaneous or related to change of position, especially sitting or standing up (orthostatic change)? Inquire for any visual impairments or difficulty walking in the dark (see Romberg test, below). Do any neurologic disorders run in the family? Are medications in use, or is there alcohol or other substance abuse?

Standards of normal

Good balance is relative. We would not insist that the average person demonstrate the balance necessary for a high-wire act, nor would we regard a lurching gait on the deck of a tossing ship as abnormal. At a more mundane level, we accept mild unsteadiness when a person first arises in the morning or first gets out of bed after an illness. Balance diminishes in the elderly.

The quality of gait clearly depends to some degree on modifying factors such as the presence of local pain or joint stiffness, age, obesity, eyesight, and general confidence in balance. As discussed in Chapter 3, what is normal for a particular patient can be evaluated in terms of past performance, ability to carry on customary functions, and reference to others of the same age and build. Everyone should normally be able to walk steadily on an even, illuminated surface, except in extreme old age. Very obese and aged patients, as well as those with mild orthopedic and arthritic conditions may have difficulty walking a line (see tandem gait) or traversing rough ground.

Preliminary observations

Informal observation reveals much about how the patient actually functions in a practical way. By the time you are to begin formal coordination testing (in the ambulatory patient), you will probably already have observed sitting and standing posture and perhaps also walking. For the patient first seen sitting in a wheelchair or lying in a hospital bed, you will not learn this information unless you insist on specific testing (provided, of course, that the patient is otherwise well enough to do so safely). In any case, always provide sufficient supervision so that the patient can be reassured and protected against falling.

Test seated posture

Observe the patient's ability to:

1 sit up straight and maintain balance without bracing arms or legs;

2 arise from bed or chair and assume a standing posture;

Stance

3 maintain a stance with feet in whatever position is most comfortable and steady (see discussion of Romberg test, below). You should observe width of base (distance between the feet) and posture of trunk and limbs.

Gait

Ask the patient to walk naturally (as if taking a stroll) and reverse direction, turning to both right and left. You should look for the following:

1 length of stride (and base, as above);

2 symmetry and extent of associated arm swing;

3 any tendency to veer to one side, to shuffle, stagger, freeze (get stuck), festinate (hurry involuntarily);

4 difficulty initiating gait;

5 scuffing, stamping, or tripping;

6 swinging one leg out (circumducting) or crossing the legs (scissoring);
7 evidence of excessive wear on one aspect of the shoe soles;
8 ability to regain balance, if temporarily lost;
9 apparent need or desire to touch, hold, or hang on to another person, walls, or piece of furniture.

Stress the patient's balance by maneuvers such as the following.

Tandem gait

1 The patient walks one foot in front of the other, heel-to-toe (in tandem), as in "walking a line," which serves to narrow the base maxi-

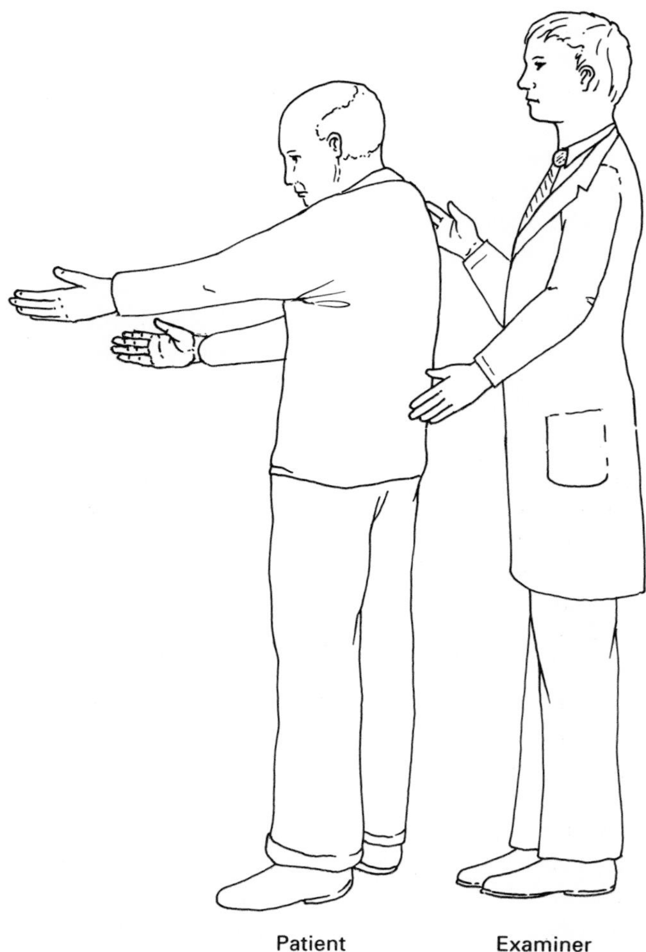

Fig. 8.1 Romberg test and arm drift/pronator drift. To provide security and minimize anxiety during Romberg testing, the examiner should stand nearby, offering reassurance, and be prepared to prevent a possible fall. For efficiency, the patient is also asked to hold the arms outstretched, palms up, to test for pronation of the forearm and downward arm drift (signs of weakness), seen here on the right. (This is not part of the Romberg test itself.)

mally. This test should be distinguished from walking on heels or toes (see Chapter 6) which is primarily intended to test muscular power.

Romberg test

2 To perform "the Romberg" (Fig. 8.1), test stance on the narrowest base that supports a steady posture, with feet completely together if possible. Encourage relaxation, especially of the shoulders, which are often held tensely if the patient is anxious. Then instruct the patient to close both eyes, indicating that you will stand close by to prevent any possibility of falling. Since most patients will sway a little, at least initially, it is helpful to indicate that a little swaying may be normal and that they should just balance themselves. If unable to maintain balance with eyes closed (having been able to do so with eyes open) then the Romberg sign is present (a positive test). For utmost clarity it is best to record an "abnormal Romberg," describing what is actually observed. (To further stress the same functions, test standing on one leg with eyes open, then closed.) Continued encouragement and protection are the keys to successful testing. For efficiency, you can test for arm drift during the Romberg test (see Chapter 6 and Fig. 8.1).

Interpretation of Romberg test

By removing the factor of visual orientation the Romberg test stresses the other systems required for balance. If stance is stable with feet together and eyes open, then the patient is presumably not vertiginous and does not lack the necessary degree of strength or cerebellar function. With eye closure, impaired proprioception that had previously been compensated for by visual orientation, is taxed beyond capacity: the patient progressively sways and would fall if not protected from doing so. Although joint position sense (JPS) does not fully reflect proprioceptive function, you should question the interpretation of an "abnormal Romberg" if JPS is good (see Chapter 7).

Pitfalls in Romberg test interpretation

1 If the patient cannot balance with the eyes open or closed, then the Romberg is untestable. (Be sure to widen the base to ascertain whether a stable stance can be maintained with eyes open. If so, then test with eyes closed.)

2 False-positive Rombergs are very common. Patients frequently sway and reach for support due to anxiety. Hold your arms out to assure the patient that you will prevent falling. Then offer continuing verbal encouragement. You will be surprised how often an apparently abnormal Romberg normalizes.

Modification of stance and gait testing

By thinking about the entire test system involved in assessing gait, you will be able to adapt your approach to the individual patient. Are there any orthopedic deformities or sources of pain, such as shortening of a leg or limitation of range of motion? To what extent can you neutralize such factors? For example, if left ankle pain with weight-bearing prevents walking, you can still assess the ability to balance on the right foot. If gait appears stiff, recheck tone (see Cases 6B and 14A). In case of visual deficits that could be interfering, test stance and gait with eyes closed. (The disorientation associated with double, blurred, or distorted vision may interfere with gait more than does absence of vision. If double vision is present, merely cover one eye—preferably the eye with the poorer acuity.) Should the patient's condition preclude standing, assess sitting balance with the thighs held close together.

If the patient has depended on a brace, cane, or walker, observe first how well the patient functions in stance and gait utilizing the accustomed aid. If a cane, walker, or other aid is not available, supply the equivalent degree of support with your hands, which will help you to assess the degree of dependence. Some elderly persons, and patients with sensory deficits in the feet, perform better with shoes on. From the standpoint of evaluating disability, determine the best level of current function and whether a chronic disorder has deteriorated.

Dizziness and ataxia

Vertigo, faintness, or other forms of "dizziness" can be expected to cause imbalance. Try to manipulate the testing situation so as to minimize factors that might induce some form of dizziness: if the patient has been on bed rest, progress slowly from sitting to standing to obviate postural hypotension. Since rapid head turning may cause vertigo in susceptible patients, avoid sudden positional changes during testing: the object is to determine their best gait when not dizzy. (You may then go on to provoke imbalance by quick turns, etc., which must be carefully supervised.) Disequilibrium or ataxia in the absence of vertigo or other illusion of motion at the time of testing is probably not a peripheral vestibular problem, such as labyrinthitis.

Other gait ataxias

Some patients have even more complex reasons for gait ataxia: deficits not seemingly explained simply by cerebellar dysfunction or by weakness, rigidity, or proprioceptive, peripheral, vestibular, or visual disorders. Ataxia in the context of hydrocephalus is not adequately characterized by any of these factors in isolation or in readily understandable combination. More rarely, you will hear of gait (or limb) apraxia, a term signifying an inability to "put together" an act, such as gait, when all the particular ingredients seem to be working. Before coming to the conclusion that a patient has either a gait apraxia or a psychogenic gait disorder, be sure that you have completed a thorough analysis by testing all component functions. Ask for help with pattern recognition, seek positive symptoms and signs of a psychologic disorder (if that category is suspected), and request appropriate neurodiagnostic tests for localization.

LIMB COORDINATION

Relevant symptoms

Patients usually recognize upper extremity incoordination as such, often referring to their difficulty as clumsiness, awkwardness, or lack of control, although occasionally a term such as "weak" will be applied. Frequently they describe their problem in operational terms, such as difficulty putting a key in a lock, making mistakes typing, or losing good penmanship. Such deficits may come to attention earlier in the dominant hand.

In the lower extremities difficulties with control are typically expressed in terms of the effect produced on walking or running. While leg incoordination is virtually always manifest in gait, gait disorders can occur without any symptoms or signs being recognizable in the legs considered individually.

Levels of assessment

The efficiency and effectiveness of coordinated movement is judged at a number of levels: highly skilled activities (like many sports or playing an instrument) that are discribed in the history; functional tests that can be reproduced (like writing or doing buttons); standard neurologic tests (like the finger–nose test described below), and special maneuvers which particularly stress coordination abilities (such as rapid clapping in triplets or other more complex rhythms).

Normal standards

Normal individuals differ quite dramatically in the speed, fluidity, accuracy, and rhythm of their gross and fine limb coordination, making recognition of subtle abnormalities difficult. As discussed in Chapter 3, you will need to rely partly on the patient's own baseline, as previously observed or reported to you. In addition, handedness is well recognized to play an important role in upper extremity coordination: dexterity (referring to the right, usually dominant hand) is synonymous with good coordination, and the word "gauche" (referring to the left) conveys (social) awkwardness. Clearly, if the nondominant upper extremity can perform better than the dominant, suspect an abnormality of the latter. Interpret mild and symmetric unsteadiness of controlled movement cautiously in the presence of marked anxiety, debilitating systemic illness, or old age.

Definitions

Dysmetria: inaccuracy of "measured" movement; misgauging a desired target, as by overshoot.

Past-pointing: a systematic drift (to one side) of a directed movement. It does not mean simply missing a target (See description of testing, below).

Intention tremor: irregular, unintentional side-to-side movements that interrupt progression of a limb towards an intended target; a form of limb ataxia.

CASE 8A
A fumbling hand

Roberto Volla, a 60-year-old right-handed executive, consulted his physician because of clumsiness – a tendency to fumble with the button on his right shirt cuff and awkwardness in closing the car door with his left arm. His wife had also observed unsteadiness when he turned quickly while walking.

Before presenting the findings of this case the methods of testing limb coordination will be described.

Testing: upper extremities

Finger–nose testing: this serves as the mainstay of upper extremity evaluation, but the other tests, below, each add something. Instruct the patient to reach out to arm's length to touch your finger, then to touch his or her own nose, then back and forth between these targets quickly and accurately. In routine examinations I find little advantage in repeating the test with patient's eyes closed. If any visual impairment interferes, ask the patient to touch the nose, starting from an outstretched position. Alternatively, the patient can approximate the index (or other) fingers of the two hands, starting with the arms outstretched to each side. Inaccuracy in touching finger, nose, or other targets qualifies as dysmetria.

Target pursuit: facing the patient, hold out your finger and have the patient place his or her finger just opposite. Then suddenly and quickly move your finger (or other limb part) 10–20 cm laterally; the patient shadows this, trying to end this single lateral movement just opposite your finger, with neither overshoot nor undershoot (dysmetria). (Adapted to the lower extremities, the patient pursues the target with the foot.)

Fingertapping and opposition: the patient taps the end of the index finger on the adjacent side of the thumb with increasing rapidity. Or, the patient opposes the tip of each finger in turn to the end of the thumb, up to maximum speed. Look for imprecision or irregularity of rhythm.

Rapid alternating hand movements: the patient supinates and pronates the hand as crisply and rapidly as possible on the anterior thigh or any other convenient surface. Alternatively, ask the patient to pretend to screw in a light bulb quickly. (For any of these tests I personally favor examining the right and left hands sequentially rather than simultaneously.) The cumbersome term, dysdiadochokinesia, has traditionally been used to refer to inability to perform rapid alternating movements precisely, and rhythmically.

Hand slap (impedance): the patient gives a quick slap to the other palm (alternatively to a thigh or to your hand). Is it done briskly, with a sharp clap, or sluggishly, with a dull thud? The purpose is to reveal impaired acceleration, which, in the absence of weakness or limb ataxia, suggests an extrapyramidal type of awkwardness or clumsiness (see Chapter 14).

Finger waggling: demonstrate for the patient a rapid waggling or trilling movement of the index (or other) finger. Difficulty reveals impedance or impaired rapid alternation. These tests are similar to finger tapping (described above), but finger tapping emphasizes precision.

Past-pointing: as defined above, past-pointing is not synonymous with dysmetria, a more general term. Most neurologists do not include specific tests for past-pointing, but do observe for systematic deviation to one side on finger–nose examination. To test past-pointing formally, ask the patient to reach out straight ahead to arm's length and touch your finger; then, with eyes closed, raise (or lower) the arm vertically and return it to the horizontal. Past-pointing manifests itself as a consistent deviation (or pointing away) to one side as a result of vestibular dysfunction.

Testing: lower extremities

Heel–shin: the heel is placed on the opposite shin and run up to the knee and back to the ankle. This should be accomplished quickly and without interruption or side-to-side wavering. Proximal weakness interferes with performance.

Heel tapping: one heel is gently tapped on the other shin, increasing the rate until the steady rhythm is broken.

Foot tapping: in a comfortable seated or standing position the patient taps the foot (toes, heel, or whole foot) in a steady, increasing rhythm.

"Check" responses

Other traditional, so-called cerebellar tests: several tests assess the patient's ability to check or stop a motion or effort suddenly. (Failure to "check" normally has been regarded as a manifestation of hypotonia which has been associated with cerebellar disease. Thus, by convention, these tests are described with coordination assessment.) An inability to check (or "put the brakes on") is sometimes referred to as abnormal "rebound" (whereas actually the difficulty is in checking further motion in the same direction). The problem is illustrated by pulling a tight cork from a bottle: when the cork suddenly pops out, releasing resistance, you must check your pull. Since in testing the check response it is hard to quantitate how much overshoot there should be, mild abnormalities will only be evident from right–left asymmetry.

Testing

In the best-known (but least desirable) form of the check test the patient flexes the forearm as you resist, holding the patient's wrist. If you let go suddenly, the patient's hand flies back and, if not checked, would hit his or her own body. (Protect against this actually happening by guarding with your other arm.)

In another, usually better, version the patient holds both arms rigidly outstretched and is asked to try to maintain the arms in that position. Tap one hand or forearm forcefully enough to displace it downward. Since the patient is exerting effort to keep the arms in their original position, the arm will usually bounce back up to, or a little beyond, the original level and then stabilize in the initial position. If the check response is impaired, the arm may bounce further up and oscillate excessively before achieving a steady posture.

In yet another variation, the patient starts with the arms outstretched and supine (palm up), then pronates one forearm suddenly, maintaining the arm in a level position. If the check response is deficient, the force of pronation will carry the whole arm down below the original plane. As in the previous test, compare the two sides, since small deviations from normal are hard to judge.

Modifying tests of limb coordination

In some instances performance cannot be evaluated because of some block to testing: arm movement causes pain; the fingers are stiff from arthritis; one leg is in a cast; there is an intravenous (IV) drip in one arm. Almost always you can devise a way of getting at least some information about coordination despite such obstacles: if the finger–nose test cannot be done or adequately evaluated because of pain from bursitis or a proximal weakness, be sure to test fine finger movements carefully. The results are not equivalent, but you can derive some useful information, which is better than settling for "untestable."

CASE 8A
Fumbling hand (*continued*)

Mr Volla had presented with a problem of control of his left hand and arm, as well as a slight change in his walking. Since the doctor had not had the opportunity to see him walk into the clinic, his stance and gait were tested before evaluating his limb coordination and other parts of the examination. Mr Volla hesitated slightly in arising from the chair, but had no difficulty with balancing while standing with feet together and eyes open and closed. His posture seemed rather stiff as he walked, holding his arms slightly flexed at elbows and wrists, and lacking a full, natural arm swing.

Examining Mr Volla's motor status in the extremities, the doctor found normal muscle bulk, full strength, and no extraneous movements. However, a perceptible increase in tone was evident on passive movement at the left wrist and elbow. The sensory examination, including JPS, was normal. On testing limb coordination, rapid finger movements and alternating hand movements were slower on the left – more so, she thought, than would be attributable to the patient's right-handedness. No oscillation or dysmetria on finger–nose testing was found. The impact of a slap delivered with either hand was rather dull and distinctly less crisp on the left. Heel–shin and heel tapping maneuvers were also rather sluggish, but not wavering. In order to reproduce further his presenting complaints, the doctor asked him to do and undo a button on his shirt. He was clumsy and slow with his left hand.

In this case Mr Volla demonstrated clumsiness and slowness of left hand motor performance. He also evidenced a disorder of posture, of the fluidity of gait, and of his ability to right himself after losing his balance. Specific testing revealed increased tone. These problems could not be attributed to weakness, decreased JPS, or visual loss. A process of exclusion through systematic testing served to narrow the diagnostic possibilities. In this case a further process of pattern recognition identified the problem of clumsiness as an extrapyramidal type of disorder. Treatment with a levodopa/carbidopa combination resulted in marked improvement in Volla's parkinsonism.

The following list summarizes symptoms and signs associated with different neurologic systems which may contribute to incoordination:

Analysis of incoordination

Motor	Weakness of voluntary movement (upper motor neuron–pyramidal system)
	Slowness, impedance, rigidity (cogwheel), adventitious movements, such as tremor (extrapyramidal system)
Sensory	Decreased proprioception (JPS, Romberg test) and touch
Vision	Decreased visual acuity, depth perception, visual fields, eye movements
Vestibular	Dizziness
Cerebellar	(See below)
Other	Musculoskeletal limitations, pain, psychologic disorders

COORDINATION OF SPEECH AND EYE MOVEMENTS

Both the coordination of speech and the coordination of eye movements with other bodily or mental activities are very complex functions and not easy to analyze at the bedside. Once again, listen and look carefully, observing how the patient functions minute by minute throughout the examination.

Speech

Impaired articulation of speech (briefly discussed under CNs 9 and 10 in Chapter 5) may result from cerebellar lesions. Disruptions of speech rhythm are more characteristic. You can stress the patient's speech rhythm by requiring rapid repetition of syllables like "la la la la la. . . ." A disintegration of the natural flow of speech due to altered rhythm and inappropriately accented syllables is called scanning speech (with tenuous reference to the rhythmic meters of poetry). Incoordination of speech and dysarthria need to be distinguished from a language disorder, which would involve mistakes in word choices, syntax, etc.

Eye movements

Patients with an impairment of eye movement coordination usually first notice practical difficulty in everyday activities such as reading, reaching, or walking. Ocular overshoot (dysmetria) occurs in cerebellar disorders and is tested like finger pursuit. Instruct the patient to follow your finger visually, stopping the eyes exactly where your finger stops. Look for the eyes overshooting the mark and then readjusting.

Nystagmus

Nystagmus occurs in many cerebellar disorders, especially those involving the cerebellar–brainstem vestibular connections. Observe and document eye movements (see Chapter 5, section on CNs 3, 4, and 6); seek expert help with interpretation of nystagmus.

CEREBELLAR PATTERNS OF INCOORDINATION

What kind of data tend to implicate the cerebellum and its direct connections as the source of incoordination? From the clinical point of view, a cerebellar problem is suspected in the following cases:

Exclusion

1 no sufficient defect in another relevant system (such as proprioception) can be found – a process of elimination;

Risk factors

2 there is a strong family history of confirmed cerebellar disease or risk factors for cerebellar degeneration (like severe alcoholism);

Pattern recognition

3 the specific signs of incoordination appear to have "cerebellar" characteristics, as summarized below. Experts often disagree as to whether observed signs are "cerebellar" or not;

4 imaging techniques point to a cerebellar lesion; if the lesion is consistent with the clinical signs, then the correlation is validated. This relevance of signs to imaged lesion gains support not only from the first three criteria described above – which is circular reasoning – but from the changes in signs and lesion appearance over time.

Findings that are compatible with, but not unique to, a cerebellar pattern include the following.

Sitting and standing: the inability to maintain balance with eyes open (in the absence of dizziness, weakness, etc.)

Gait: wide-based gait, with a tendency to stagger, especially if the base is narrowed.

Limb movements: dysmetria, intention tremor (see below), hypotonia, and decomposition of rhythmic movements.

Speech: disruption of the normal rhythm of speech, scanning speech, and dysarthria (see speech).

Eye movements: overshooting of the intended point of fixation (ocular dysmetria); nystagmus (see Chapter 5).

Intention tremor

Intention tremor is a decomposition of controlled movement, best thought of as a form of limb ataxia, analogous to erratic staggering of gait. The term "intention" in intention tremor simply means that the irregularity becomes maximal as the movement nears an intended target. (In contrast, an action tremor is a more regular, less chaotic tremor that occurs with sustained posture, such as outstretched hands, as well as with active movement.)

Cerebellar system

The peripheral and brainstem components of the vestibular system are closely linked to the cerebellum, so that a distinction between vestibular and cerebellar disorders is not always justified. Moreover, cerebellar dysfunction, in general, does not necessarily signify a lesion in the cerebellum itself, but rather a problem in the cerebellar system – including also its brainstem, spinal, and thalamic connections.

RECORDING THE COORDINATION EXAMINATION

Analysis of coordination presumes examination of component motor, sensory, and other functions that are usually recorded separately: strength, tone, adventitious movements with "motor" (see Chapter 6), and JPS testing with "sensory." The documentation of the co-ordination examination should include the following categories:

The core examination

1 postural stability, sitting (if stance is untestable);
2 stance – placement of feet (base), posture of body and limbs;
3 Romberg test (since this test distinguishes proprioceptive deficits, it can be recorded with "sensory," if you prefer);
4 gait – base, stride, rhythm, and associated postures and arm movements, tandem gait;
5 limb coordination – finger–nose, heel–shin, or heel tapping, and rapid rhythmic and alternating hand movements;
6 speech – rhythm, articulation, and phonation (these may be recorded under CNs 9, 10, and 12, but if abnormalities are present, note under "coordination");
7 eye coordination – abnormal findings, including nystagmus, are usually recorded under cranial nerve functions (CNs 3, 4, and 6), but may be summarized with the coordination examination for emphasis.

The coordination findings in the following case will be documented according to this format.

CASE 8B
Severe headache and inability to walk

Sam Hopper, a 54-year-old right-handed hypertensive mechanic, was driving home on Christmas Eve and, while stuck in a traffic jam, experienced severe left-sided occipital and supraorbital headache and felt nauseated. He managed to drive his car (which had automatic transmission) the remaining short distance home, but when he got out of the car he staggered and fell. He was helped inside and put to bed because he refused to go to the hospital. For the next 24 hours he stayed in bed, vomiting repeatedly and complaining of dizziness and headache. Finally, his family called an ambulance which took him to the hospital. The doctor did not see Mr Hopper arrive, but confirmed that he had been carried in on a stretcher and had refused to walk himself.

Neurologic examination revealed a man in great distress, repeatedly retching and holding his head in pain. (He no longer complained of dizziness when still, but grabbed to hold onto something with any sudden change in position.) Blood pressure was 190/110 in the right arm, supine. As best as could be tested under the circumstances, his resistive strength was not diminished and there was no increase or obvious decrease in limb tone. JPS and other sensory tests were normal. Reflexes were 2+ symmetric throughout and were not recognizably

Normal strength, tone, sensation

pendulous (see Chapter 9); plantar responses were flexor (normal). Examination of cranial nerve functions was normal with the exception of eye movements, as noted below; corneal reflexes and facial movements appeared symmetric. Mr Hopper appeared exhausted but was not somnolent or disoriented. No other abnormal findings were evident, aside from his coordination tests which are described below.

Posture

1 No abnormality when lying in bed; barely able to maintain a seated posture.

Stance

2 Needed help to stand up and could not maintain standing balance, even on a wide base, eyes open (not vertiginous at the time); tended to topple to the left and backward.

3 Romberg test not carried out.

Gait

4 Could take a few steps on a very wide base, but showed a strong tendency to fall to the left.

Limbs

5 Normal on the right; on the left, severe, coarse, jerky "tremor" across the line of intended motion on finger–nose and heel–shin testing; poor rhythm and accuracy on finger tapping or serial opposition of thumb to fingers; jerky and uncontrolled attempt at hand pronation–supination; marked overshoot (impaired check) with sudden pronation of outstretched forearm (vs. right side).

Speech

6 Thick, dysarthric speech, but understandable with difficulty; poor rhythm and articulation of test syllables (mi, la, go).

Eyes

7 Did not achieve final 3–4 mm of left horizontal gaze; fine horizontal nystagmus beating toward right on right gaze and upward gaze; also upbeating component on upward gaze; full range of upward and downward gaze.

Case summary and diagnosis

The patient's examination showed severe disequilibrium of the trunk (even when he was not actively vertiginous), nystagmus, severe incoordination of the left limbs, and no weakness or sensory deficits. The clinical formulation pointed to an acute left and midline cerebellar dysfunction, probably an acute hemorrhage into the left cerebellar hemisphere and vermis. After computerized tomography (CT) scan confirmation, operative therapy was successfully undertaken.

In contrast to Mr Volla's slow and clumsy type of motor problem, which had elements of limb and gait incoordination due to an extrapyramidal disorder, Mr Hopper's signs suggested a cerebellar pattern (see Chapter 13, Fig. 13.18, for clinical–anatomic localization, especially the occurrence of limb ataxia ipsilateral to the cerebellar hemispheric lesion).

SUMMARY

Priorities

1 *Stance and gait*: do not make any assumptions but actually test getting

up and walking. Equip the patient with shoes, glasses, and any other aids to maximize performance.

2 *Upper extremity coordination* (finger–nose test, etc.): whereas lower extremity ataxia is usually reflected in abnormal stance and gait, hand and arm incoordination may not be evident upon simple inspection. Disorders of the nondominant limb may not be noted as soon symptomatically.

3 *Speech articulation and swallowing*: dysarthria will be evident, but ask specifically for swallowing difficulty in the review of neurologic symptoms. Test swallowing directly (but cautiously); it is a complex coordinated act, the success or failure of which can be witnessed. Do not rely merely on the gag reflex. Dysarthria and dysphagia are often neglected, not only in examination but also in the medical record, appearing neither with lower cranial nerves nor with coordination.

Pitfalls

1 Misinterpreting an "abnormal" Romberg test which, in fact, is false-positive. Many so-called abnormal Rombergs are correctable with reassurance, relaxation, and protection against falling. True positives are quite unusual.

2 Guessing about gait: accepting the patient's attribution that ataxia is due to dizziness (but actual vertigo and faintness are absent); or assuming that the unsteadiness is due to pain of arthritis or minor weakness (which are inadequate to explain the degree of difficulty).

3 Relying only on finger–nose testing for coordination: unless you observe that gait is truly normal (and there are no symptoms of incoordination), test the lower extremities specifically, as well.

PROBLEM FOR SELF-STUDY

Problem

1 A 53-year-old man is evaluated for sudden onset of clumsiness on the left side, 2 hours earlier. An immediate CT scan shows a well-demarcated, low-density lesion in the right internal capsule. What additional parts of the examination would be most productive?

Comment

1 Look for left-sided weakness, changes in tone and deep tendon reflexes, and a Babinski sign. The purpose would be to see whether a lesion in the corticospinal tract on the right side of the brain might have caused a mild left-sided upper motor neuron syndrome manifest as clumsiness. Test JPS on the left. Check finger–nose, heel–shin, rapid alternating hand and finger movements, etc. In this case, the only abnormalities were intention tremor and dysmetria on the left. The well-demarcated low-density lesion (presumptive lacunar infarct) on immediate CT had to be older than the acute symptoms (see Chapter 15). Most likely an ischemic lesion in the left cerebellar hemisphere (or brainstem connections) would appear on a later,

repeat scan. Cerebellar signs are ipsilateral to the cerebellar lesion because of the "double-cross" of pathways (see Fig. 13.18).

FURTHER READING

Gilman, S., Bloedel, J.R., Lechtenberg, R. *Disorders of the Cerebellum*. F.A. Davis, Philadelphia (PA), 1981. An older reference, but still the major text on the cerebellum for neurologists, as a source of clinical, anatomic, and pathologic information.

Kandel, E.R., Schwartz, J.H., Jessell, T.M. *Principles of Neural Science*. 3rd edn. Elsevier, New York (NY), 1991. This account of the cerebellum (Chapter 41) builds upon prior knowledge of the anatomy to offer modern insights into physiology and function.

Landau, W.M. Clinical neuromythology V. Ataxic hindbrain thinking: the clumsy cerebellum syndrome. *Neurology* 1989; 39:315–23. Provocative and acerbic critique of common clinical assumptions about "cerebellar" signs.

Schmahmann, J.D. An emerging concept: the cerebellar contribution to higher function. *Arch Neurol* 1991; 48:1178–87. The relationship of the cerebellum to behavior and mental processes, with details of the cerebrocerebellar pathways.

Simon, R.P., Aminoff, M.J., Greenberg, D.A. *Clinic Neurology* Appleton Lange, Norwalk (CT), 1989. Clinical correlations and work-up of balance, gait, and other coordination problems are well outlined in Chapter 4.

chapter 

Reflex Testing

Reflex testing provides access to a variety of disturbances of neurologic function that are not directly reflected in symptoms. In the following case, the only distinctly abnormal findings were revealed in the reflex examination.

CASE 9A
Another headache patient

Marie Dorn, a 64-year-old right-handed woman, was known in the clinic as a "complainer"—one problem after another. This time she complained of a headache that had been present for 2 or 3 weeks, "ever since my landlord turned the heat down." After taking more history that he found noncontributory, the doctor examined her. He found no abnormalities on head and neck, cranial nerve or sensory examinations. She was not quite as strong or well coordinated in her left hand, but this seemed consistent with handedness. However, on reflex testing, the left-sided tendon reflexes were all brisker than on the right. Moreover, the left plantar response was extensor: a Babinski sign. The computerized tomography (CT) scan showed a right frontal subdural hematoma, a blood clot pressing upon the brain. This was evacuated surgically.

She made a good recovery and subsequently recalled that a month before her admission she had banged her head on a cabinet. She had relieved the immediate pain with aspirin (which had a detrimental antiplatelet effect, partially inhibiting blood coagulation). For once, she "didn't make anything more of it!"

Deep tendon reflexes and pathologic reflexes

The examination of Ms Dorn revealed abnormalities in two different groups of reflexes: the deep tendon, or stretch, reflexes (DTRs) and the pathologic reflexes. (The latter, if present, are abnormal signs, whereas stretch reflexes may be abnormal in degree or in lack of symmetry.)

Superficial reflexes and corticobulbar reflexes

In addition, there are two other main groups, namely the superficial or cutaneous reflexes and the corticobulbar reflexes, as well as an assortment of miscellaneous reflexes. These groupings are somewhat arbitrary, but remain helpful clinically.

Segmental and suprasegmental pathways

All of the reflexes have segmental afferent and efferent limbs and are subject to various forms of suprasegmental control. Thus, the pathways that mediate or influence these reflexes span much of the nervous system; the reflex responses serve as markers for many kinds and locations of abnormal neurologic activity. At the same time, the range of normal for the naturally occurring (physiologic) reflexes is quite broad. Therefore, we search not so much for subtle, general alterations in the level of reflex activity as for the following patterns of change:

1 extremes of hyperactivity or hypoactivity, such as absent DTRs (as in the case of severe polyneuropathy);

2 lateralized asymmetry, as in right-sided hyperreflexia (as in a left cerebral tumor);

3 focal differences, such as an absent left ankle jerk, all other reflexes being present and symmetric (as in sciatica, a left S1 radiculopathy);

4 a major disproportion between reflexes in one region vs. another, such as normal 1+ upper extremity DTRs and very hyperactive lower extremity DTRs, illustrated by thoracic spinal cord compression from a ruptured disc;

5 presence of a definitely pathologic type of reflex, a right Babinski sign (extensor plantar response) – as in a left cerebral stroke.

Lay notions about reflexes

You should be aware in evaluating reflexes that many patients have surprising ideas about their significance. The level of DTRs does not correlate with reaction time, in the sense that a person may, in lay terms, have "quick reflexes" or "fast reflexes." Many athletes with very quick reaction times have hypoactive (less brisk than average) DTRs. In addition, within the broad range of normal, more or less brisk reflexes are neither good nor bad – so that when one speaks loosely of a patient having "good reflexes," it merely implies that they are not hard to elicit (or not reactive to an extreme degree). Some patients also have heard, or even believe, that reflexes are tested to determine craziness. In any case, patients are intrigued by the mystique of a sudden body reaction which can be easily elicited but is seemingly beyond their own control.

TENDON (STRETCH) REFLEXES

Testing

Examination of the DTRs (Fig. 9.1) is easiest in the sitting position, but can also be readily accomplished with the patient lying down. Either way, the tendon to be tapped should be in a state of partial passive stretch. Alter the limb position empirically to find the position that produces the best responses. The steps to eliciting the reflex can be summarized as follows.

Explanation

1 While you position the patient and yourself comfortably, explain that you will be checking reflexes by gentle tapping. (Check for any tenderness before tapping.)

Relaxation

2 In addition to setting the patient at ease, fully support the limb to be tested, so that the patient need not actively maintain the posture of the limb at all. (See further discussion below.)

Eliciting the reflex

3 You can either tap the tendon directly or tap your finger or thumb placed on the tendon. The latter may be preferable if the tendon is

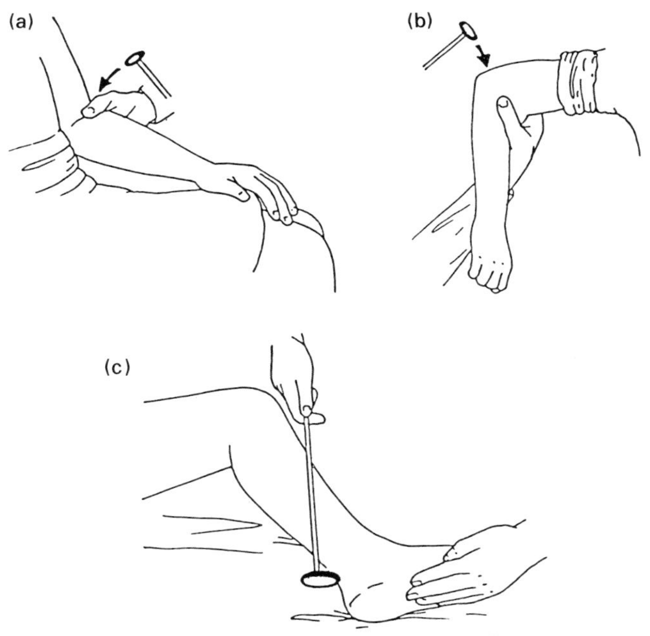

Fig. 9.1 Eliciting deep tendon reflexes. (a) Biceps jerk; (b) triceps jerk. The limb should be supported and relaxed, but the tendon should not be lax. (c) Ankle jerk, when recumbent. Note the examiner's gentle dorsiflexion of the foot.

mobile, like the biceps tendon. (Either the point or blade of a hatchet-shaped reflex hammer may be used.)

4 To identify the tendon, in case of doubt, have the patient tighten the muscle that attaches to the tendon in question: to find the triceps tendon, the forearm should be forcefully extended against resistance, while you palpate the arm just above the point of the elbow (olecranon); you will feel the tendon tighten.

5 Flick the reflex hammer quickly, but lightly to produce a brief, discrete stimulus.

6 The reflex may be noted as a jerk of the limb, a visible twitch of the muscle, or felt as a slight twitch of the tendon under your finger or of the muscle under your hand (Table 9.1).

Table 9.1 Reflex techniques: "tendon jerks"

Reflex (roots and nerve)	Positioning	Response
Biceps (C5, C6) (Musculocutaneous nerve)	Forearm partly bent and resting against the patient's body or cradled in your arm. Tap your thumb or finger placed on the tendon in the antecubital fossa	Forearm flexion; visible or palpable contraction of the biceps tendon and muscle
Triceps (C7, C8) (Radial nerve)	Forearm hangs freely (as you support upper arm) or rests partially flexed on the abdomen. Tap the tendon directly, above its elbow insertion	Extension jerk of the forearm or just a visible twitch of the triceps muscle
Brachioradialis (C5, C6) (Radial nerve)	Lightly tap lower third of the radius (do not strike the forearm muscles directly, as local muscle contraction may occur)	Radial dorsiflexion of hand; slight flexion, supination of forearm
Knee jerk (Patellar); (L3, L4) (Femoral nerve)	In the supine patient buckle the knee 30, 60°. When sitting, dangle the leg freely. Carefully palpate the tendon between the kneecap and the tibial bone below	Extension of leg; visible or palpable contraction of quadriceps muscle
Ankle jerk (Achilles); (S1, S2) (Sciatic nerve)	Easiest with the patient in the sitting position, but can be done supine by externally rotating the leg and flexing the knee. With one hand under the foot, gently dorsiflex it to partially tighten the Achilles tendon (see Fig. 9.1)	Plantar flexion of the foot felt or seen; sometimes only slight contraction of calf muscles

False response

Distinguish the tendon jerk from the immediate mechanical effect of deforming the tendon. (Simply indenting the Achilles tendon, for example, causes a slight plantar flexion of the foot.) Patients sometimes react nervously by a semivoluntary jerk of the limb that occurs later than a reflex. If you suspect this type of reaction, ask the patient again not to "help"; restart with the patient's eyes closed, so that the stimulus will not be anticipated.

If you have difficulty

If you cannot at first elicit the reflex, the following steps may be helpful.

1 Experiment with different limb positions and degrees of tendon stretch (and recheck the place you are striking).
2 Try to induce proximal relaxation which may help more than focusing on the joint you are testing. For example, if the patient's forearm seems tense as you attempt to elicit the biceps jerk, ask the patient to relax the shoulders. Also, try again later when the patient may be more at ease.
3 Try a totally different body position, such as sitting (if you are unable to elicit the reflexes with the patient lying).
4 Try striking less hard – often "less is more."
5 Always try "reinforcement" before concluding that a reflex is absent (see below).

Reinforcement

Reflex responses can be reinforced or augmented by means of the patient exerting other muscle groups while you deliver the stimulus. Pulling (isometrically) with one hand against the other is often used, but any exertion (away from the area being tested) will suffice: clenching a fist, the jaws, and so forth. For maximum effect, tap the tendon immediately after saying "pull"; if the patient has responded to the order quickly, the pull will come just as your hammer strikes.

Pitfalls and priorities

Probably the most common error in reflex testing comes not from wielding the hammer, but from an exercise of the imagination! Since you are likely to be very invested in obtaining reflexes, you may be susceptible to a very widespread tendency to observe or record at least a 1+ response, even when you are not absolutely sure a real reflex jerk occurred. (The mental game-playing sometimes goes like this: "I thought it might have been there, and I'm not really sure it wasn't.") This pitfall is especially common with ankle jerks which are frequently absent, in fact. Far better to miss a minimal reflex than to record a false positive.

The usefulness of the brachioradialis reflex is extremely limited. It is often hard to elicit, especially in a relatively hyporeflexic person: bilateral absence in such a situation bears no significance. The truth is, if you never performed another brachioradialis reflex, your patients would probably be none the worse for it. In contrast, always check ankle jerks (see Chapter 19 on the screening neurologic examination).

Clinical correlation

DTRs are affected by dysfunction in the segmental reflex arcs or in the suprasegmental control pathway (Fig. 9.2). Pathology in the afferent or efferent limb of the segmental pathways may decrease the reflex, but will

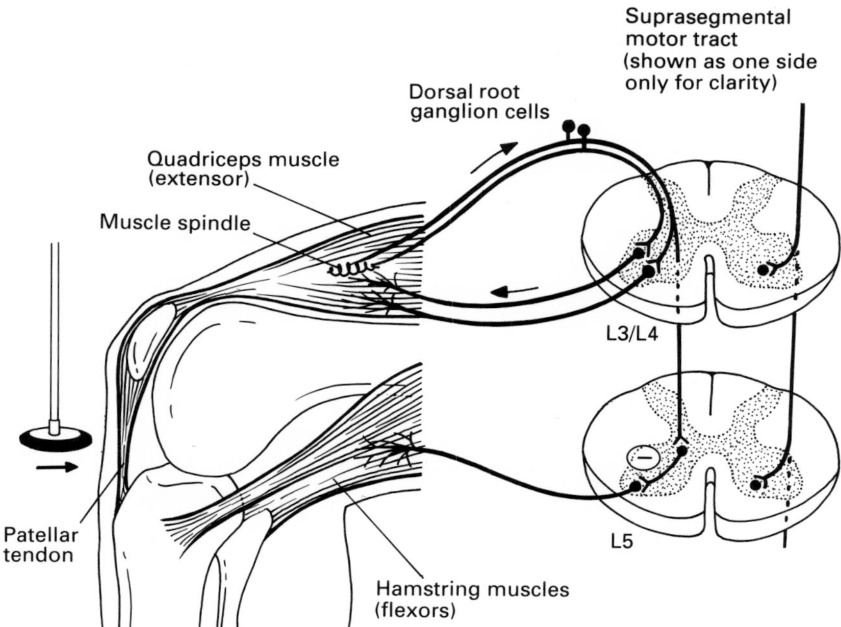

Fig. 9.2 The knee jerk (patellar reflex). Striking the patellar tendon initiates the monosynaptic reflex arc. Afferent impulses are conveyed from the muscle spindle to anterior horn cells which innervate large muscle fibers of the quadriceps. A parallel (or branch) pathway innervates interneurons in another segment (L5 shown here) which inhibit anterior horn cells, thus relaxing the antagonist muscles, the hamstrings of the posterior thigh. Multiple suprasegmental descending tracts (represented here by one tract on the other side) influence the anterior horn cell pool of each segment.

not increase it. On the other hand, suprasegmental disorders, such as lesions of the corticospinal and other descending tracts that influence the spinal cord segments, ordinarily increase DTRs (see Table 9.2 and Chapter 13). At times, especially in the acute stage of injury (as in the initial hours after a cerebral stroke), the contralateral DTRs may be diminished, usually increasing subsequently. The extreme example of a paradoxic, acute pattern is in the flaccid, areflexic state of "spinal shock" below the level of sudden, severe spinal cord damage.

The segmental reflex arc is particularly sensitive to disorders of the afferent limb. Polyneuropathies which are predominantly sensory tend to cause early and profound decreases in DTRs, beginning with the ankle jerks, then progressing to the knee jerks, and eventually the arm reflexes, while strength may be normal or relatively preserved. (The ankle jerk reflex traverses the S1 roots within the longest nerve in the body, the sciatic.) Lesions affecting only components of the efferent arc, such as the anterior horn cells or anterior roots, do not characteristically obliterate the reflex response until substantial weakness develops: if the motor

Table 9.2 Clinical correlation of superficial and deep tendon (stretch) reflexes

	Deep tendon reflexes (stretch reflexes)	Superficial reflexes
Segmental arc lesion		
Afferent limb lesion	Decreased or absent (ipsilateral); (reflex sensitive to afferent limb dysfunction)	Decreased or absent (ipsilateral)
Efferent limb lesion	Decreased or absent (ipsilateral); (reflex less sensitive to partial dysfunction)	Decreased or absent (ipsilateral)
Suprasegmental lesion		
Acute	Increased, unchanged, or decreased (contralateral)	May be decreased or absent, never increased (contralateral)
Subacute, chronic	Typically increased – occasionally unchanged or decreased	Reflex may normalize, depending on pathology

outflow at that level is working well enough to permit movement, it may well sustain at least some stretch reflex activity.

Range of normal

As earlier noted, the general state of DTR activity (from barely present to very brisk) varies greatly from one normal individual to another. Moreover, some variation occurs within a given person from one time to another. Thus, you should not necessarily be surprised (or assume that your technique is to blame) if you find reflexes to be brisker (or less brisk) than previously recorded. Suspect a pathologic condition, however, if the reflexes show a progressive change, if they have undergone an extreme change, have disappeared entirely (even when tested with reinforcement), or show a major disproportion (comparing ankle jerks to knee jerks or legs to arms). Of course, consistent right–left asymmetries always require an explanation.

Recording DTRs

Reflexes are usually graded on a semiquantitative scale (0–4) according to the briskness of reaction. The conventional use of "plus" (+) creates confusion, since 3+ might mean either three plusses (+++) or "greater than 3." Unlike the 0–5 scale for grading strength, in which 3+ or 4− are intermediates between 3 and 4, DTRs are usually graded on a scale of 0–4 with no intermediates: + = 1+, ++ = 2+, etc.

0	absent response
1+ or (+)	a slight jerk or a palpable or visible muscle contraction without actual movement at the joint

2+ or ++	a moderate, average jerk
3+ or +++	a very brisk jerk
4+ or ++++	an extremely hyperactive reflex, conventionally understood to have associated, sustained clonus

Specify reinforcement, if applicable. Also, document any concern you have as to the role of pain or poor relaxation that may have affected the observed result. You should be aware that the terms hyperreflexic or hyporeflexic do not necessarily indicate pathologic states (unlike the terms hyperthyroid or hypothyroid). 3+ reflexes may be called hyperreflexic, but are probably normal if symmetric and associated with no other abnormalities. Similarly, generalized, 1+ hyporeflexic responses are usually perfectly normal.

Pendular reflexes

Rarely, you may see the leg (using the knee jerk as an example) swing unusually freely back and forth, before coming to rest—a so-called pendular reflex. This suggests hypotonia, usually associated in adults with cerebellar disorders.

Relaxation phase

The relaxation phase of any reflex is characteristically delayed in hypothyroidism, creating what is called a "hung-up reflex." Observe the limb for a delayed return to resting position, or feel the slow relaxation of the tendon under your finger. With the ankle jerk, you will feel the tempo of relaxation with your hand applied to the sole of the foot.

Clonus

Clonus is an oscillation at a joint, due to a reverberating mechanism of rapid contraction and relaxation, associated with upper motor neuron (UMN) dysfunction. You can elicit clonus by stretching a tendon, such as the Achilles tendon at the ankle: dorsiflex the patient's foot quickly but with only mild force, maintaining it in the dorsiflexed position. This maneuver may cause a flexion–extension oscillation that is both visible and palpable. Clonus, if it is symmetric and unsustained (only several beats despite continued stretch) may not be pathologic.

CORTICOBULBAR REFLEXES

Overview

The corticobulbar reflexes are related to the tendon reflexes since both are elicited by stretch. However, the jaw jerk and snout reflexes are cranial and we do not tap the tendons directly. The UMN pathway is corticobulbar (the cortical motor neuron fibers synapsing at brainstem nuclei) instead of corticospinal.

Jaw jerk

Elicit the jaw jerk by placing your finger on the chin (jaw relaxed) and tapping downward, which may result in an upward jerk (Fig. 9.3a). Both the stretch stimulus and the jerk are mediated by CN 5. You may observe a mild jaw jerk normally in a person with very brisk DTRs, but a brisk jaw jerk raises suspicion of abnormality, as discussed below.

Snout reflex

To elicit the snout reflex (as most commonly defined), place your

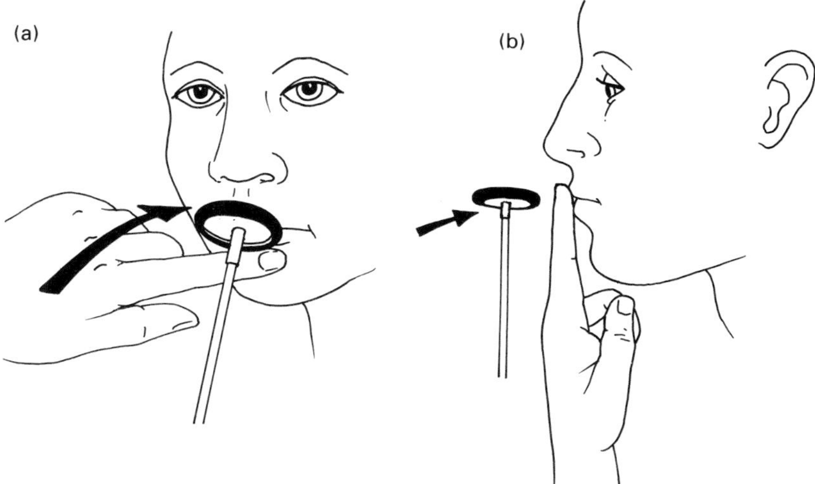

Fig. 9.3 Jaw jerk and snout reflexes. (a) The jaw jerk. The downward tap on the chin may elicit an upward jerk of the chin due to contraction of the masseter muscles. Normally absent or slight, the jaw jerk is exaggerated when there is bilateral corticobulbar dysfunction involving control of the motor nucleus of CN 5 in the pons (see text). (b) In present usage, the snout reflex is elicited by tapping the lips. An abnormal response is an outward pouting of the lips, due to bilateral corticobulbar dysfunction affecting the segmental response of the facial (CN 7) nuclei.

(gloved) finger or tongue blade vertically against the patient's lightly closed lips and tap gently with your reflex hammer or finger (Fig. 9.3b). The reaction is a pouting out of the lips, as in forming a snout. When marked, this response can also occur with light tapping at any point around the lips that stretches the orbicularis oris muscle (innervated by CN 7). A snout reflex suggests corticobulbar dysfunction at a level above the pons. (Note that "snout reflex" is also used by some to refer to a stroking across the lips, akin to the suck reflex – see section on "pathologic" reflexes.)

Localizing value

One of the main uses of the jaw jerk and snout reflexes is to help establish a level of abnormal reflex activity, that is, whether cranial as well as spinal structures are involved (see Fig. 14.7). If a patient has hyperreflexia in the arms and legs and Babinski signs, we would like to determine whether the UMN pathology is at a cervical level or in the brain. Lack of a jaw jerk or snout reflex in this situation suggests that a lesion is at or below the pontine location of the relevant nuclei of CNs 5 and 7, respectively, and therefore may well be cervical. Conversely, a pathologically brisk jaw jerk or snout reflex would suggest a level of dysfunction above the pons.

Since the jaw jerk and snout are controlled at a suprasegmental level by corticobular motor fibers that are both crossed and uncrossed, an abnormally brisk response is typically associated with a bilateral pathologic process.

"Pseudobulbar palsy"

Dysarthria, dysphonia, trouble swallowing, increased jaw jerk and snout reflexes, and (interestingly) lability of affect, comprise the syndrome of "pseudobulbar palsy" (see Chapter 5, section on CNs 9 and 10).

SUPERFICIAL REFLEXES

Overview

Reflexes elicited by stroking the skin or mucous membranes are considered "superficial reflexes." They are polysynaptic, having segmental arcs and also a cortical circuit, so that the response may be altered by influences operating at either a segmental or suprasegmental level. The corneal reflex and gag reflexes (see Chapter 5) provide excellent models. For example, a decreased response after corneal stimulation may be due to dysfunction in the afferent or efferent limb mediated by CNs 5 and 7, respectively, or may be due to suprasegmental factors, such as a lesion in the contralateral frontoparietal lobes.

Testing of superficial abdominal reflexes

The superficial abdominal reflexes (Fig. 9.4) are elicited by stroking the skin of the four quadrants of the abdomen; the response is a contraction of the abdominal muscles of that quadrant, which has the effect of pulling the umbilicus to that side. This reflex shoud not be tested immediately after the abdomen has been palpated or otherwise handled and the patient should be warm and relaxed for best results. Using a slightly rough object, such as the wooden end of a throat swab or a broken tongue blade, gently stroke the skin diagonally in toward or out from the umbilicus or in an arc across the quadrant, each quadrant in turn. Observe closely each time you stroke the skin, since repetitive stroking in the same area will lead to fatiguing (disappearance) of the response.

Responses are usually easier to obtain in young people. The abdominal effects of pregnancy, operation, or painful internal pathology interfere with the reflex response. Lack of abdominal reflexes is not necessarily pathologic.

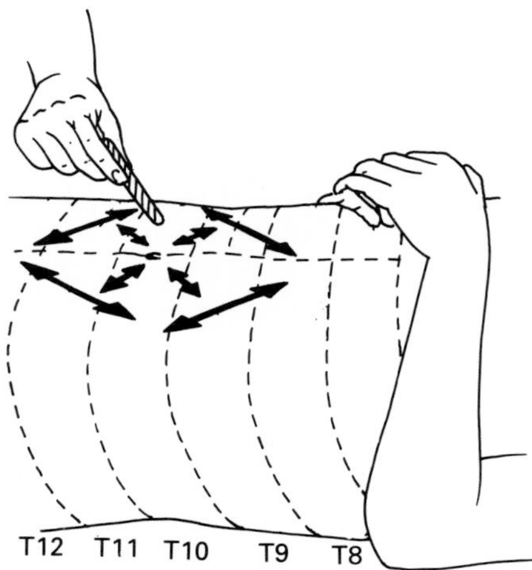

Fig. 9.4 Superficial abdominal reflexes. These reflexes are elicited by stroking rather lightly with a blunt object such as the wooden end of a throat swab. Each quadrant around the umbilicus (T10 level) should be tested by stroking in toward or out from the umbilicus or by stroking diagonally across each quadrant.

Clinical correlation

The superficial abdominal reflexes are mediated at a segmental level by spinal roots and nerves, T7–T12. Since the umbilicus is a marker for T10 dermatome, the upper quadrants are served by T7–T10 and the lower quadrants by T10–T12, for both the afferent and efferent limbs. A lesion of the spinal cord, roots, or intercostal nerves at these levels may decrease or obliterate the response on the same side as the lesion (see Table 9.2). More commonly, acute suprasegmental lesions will temporarily decrease superficial reflexes at all lower segmental levels. Thus, a lesion of the corticospinal tract on the left at T10 cord level (abolishing descending input to T11 and T12 segments) would be expected to result in the absence of a superficial abdominal reflex in the left lower quadrant.

Cremasteric reflex

A stroking stimulus of the inside of the thigh of a male will cause retraction of the testicle on that side. This reflex (at the L1–L2 segmental level) is little used.

Anal reflex

Testing anal reflexes (sacral segments S3–S5) is part of the special examination of the perineum which is specifically indicated only in selected cases (see Chapter 19). However, when you perform a rectal examination, you will typically notice a reflex contraction of the anal sphincter when tactile contact is first made. The bulbocavernosus reflex (anal/perineal contraction upon squeezing the glans penis) rarely provides additional useful information.

Summary of superficial reflexes

1 With the exception of the gag reflex in patients with major cerebral or brainstem deficits, these superficial reflexes will not contribute to most of your neurologic evaluations. They need not be performed routinely.

2 A decreased or absent superficial reflex, whether at a spinal level (superficial abdominal) or cranial level (corneal, gag) does not necessarily mean that the lesion is in the spinal cord or brainstem, respectively, (or their roots and nerves). Consider both a segmental and a suprasegmental localization.

3 Superficial reflex responses are subject to a wide range of individual variation, to many systemic and local influences, and to difficulty of quantitation. Therefore, beware of overinterpreting results that are not distinctly abnormal.

"PATHOLOGIC" REFLEXES

Overview

A number of reflexes are most conveniently grouped as "pathologic," because we focus on a response that is abnormal in and of itself (rather than issues of degree, asymmetry, or major disproportion). The DTR examination is pathologic if arm reflexes are 1+ with reinforcement, while leg reflexes are 4+, but a definite Babinski sign is pathologic regardless of other findings. Many other pathologic reflexes do, however, have degrees of abnormality that affect their clinical significance. Only a few of the many pathologic reflexes that have been described will be mentioned here (for more information see Further reading section).

Plantar response

Babinski

The normal plantar reflex (after infancy) consists mainly of flexion of the great toe in response to plantar stimulation (flexor plantar response). The pathologic response (Babinski sign) is extensor and signifies UMN dysfunction at any level. Many physicians refer to the plantar test as the "Babinski," which purists decry but in fact has crept into wide usage. Just specify clearly whether the test is abnormal (extensor, toe up).

Testing

To elicit a plantar response, stroke the lateral sole with a slightly rough object, such as a key, or even a thumbnail (Fig. 9.5). (The stimulus is usually somewhat disagreeable, producing an uncomfortable, semiticklish feeling, but it should not be painful or abrade the skin.) The usual method is to stroke the lateral aspect of the sole from about the midpoint of the foot forward towards the base of the 5th toe and then in an arc across the ball of the foot. You may find in some cases, however, that the full, curving stroke will provoke evasive movement (see below) and a limited, short stroke, very laterally on the sole, will produce a more definitive response. Some neurologists emphasize fanning of the toes and other details of the Babinski sign, but I would recommend concentrating mainly on the extensor action of the great toe.

There may be very little flexor or extensor movement at all. This neutral or equivocal response is quite likely to be normal, if symmetric, especially if a similar response had previously been recorded as a base-

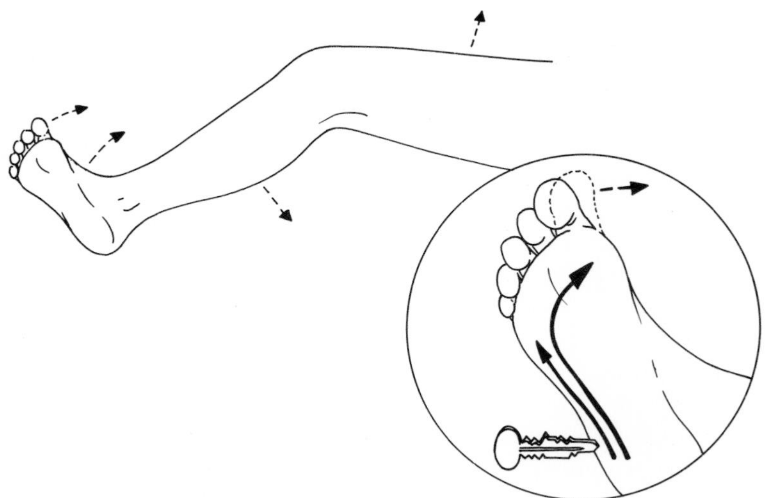

Fig. 9.5 Plantar reflex ("Babinski") and triple flexion response. The detail (in the circle) shows the path of stroking the sole and the pathologic extensor plantar response (upgoing toe, Babinski sign). The lower limb drawing depicts the pathologic triple flexion response (dorsiflexion of foot and flexion of leg and thigh) in addition to the extensor response of the great toe.

line. More confusing is the distinction between a pathologic, reflexive pulling back of the foot and leg (that may accompany an extensor plantar sign) versus semivoluntary withdrawal.

Nonpathologic withdrawal

Lateral plantar stroking, since it is a disagreeable stimulus, often provokes an evasive pulling away of the leg, foot, and toes – a withdrawal response. This type of withdrawal, which is regarded as semivoluntary because it can be partially resisted by act of will, is always nonstereotypic. Each repeated stimulus causes a different variation in the way the foot is withdrawn; there is usually an aspect of "shaking-off" the stimulus.

Triple flexion

The patient with an UMN lesion may evidence not only an extension of the great toe but any degree of dorsiflexion of the foot, flexion at the knee, and flexion (perhaps with slight abduction) at the hip. Although variable in degree, the triple flexion response is stereotypic in form. A definite triple flexion response (flexor withdrawal reflex) is equivalent to the Babinski sign. The patient, if asked for a subjective response to the stimulus, will usually express relatively little discomfort and display little annoyance. In fact, you may be surprised by the disparity between the vigorous triple flexion and the minimal affective reaction – showing that this is not a "ticklish" response.

If you remain in doubt as to whether the plantar response is strongly pathologic or merely an exaggerated nonpathologic withdrawal, the first approach is stimulus reduction. A very lateral, short stroke that does not extend across the ball of the foot may produce an upgoing (extensor) or downgoing (flexor) plantar response without provoking withdrawal. Other ways of eliciting the extensor plantar sign should also be tried. Such tests (which are burdened with eponymic designations) include stroking the ankle posterior to the lateral malleolus (probably the most useful), stroking firmly downward on the shin, squeezing the calf, or lightly pricking the dorsum of the great toe with a pin. Each of these more remote stimuli depends on a widened receptive field (a larger area in which the stimulus is effective).

In instances of peripheral inability to dorsiflex the great toe (as in deformity, denervation, bandaging, or absence) the triple-flexion response signifies pathology. Misinterpretation of the triple-flexion response as withdrawal is less of a problem when unilateral than when it is bilateral: in the latter case, the result is often erroneously recorded as bilateral "withdrawal" (implying lack of abnormality).

Frontal release reflexes

The so-called frontal release reflexes are normal responses in infants, but reappear in adults only under pathologic conditions. They should be differentiated from the corticobulbar reflexes, such as the jaw jerk, that involve frontal motor pathways, but do not involve a return of the "primitive" infantile responses. A frontal reflex suggests pathology in an area of a frontal lobe anterior to the primary motor cortex, but may be seen in diffuse cerebral disease without specific frontal lesions.

Grasp

To elicit the grasp reflex, draw two or three of your fingers across the patient's palm from the heel of the palm towards the base of the index finger. A positive, abnormal response consists of a grasp, or closure of the patient's hand on your fingers. If this is sufficiently strong, the patient's fingers may flex sufficiently to hook on to yours – a traction or hooking response.

An involuntary grasp reflex should be clearly distinguished from the strength of a grip, such as the handgrip that you may test as part of your motor evaluation. Also, differentiate it from hand-holding, a patient's comfort-seeking grasp. The involuntary character of the grasp reflex is relative; some alert patients may be able to release it with urging. Spontaneous grasping or exploratory manual behavior are often associated with the grasp reflex. Like the other frontal reflexes described below, the grasp reflex is usually contralateral to the frontal lesion, but the sign has also been reported ipsilaterally.

Suck and rooting reflexes

Suck and rooting reflexes mimic the responses of an infant whose lips and cheek are stimulated by a nipple. With a light touch or stroking of the lips, sucking motions may be observed. A light stimulus to the cheek near the corner of the mouth may evoke turning in that direction and groping with the lips (rooting) for the source of the tactile stimulus. These pathologic reflexes are uncommonly seen.

Miscellaneous reflexes

Glabellar reflex

The abnormal glabellar response consists of a tendency to blink repeatedly when you tap repetitively just above the bridge of the nose. Particularly since the testing is near the eyes, briefly explain that you will just be tapping gently between the eyes to test a reflex. Normally, a person will blink with the first few slow, light taps and then accommodate to this stimulus. Patients with extrapyramidal disorders, such as parkinsonism, fail to suppress the blink reaction normally. Often the eye blink is incomplete, but the continued reaction to each new stimulus is evident.

Chvostek

Nerves that lie near the surface can be stimulated by percussion. With your finger percuss the facial nerve as it emerges anterior to the ear lobe; you can also stimulate any of its branches that arborize to the various muscles of facial expression. In the normal person you will elicit no twitch or only a minimal one. In the presence of decreased ionized calcium in the serum (or other situations of neuron hyperirritability) you may observe a distinct twitch of the innervated muscles. (An analogous hyperreactivity can be demonstrated by tapping the peroneal nerve at the head of the fibula, causing a dorsiflexion and eversion of the foot.)

SUMMARY

Priorities

1 The plantar response ("Babinski test"): if the patient's reaction is to pull away, apparently out of ticklishness, reduce the stimulus, applying a shortened, lateral stroke without coming across the ball of the foot. Observe for the pathologic, stereotypic triple-flexion (flexion

withdrawal) response that frequently occurs in fragmentary form. Often normal patients exhibit a neutral or only minimally flexor response; do not expect to see marked flexion in every instance.

2 Ankle jerk (Achilles reflex): this is by far the most important DTR for screening; practice it at every opportunity, so that when you cannot elicit it, even with reinforcement, you will feel quite confident of your finding. Ankle jerks are symmetrically decreased early in most polyneuropathies and polyradiculopathies. A focal decrease in an ankle jerk may be seen on the side of a sciatic nerve lesion or lumbosacral radiculopathy (e.g. disc disease) involving the S1 root.

3 Understand major disproportions between DTRs at different levels: for example, 0–1+ ankle jerks in the face of 2–3+ knee jerks, biceps, and triceps jerks strongly point to a distal polyneuropathy. Or, 1+ DTRs in the arms, but 3–4+ at the knees and ankles, suggest bilateral UMN dysfunction above the midlumbar spinal cord (see Fig. 13.9).

Pitfalls

1 Mistaking pathologic triple-flexion responses (to plantar stimulation) for "ticklish" semivoluntary withdrawal, especially if bilateral.

2 Imagining the presence of ankle jerks or other reflexes because of slight, mechanically induced movement when, in fact, the absent reflexes constitute an important sign. (Symmetrically decreased or absent ankle jerks bear little clinical significance in far advanced age.)

3 Not reproducing apparent reflex asymmetry (noted on initial testing). Often the DTR on one side may appear slightly less brisk than the opposite one because of differences in position, relaxation, guarding against pain, etc. Any significant asymmetry should be reproducible.

PROBLEMS FOR SELF-STUDY

Problems

1 A 20-year-old woman complains of 4 days of increasing fatigue while walking, as well as aching and diffuse pains in her legs. Examination reveals absent ankle and knee jerks, while arm reflexes are definitely, but barely present (trace). What additional clinical information would you most like to have?

2 A patient suspected of hysteric weakness has 3–4+ DTRs throughout her arms and legs. What additional reflexes would you wish to test in particular, and how would the result help you to localize a possible lesion?

Comments

1 Establish whether prior records contain a baseline on DTR activity. The current findings could be normal for her, and the symptoms unrelated, but you would need to be concerned. Check for limb weakness, abnormal tone, sensory loss, and Babinski signs to start with. Acute bilateral loss (or progressive decrease) of DTRs is usually

due to an acute polyneuropathy or polyradiculopathy. The most common acute condition is the Guillain–Barré syndrome, an acute polyradiculoneuropathy with weakness that often follows an ascending pattern. Sensory loss is minimal (usually limited to slight vibratory impairment). Since this is a peripheral nervous system problem, plantar responses are flexor.

2 Even extremely brisk, symmetric DTRs with unsustained clonus can be normal, but should not be presumed so, especially in a patient with "weakness." If the patient does have a central nervous system lesion, the corticobulbar reflexes (jaw jerk and snout) would be of particular relevance in helping to establish a reflex level. If these were absent or minimal (as is normal), and no other brainstem localizing signs were present, then one would hypothesize a possible cervical spinal cord problem causing UMN signs below. If jaw jerk and snout were brisk, attention would turn to a bilateral lesion affecting both corticobulbar and corticospinal tracts in the upper brainstem or cerebral hemispheres. Extensor plantar responses would be confirmatory of corticospinal pathology; superficial abdominal reflexes would probably have disappeared.

FURTHER READING

Davidoff, R.A. Skeletal muscle tone and the misunderstood stretch reflex. *Neurology* 1992; 42:951–63. Deep tendon reflexes are useful markers clinically, but the physiologic role of stretch reflexes is not what many physicians think. Current concepts are reviewed in considerable detail.

Haerer, A.F. *De Jong's The Neurologic Examination*. 5th edn. Lippincott, Philadelphia (PA), 1992. Testing and anatomy of the principal reflexes, their less familiar variations (with eponyms), and other reflexes rarely used and little known (Chapters 33–39).

chapter 10

Assessing Mental Status, Language, and Other Higher Functions

Overview

Evaluation of mental status is the part of the neurologic examination that touches closest to the patient as an individual. Therefore, mental status and behavior (and their accurate assessment) are major determinants of the success of the clinical relationship. This assessment is also the most open-ended part of the neurologic examination. As you are already aware, the entire encounter provides you with information on mental status and behavior. You learn facets of it from the history, both from the substance of it and from the process of eliciting the patient's account. You learn from the way the patient responds and acts during the general examination and during other parts of the neurologic examination. You will typically learn even more in subsequent encounters, as you work with the patient over time, through diagnostic procedures and therapy, stresses and strains, success and disappointment.

The purpose of this assessment, of course, is to determine whether or not mental status and behavior are normal.

1 Is there any abnormality?

2 Can the abnormality be described and categorized in neurologic (or psychologic) terms?

3 Can the neurologic dysfunction be localized?

But what is normal? What are the mental and behavioral attributes that enable a patient to function in his or her job, in family and society, in recreation and reflection, and in managing personal health? And what is the patient's own concept of normal function?

The goal of this chapter is to help you acquire skills for obtaining relevant data at the bedside or in the clinic. The first section will emphasize practical and common sense aspects of mental status evaluation in the context of the conventional, systematic examination. Subsequent sections will introduce you to a more integrated, less formal approach, and then to the evaluation of language and other so-called higher cortical functions.

MENTAL STATUS AND BEHAVIOR

Sizing-up function

One way to identify mental and behavioral attributes is to stand back from the medical model and consider the following situation: you are interviewing a person for a job, or for admission to college or medical school. Aside from the formal requirements of prior education, training, and skills, what would you like to know about the person's attributes? Your charge is to "size-up" the candidate – in this case not physically, but mentally, emotionally, and in social interaction. Is the person lively, attentive, and perceptive? Does he or she make sense, stay on the track, have something informative to say, and say it clearly? Is there humor or gravity that is right for the subject and occasion? Does the person display an interest in and memory for events? Are plans realistic and coherent, etc.? The first step in evaluation is to take a real interest in the person.

Empathy and scrutiny

This approach requires both empathy and objectivity. The interviewing skills that you are developing in history taking are just the skills you need to obtain mental status data while building a rapport – and, as a rule, the more rapport the better the data. It is essential to distinguish uninformative chatter from answers that reveal the attributes in which you are specifically interested: has the patient actually demonstrated an active mind or, conversely, is there a poverty of thought that bores you as you listen? Of course, good mental status does not require scintillating conversational ability, but even the most laconic, down-to-earth individuals will normally have something sensible to say, especially if you approach them on their own terms.

To summarize the kinds of general qualities that have been mentioned, we wish to know whether a person:

1 conducts himself or herself appropriately for the occasion;

2 pays attention to questions or a line of thought and is not easily distracted;

3 has a retentive mind and is not forgetful;

4 is perceptive;

5 is well-informed;
6 thinks straight, makes sense; can grasp principles;
7 shows good judgment;
8 comprehends written and verbal information and nonverbal messages;
9 communicates understandably, etc.

For comparison, the following are standard components of the conventional mental status examination:

Conventional format

1 general appearance and behavior (including level of consciousness and affect);
2 attention and concentration;
3 memory;
4 orientation;
5 thought processes (including abstract thought, judgment, and insight);
6 thought content (including fund of knowledge);
7 calculations.

(Language and other "higher functions" are considered separately later.)

Given that the two lists have so much in common, you can begin the mental status evaluation with the confidence that a useful examination is readily accessible.

GENERAL INDICATIONS OF IMPAIRED MENTAL STATUS

The three major criteria for clinical concern are listed below.

Baseline

1 Has the patient deteriorated from his or her usual state or baseline? Acceptable performance for an adult with congenital mental retardation would obviously differ from that of a previously successful lawyer who had just recently begun to display forgetfulness. (Here we will not consider developmental abnormalities or chronic, static deficits.)

Daily function

2 Is mental acuity no longer sufficient to enable adequate function in job and family? Along the same line, is a patient able to take responsibility for managing any health problems by keeping appointments, complying with medication schedules, and participating in decision making?

Mood

3 Has the patient become mentally distressed beyond normal responses to adversity? Even if able to function at work, a patient cannot be considered normal mentally if wracked with anxiety, panic, pain, or depressive moods, etc. These emotional aspects are not always fully revealed in mental performance, but sooner or later affect it.

THE FORMAL MENTAL STATUS EXAMINATION

Appearance, behavior, and level of consciousness

Appearance

While real insight requires looking beyond the clothes and probing more than skin deep, appearances are often revealing. A patient's ability to understand bodily needs is reflected in signs of personal care. Allowing for broad cultural, economic, and generational differences (as well as some individual eccentricity), the dress and personal hygiene of a patient coming to an office or clinic provides clues to the patient's self-image, judgment, and any disinhibitions.

Level of consciousness

The alertness of ambulatory patients is readily perceived, but the mere appearance of the hospitalized patient in bed does not always reflect the state of consciousness. Alertness needs to be distinguished from mere wakefulness, and sleepiness from stupor. Is the unresponsive patient comatose or simply unable to communicate cognizance? The examination of the "unresponsive patient" will be introduced in Chapter 18.

Affect

Affect is the outward expression of mood or emotions. We ask the patient what his or her mood is like, but we observe the patient's affect—whether the patient appears happy, sad, subdued, angry, etc. The overused term, "flat affect" describes a rather wooden, or even stony countenance that gives little clue as to inner mood. You should try to characterize affect more specifically, looking for hints of the patient's emotional tone, even if expressed within a narrow range of affective responses. Your own emotional reaction to the patient also serves as a clue to the patient's affect.

Behavior

Behavior is universally noticed, not always well observed, and frequently not described specifically. Behavior, in common parlance, connotes social comportment—how well a person complies with social rules and cultural expectations. In neurology, all outward activity is studied as behavior. Some behavior is associated with important changes of affect (emotionally charged behavior), some is affectively neutral, some is purposeful, some idle or involuntary, some is instinctual or reflexic, and some is regarded as creative.

Too often the behavioral assessment tends to fall through the cracks between the physical part of the neurologic examination and the circumscribed questions of the formal mental status examination. While we do not customarily set aside a part of the examination as behavioral, we try to make observations on behavior throughout the encounter—the history, general examination, neurologic examination, and in follow-up. Particularly important behavioral information is conveyed in facial expression, tone of voice, manner of speech, posture, use of hands and other body language, characteristics of gait, nature and degree of spontaneous and restless movement, quickness and modulation of responses to outer stimuli (passivity, irritability, etc.). How telling is a slumped posture or hand wringing, or the subtler signs of a curled lip or an arching of the eyebrows!

Dress and personal hygiene reflect behavior, but like behavior in general, should be understood in terms of cultural relativism; what is deemed appropriate in one context may not be in another. In any case, as you assess behavior you should avoid being judgmental.

Approach to formal questioning

As you come to the part of the examination that requires specific test questions, you may wonder how to introduce them in a way that will seem least awkward. I often broach the issue in this general way: "I am now going to ask some routine questions to test your memory and other mental functions. This might seem a little silly but it will help my understanding, so please bear with me." Of course, I vary the explanation for different patients, so that it will seem neither too complicated nor condescending.

Attention and concentration

Testing

Attentiveness is the keystone of the whole edifice of mental status testing. Evaluation of cognitive function is dependent upon patient participation. To test memory, the ability to think abstractly, calculation skills, etc., you need the attentive cooperation of the patient, which means that the patient adheres to your agenda.

Digit span

To test attention by digit span performance, give a series of digits at an even rate of about one per second. Ask the patient to repeat them in the same order. Provide an example for the patient: "I am going to give you a series of numbers to repeat in the same order that I give them to you: 1, 8, 3 . . ." and you repeat 1, 8, 3 . . . The usual norm is quoted as seven digits forward. Such a test requires only what is called immediate memory or registration – what you can hold actively "in mind." Repeating the digits in reverse order adds little of value.

Serial subtractions

Ask the patient to subtract a number repeatedly, such as 100 minus 7, then the answer minus 7, etc. The most important aspect of the test is whether the patient will be able to concentrate sufficiently to keep track of each subtraction in turn and to continue on down until asked to stop. If difficulty is encountered, try to determine whether it is the result of unfamiliarity with the arithmetic operation or an inability to persevere in the task. Arithmetic difficulty, whether from lack of schooling or disuse, can be minimized by requiring subtraction of 3 rather than 7, or even counting backward by 1s.

Other attention tests

Another test requires the patient to signal when a predesignated letter of the alphabet is heard. Start naming letters (in no particular order) and when the designated letter comes up, the arranged signal (such as holding up a hand) should be given. Obviously, you can easily devise further tests of your own that will serve just as well, if you recognize and control the variables involved. The advantage of a traditional test like digit span is that you need not describe the procedure when you record the results.

Interpretation

If performance is poor on a test of attention, ask the patient to restate the task. Perhaps the patient misunderstood the task, or was inattentive to the instruction, or started out correctly but wandered. Try the task again, or turn to a different one. There are many reasons for distractability and impaired concentration – from metabolic delirium to pain, anxiety, and focal brain lesions.

Remember that it is the perseverance in a clearly defined, sustained task that challenges concentration; any test meeting that objective will be likely to suffice. Whatever the cause of inattention, its recognition as a problem is essential: inattention will affect other aspects of testing, as well as participation in general care.

Evaluation of memory

The patient's success with memory testing depends upon several components of the test system:

1 attention to the task: registration of test items (immediate memory);
2 processing and storage;
3 ability to access the test items retained in memory;
4 sufficient communicative capacity to express the answer (or understand the question).

From this view of the whole system you can see that complaints of memory difficulty do not always originate in a declining memory storage and recall capacity. A patient may have holes in past memory resulting from blocks to attention, processing, or communication and yet have normal ability to form new memories at present.

Testing recent memory

Three objects

When giving any memory task, first be sure that the patient registers the information to be retained, that is, the patient must be able to hold the task in so-called immediate memory. If you assign three items, such as "ball," "seventeen," and "purple," ask the patient to repeat them back to you immediately, so as to assure that attention was adequate to apprehend the task. (This is really just a further confirmation of what has already been learned about attention and concentration by such means as the digit span test or serial calculations.) You should feel free to give any test items you like, although they should not be so complex or unusual as to intimidate the patient. A better performance will sometimes be facilitated by giving a short "story" – a one or more sentence description of some occurrence that might engage interest, arouse amusement, or convey a cultural overtone with which the patient can identify: "Angelo went to the market to buy two pounds of spaghetti for his grandmother." No matter how homespun the example, your purpose will be served if the patient can repeat it correctly after a few minutes – we often try to approximate 3 or 5 minutes, but the exact timing is not important.

Brief "story"

If the patient does not recall the items given, you can try several tactics. Since some patients are inhibited by a fear of error, encourage them to take a guess, even if unsure. Next you might provide hints, such as giving the category of the test item (a "number" for the item "seventeen") or "it was about food" for the story of Angelo's errand. If necessary, narrow down the range of options, such as, "It was a number between 10 and 20," or more specifically still, give a multiple choice: "Was the story about getting potatoes, noodles, or spaghetti?" Recall elicited by prompting does not confirm normal memory, but does demonstrate at least partial capacity.

Misleadingly poor performances generally come from patients who do badly in a formal testing situation but who obviously have well-preserved functional capacities. They are the patients who recall only two out of three test items but the next day remind the examiner of some minor point of amusement that had been shared together the day before.

CASE 10A
A memorable piece

An 88-year-old former concert pianist, Emil Langhans, was undergoing hospital treatment for pneumonia. As his illness resolved and plans were being readied for his return home, his care-givers became aware that he was quite forgetful: he did not recall the date and seemed unable to keep in mind the schedule of medication that he was to follow at home.

Assessment of mental status disclosed a friendly, cooperative, elderly man who was somewhat deaf, but nonetheless remained attentive. His social graces were well preserved. He knew he was in a hospital, but could not name it.

When asked to recall three objects, he repeated them back immediately, but did not recall them, even with clues, a few minutes later. His examiner then asked him to remember a two-sentence story about fishing, but he failed. When then asked to remember "Chopin Polonaise" he broke into a big grin and described his lifelong devotion to Chopin's music. He then elaborated on details of several Chopin recitals he had given in Europe 40 years before (and his family verified the facts). Five minutes later he promptly recalled the test item. The remainder of the examination disclosed no other very severe deficits.

This patient obviously had a major impairment of recent memory, but was capable of recalling a test item that sufficiently ignited his enthusiasm – revealing the relativity of memory performance and its affective component. Operating within a familiar frame of reference and without novel demands, he had been able to manage at home previously (and, indeed, was able to return home and function as he had before). His far better recall of selected events in the remote past was consistent with the pattern often encountered in cases of senile dementia of the Alzheimer type (compare with Case 1B).

Remote memory

As indicated above, you will often find some degree of dissociation between the ability to form new memories (recent memory) and the ability to recollect events from the distant past. In testing remote memory, you must be able to verify the patient's responses. Therefore, you will often need to inquire about specific events in the public realm. Depending upon the age and background of the patient, you might ask, "Whom were the Allies fighting in World War II?"; "What happened to John Lennon?"; "Who gave the speech, 'I have a dream'?"; or "Who was involved in Watergate?" The accuracy and amount of detail supplied with each answer speaks not only to the issue of remote memory, however, but also to fund of knowledge (as will be discussed below). Overall, testing of remote memory usually adds rather little, if recent memory is intact.

Pitfalls

The main pitfalls to memory testing and interpretation are as follows.

1 Not being sure that the patient has registered the task. (Check on attention and comprehension.)

2 Not knowing how to assess wrong answers. If the patient recalls only two out of three items, does that mean that there is a one-third memory deficit or that good capacity for recall has been demonstrated by two correct answers and the third just represented a "slip"? In other words, is the "bottle two-thirds full or one-third empty?" (In general, accurate recall of at least some items tends to suggest quite good memory capacity. Since the "slip" may be due to extraneous factors, be sure to retest in other ways before postulating any major memory deficit. Try to engage the patient's interest and ease anxiety.)

3 Not distinguishing deficits in memory capacity from isolated or episodic memory lapses. The inability of a patient to remember a particular event or period of time, such as the hours surrounding a concussive head injury, the minutes after a convulsion, or the days in an intensive care unit when obtunded, does not signify an ongoing problem with memory capacity.

Clinical correlations

Relatively consistent impairment of recent memory capacity, associated with better remote memory performance, suggests a limited number of organic disorders (such as Alzheimer's disease). In contrast, hysteric amnesia (which is extremely rare) is typically all-encompassing, even to the point of not remembering one's own name. Focal brain diseases that involve the hippocampus and/or its thalamic and hypothalamic connections in the memory circuit include the Wernicke–Korsakoff syndrome (seen in alcoholic–nutritional disorders), infarction in the temporal territory of the left (or left and right) posterior cerebral arteries, and herpes simplex encephalitis. Memory deficits are common after episodes of hypoxic encephalopathy but, as with Alzheimer's disease, other cognitive deficits typically are associated.

Orientation

A patient's orientation as to person, place, and time is an important measure of mental status, but reflects more than one type of mental processing. (Try to list the elements that together maintain a sense of orientation.)

Testing

1 Person: you should confirm the patient's self-identification as you introduce yourself and elicit the patient's name in return. Personal identity is rarely lost in an alert and responsive patient.

2 Place: if orientation to place is not fully evident from foregoing conversation, ask directly, "Do you know the name of this place?" or "Have you been able to keep track of your location now? Where are you?" Adjust the phrasing of the question to the context of the situation, so that it does not sound demeaning, but do not fail to confirm the answer because of a sense of awkwardness. If the patient is attentive, but does not recall the place by name, encourage deductions from environmental clues: "Look around you and tell me what kind of place you think this is." (This opener occasionally elicits amusing replies.) More pointedly, you might draw the patient's attention to items such as medical clothing, instruments, hospital beds, an intravenous line, as clues. If unsuccessful, you could offer a multiple choice, such as hotel, school, hospital, post office, or doctor's office.

3 Time: orientation to time can be approached in the same general way as sense of place. If unaware of month, date, and day of the week, you can focus in by asking the season, perhaps by way of reference to recent or upcoming holidays. By looking out the window the patient ordinarily should be able to deduce the season. For a hospitalized patient, knowledge of the exact date may not be very meaningful, but most patients should ordinarily be able to state the day and date (and remember them once given). Very sick patients frequently lose track of elapsed time, so that asking "How long have you been here?" tends to be useful only if the answer is correct or implausibly wrong. When the patient is initially disoriented to time, try to assess (as with all errors) how well clues are utilized to approximate the correct answers. In short, explore mistakes.

Interpretation

A variety of mental status abnormalities (or information deficits) result in some degree of disorientation. The proper interpretation depends upon establishing the type of disorientation – such as that arising from global confusion vs. that from memory loss. Disorientation is commonly taken as a sign of confusion or clouding of the sensorium, which points to an organic as opposed to psychologic basis, but this can only be supported by dissecting out the mechanism.

If the patient is obviously entirely oriented and no need for details is likely to arise, then the common notation "oriented times three" suffices. (Remember, "O × 3" is normal and does not mean zero for three.) Specify any abnormalities. For example, "Mr Langhans did not know the year, date, or day of the week." (Clearly, a response as to year that is one year off and self-corrected carries a different significance from an answer that is 40 years off and is defended by the patient even when clues or contradictory evidence are offered.)

Thought processes, including abstractions, judgment, and insight

Making sense

Thought processes include many aspects of cerebral function that are not readily separable from one another. The essence, however, is whether the patient makes sense and can grasp relationships. Does he or she think logically and stay on the subject at hand? Is there "rhyme or reason," organization, and purpose to what is expressed? Admittedly, people think in somewhat different ways – some more linearly and verbally, some more through images, etc. Brilliant thinkers have, on occasion, been passed off as weird or even crazy. Nonetheless, in most clinical encounters you can readily assess at least the most overt features of the patient's thought processes.

Ability to abstract

As you know, the ability to deal in abstract thought involves generalizing or recognizing an underlying theme or principle that can then be applied to other situations. Common ways to test this capacity include the following.

Proverbs

1 Interpretation of proverbs. Because of variations in educational level and sophistication, I usually test with rather plain, homespun examples, such as "Too many cooks spoil the broth" or "A stitch in time saves nine." Ask the patient whether the proverb is familiar and what it means. How could the meaning be explained to somone else? An abstract interpretation of "stitch in time" might be that "prompt action prevents the need for more work later." A concrete reply usually adheres to the particular example, often reiterating the words of the proverb, such as, "If you take a stitch now, you won't have to do a lot of sewing later." A reply of this type is not wrong, but fails to capture the point that the message can be generalized. You might then ask further, "Is this proverb necessarily about sewing – could you apply it to another situation? Would you give me an example?" Do not diagnose an abnormality of thought on the basis of a single proverb; try others. When a patient resists interpretation because he or she "hasn't heard that one," it is usually a clue to impaired thinking, but you can ask the patient to supply a proverb and interpret it for you. Certain proverbs (like "A rolling stone gathers no moss") have more than one reasonable interpretation; the point of the test is not the precise content but rather the process of abstracting or generalizing. (Many younger people take moss to be an impediment to freedom while many older people see moss as wealth that eludes the shiftless. What do you think?)

Similarities

2 Another application of abstract thinking is the identification of similarities or common features among a series of items: what do an apple and an orange have in common? What are the similarities between a ship and an airplane? Occasionally, the patient will start off by telling you the differences, but you can then reemphasize your objective of identifying qualities that they share, and even give an example (such as "an apple and an orange both have seeds").

Interpretation

You may read different accounts of what concrete answers signify. In general, concrete or reiterative answers, usually restricted rather than expansive, suggest an organic dysfunction, such as a dementia. Some psychotic patients will give answers that may have some concrete characteristics, but are more idiosyncratic, and may be clever, expansive, or symbolic. Occasionally, a patient will quote you back another proverb; if it is highly pertinent to the idea of the test proverb, the reply can be taken as evidence of the ability to abstract. Otherwise, it probably represents an unfocused response to the topic of proverbs and does not demonstrate understanding.

Tangential thinking

A person's tendency to stray from the topic at hand, to veer off in another direction (tangential thinking) becomes evident from conversation. Some patients may simply have poor attention and concentration. Others will seem pulled off the subject by issues that are dominating their thought and, hence, reemerge at the flimsiest connection. "Loose associations" represent a propensity to make connections that are not evident to others or do not appear germane. Both tangential thinking and loose associations occur in psychosis, but may also arise in confusional states. However, associations that seem loose to one observer may appear brilliant and creative to another.

Insight

Insight is a hard characteristic to define, as it depends upon intelligence and psychologic factors and can be impaired by focal neurologic lesions (see Chapters 1 and 12). The latter type of derangement is, most typically, the lack of recognition of a clinical deficit (such as a left-sided weakness) and failure to apprehend its personal significance. A more general kind of defective insight involves an inability to perceive the implications of a situation or what a person is "driving at." You will tend to pick up failures of this type when taking a history or explaining your diagnostic impression and plan of management. (Of course, you could pose a situation, real or artificial, for the patient to analyze: "A young man with a history of arrest for disorderly conduct encounters a fight between two individuals. How might he respond and what might be the consequences?")

Judgment

Tests of judgment, while depending on insight, usually require making an actual decision ("What would you do or what conclusion would you reach?"). The tests that are traditionally suggested for evaluation of judgment certainly do not probe the depths of this process, but can screen for grossly abnormal responses. Two of these tests are as follows: "You find a stamped, sealed, addressed envelope on the sidewalk. What would you do with it?" "You are in a theater and someone yells 'Fire'; what would you do?" Be aware that patients with normal mental status may make light of such a test and give a bizarre or contrary response. In addition, all matters of judgment are subject to cultural and other value-laden relativity. (What would you do if you found an envelope of money on the sidewalk?)

Overall, the best initial source of data on judgment is the history that family or friends provide, although you may need to seek multiple sources for verification. Abnormal judgment is usually best revealed in real-life activities. As you get to know a patient and participate in health mangement over time, you will have considerable opportunity to witness, first-hand, the judgment that a patient exercises with respect to participating in a program of care.

Calculations

As previously noted, the serial 7 test assesses both concentration and ability to subtract. Calculation skill can be tested with any kind of computation, but addition and multiplication, at least in their simpler forms, are often learned by rote; therefore, the answers may be remembered rather than "figured out." Be sure to determine the patient's educational level. Start with a simple problem and allow the patient to work it out on paper, if preferred. Use of a word problem adds another dimension, but allows you to put the calculation into a familiar context: "If a loaf of bread costs 57 cents and you give the cashier a dollar, how much change would you receive?" Previously attained computational ability may suffer but not vanish from disuse, whereas profound loss occurs in global, dementing processes such as advanced Alzheimer's disease, or in focal pathology (such as stroke involving the dominant parietal lobe).

Spatial relationships

Spatial relationships are discussed in a later section on other higher functions.

Thought content

How do you judge thought content – by quantity or quality? A paucity of thought should not be assumed because the patient is laconic, nor should volume be mistaken for quality. Some people are just reticent in expressing their ideas. Others who are afflicted with cerebral (especially frontal) deficits may respond slowly but ultimately divulge a surprisingly good quality of thought. Consider whether relevant information is transmitted: is the conversation hollow, is there a vacuousness, a succession of trivial phrases, sometimes called "cocktail party conversation?"

Testing fund of knowledge

Although you can usually form quite a good notion of thought content from conversation, particularly from inquiring about a patient's own interests, there are some time-honored subjects that you may wish to use for testing. Such topics include the name of the President, the names of prior Presidents going back in time, the Governor, Mayor, etc. If a person has had little education or has suffered cultural isolation or deprivation, you will learn most by asking about mundane activities that fall within the patient's sphere of daily life (defined and verified with the help of a relative or friend): the name of the local market, the minister at the patient's church, the names of the next-door neighbors, etc. Patients with little knowledge of current events may gain other sorts of information from television programs: you can ask about specific programs, such as soap operas, within the limits of your own knowledge! Testing vocabulary or itemizing within categories (types of fruit or brands of cars) is also revealing.

Interpretation

Retention of information depends upon remote memory (see above). Of course, you need to take into account the age and educational and cultural background of the patient. Most adults during the Great Depression and World War II would know the name of the President during those years, but some young people in the 1980s without much formal education might not. Similarly, almost anyone beyond childhood in the early 1960s would know some of the circumstances of the death of John F. Kennedy, since this was such a traumatic landmark of that decade.

What do data on fund of knowledge tell you? Ample factual information certifies contact with sources of information, memory (either remote, recent, or both), and ability to communicate. If the fund of knowledge appears deficient, you cannot draw any further interpretation without determining the reason. Thus, fund of knowledge does not reflect any one mental capacity, but is rather a composite product, resulting from both endogenous and exogenous influences. As such, it has some value as a broad screen, but you should avoid quick judgments based upon your own intellectually or culturally biased expectations.

PERSONALIZING THE MENTAL STATUS ASSESSMENT

The formal mental status examination may strike you as awkward. In some situations it seems so stilted and impersonal that you may wonder whether the tests are intended for real people. These perceptions are particularly unfortunate, since the patient's cognitive, emotional, and behavioral attributes are the most individual, the most truly personal parts of the neurologic assessment. Patients sometimes find the formal examination threatening to their self-esteem, or even demeaning. If handled insensitively, being tested feels like being "grilled" and many medical patients worry that their physicians think they are "crazy."

Setting a personal standard

A far better determination of mental status will eventuate if the patient is enlisted as an ally of the examiner. For this reason, I find it helpful to assess the patient's performance against a standard that the patient helps to supply. I might ask, "Are you good at figures?" and the patient might reply, "Yes, I worked for years as a bookkeeper; I ought to be able to add!" Such a response would greatly assist in my interpretation of errors of performance. If the patient did not claim any special affinity for numbers, I might inquire whether the patient does his or her own shopping and, if so, I would put calculations in the form of making correct change. In each instance, the task would proceed from the simple to the more complex.

Personalizing the examination

Rote questions asked in a perfunctory fashion accomplish little. The mental status assessment should be flexible and conducive to achieving optimal communication with the individual patient. Sometimes, down-to-earth, informal methods succeed when more structured questioning fails. Take an interest in the person by eliciting an account of daily activities and interests. Gently lead the patient along a path familiar to his or her walk of life. To learn more about the mental status, learn more about the person.

INTEGRATION OF THE MENTAL STATUS EXAMINATION INTO THE ENTIRE ENCOUNTER

The process of individualizing the format and style of the mental status examination can be extended by integrating it more thoroughly into the whole encounter. The method is less formal, but the goals are the same. This approach is, in fact, the one implicitly used in daily practice by seasoned clinicians who derive a great deal of mental status information from the history, the physical examination, and social interactions without ever asking a formal test question. Your ability to succeed in this fashion begins with two parts of the examination, namely attention and memory, which will be discussed in greater detail.

Attention

As in the formal examination, the first step is to determine the quality and span of the patient's attention and concentration. You can infer these from the patient's responses to a detailed line of questioning during the interview, or how quickly the patient responds to directions during the examination. How well does the patient sustain activity (such as maintaining the arms outstretched), or carry over the instructions for a test as it is repeated on different parts of the body?

Memory

You can often make solid inferences about recent memory and new memory formation during review of the clinical history, assuming that you possess some independent knowledge of the facts. Ask about events that led to hospitalization or the office visit, recent changes in medication, or what has been done since admission to the hospital (tests done, doctors seen, length of stay, and so on). Does the patient take an interest in the news by means of daily paper or newscast? If the patient provides a coherent account, including precise details of chronology, then memory is sure to be quite good. Further substantiation can be gained by referring back to an item discussed a few minutes before to see whether that information has been retained. In order to gain data on remote memory and fund of knowledge, extend the discussion of recent affairs to related past events.

Orientation, thought processes

You can learn quite a lot about a patient's orientation and thought processes by asking about recent and anticipated activities. "What are your plans now?" or "How do you think this illness will affect your upcoming plans?" Abnormalities of insight and judgment may become evident during discussion of the chief complaint and present illness. Compare the patient's perception of the problem to deficits found on physical examination and to the functional status reported by independent observers. Is the patient proving able to participate effectively in considering diagnostic, therapeutic, and aftercare decisions?

Limitations

Thus, important objectives of the conventional mental status examination can be incorporated into the comprehensive clinical evaluation in a way that is both revealing and nonalienating. Less amenable to this approach are several abstract tasks of the conventional examination, such as the patient's ability to interpret proverbs, identify similarities, calculate, demonstrate spatial relationships, name objects, read, comprehend multistep or contingency commands, etc. You will not be able to exercise as much control over the specific form of response during a conversational interview and the patient's response can therefore be misleadingly glib. Some patients will steer the discussion toward the familiar, while their capacity to deal with broader topics is left unchallenged. For this reason, an ability to use the formal, conventional mental status examination remains important, even as you learn to mold it to individual application. A highly structured and inherently more confrontational examination is indicated when prior techniques have not succeeded in obtaining adequate data, when the patient's thinking is so disorganized that the examiner must tightly control the interview, or when a more comprehensive survey of cortical function is required.

Recording the mental status examination

The recording of the mental status assessment should reflect with complete candor the actual mode of assessment. Ideally, the documentation of a mental status examination should include the specific test items and responses. However, as a practical economy, it will usually suffice for you to indicate the areas you have tested (such as attention, memory, and orientation) if you are fully confident that the results are normal. Rather than noting only "oriented times three" as evidence of a normal mental status (as is so often done), you might stress that "the patient recalled recent events clearly, asked well-reasoned questions, and demonstrated intact conversational language as well as normal behavior and affect." However, when particular concern has arisen about mental status or when you encounter abnormal performance, you should include pertinent verbatim recording, specific descriptions, or other raw data: "Serial 3s to 91; recalled none of three objects 5 minutes after registering the task satisfactorily; place: 'some hotel'; year '1936'," etc. A limited mental status examination is included in the neurologic examination documentation (see Chapter 11).

PRACTICING MENTAL STATUS EVALUATIONS

Once you have gained more experience in formal testing, integration of the mental status evaluation into the entire clinical encounter will be suitable for the patient without any hint of a neurologic or psychiatric problem. As a practical matter, the patient who gives a clear, detailed, informative, and internally consistent chronology of events, behaves appropriately, and has a normal neurologic screening history and examination, can be spared formal mental status testing. In order to succeed with this model, you will need to practice being the empathetic listener and counselor while at the same time critically assessing the information obtained. To listen empathetically, remaining "tuned in," while internally analyzing responses for evidence of particular mental attributes is not easy. This is the art of the method, which has much in common with the art of interviewing in general.

Avoid facile assumptions

You should not rely on appearance or intuition, but should be able to cite specific evidence, whether gained through observation or through formal testing, as to mental and behavioral status. Memory deficits, in particular, can easily escape the notice of the unwary clinician. Relate your findings in this and other areas to the reports of reliable, independent observers (such as family members) who may have become aware of an increasing inability to deal with everyday life. Has the edge of wit or intellect become blunted or a sense of enterprise been lost? These reports have particular value when cast in operational terms, relating the patient's actual activities.

Changes in intelligence, personality, and behavior will be particularly difficult to detect in the initial stages of your relationship with the patient. Serial encounters often prove helpful, but only rarely do they lead to the same kind of insight and intimacy that a family member can have.

Learn from intimate care-givers

In an institutional setting, nurses, aides, and therapists are often a great help, as they are the ones who spend the most time actually working with the patient. Their observations are based on repetitive interactions with the patient and will benefit your evaluation. To follow the patient over time, seeing him or her at different times of day, in different moods, in different settings, alone and with family, systemically ill and recuperating, avails a good opportunity to understand mental status and behavior.

Blocks to good evaluation

At one time or another you will encounter numerous obstacles along the path of assessing mental status. Certainly, one of these may well be an impatient attitude on your part, as the examiner. Quite naturally you will experience frustration at a patient's slowness, inconsistency, lapses, and errors, which are aspects of the pathology that deter you from obtaining the very data you may need to make a diagnosis (a circular dilemma).

Similarly, poor attention and concentration on the part of the patient stultify your attempts to acquire relevant information. Language barriers represent one of the most common, if mundane, blocks to mental status evaluation. Even with a good interpreter the process is cumbersome and nuances tend to be missed.

Low output

Low psychomotor output (a lack of activity and mental expression) constitutes the greatest obstacle to mental status assessment (see also Chapter 18). Here you have virtually no raw materials with which to work. The deeply depressed patient, for example, will sometimes generate so little output that the clinician may wrongly diagnose an organic dementia instead of a so-called depressive pseudodementia. At the same time, however, the sheer force of your empathetic interest can sometimes "turn on" or mobilize an increased level of psychic energy. This, in turn, enables you to reach a higher level of communication and to gain better insight into mental processes.

PSYCHIATRIC APPROACHES TO MENTAL STATUS ASSESSMENT

A psychiatrist's approach to mental status assessment has much in common with the neurologic approach, but some aspects receive altered emphasis in both history and testing. In principle we can even question any distinction between a psychiatric and neurologic mental status examination, since both disciplines work with the same mind and same brain. The practical differences in approach emanate from presumptions about diagnosis, the particular skills learned in each field, and the need to triage care.

A psychiatric interview places particular stress on personal and family history of mood and behavior, family and social interactions, function in society, and personal ability to distinguish practical reality. The historical interview and mental testing nearly merge. If a patient says, "I feel suicidal," then the patient is presumed, as a rule, to be suicidal. Yet the patient may not offer this complaint, and you will not necessarily gain any clues from observed behavior prior to an actual attempt. Direct questioning with regard to suicidal ideation, hallucinations, and delusions is essential. Pay special attention to affect and any dissociation between affect and stated mood or reported behavior. Scrutinize thought processes: tangential thinking, loose associations, flight of ideas, etc.

A psychiatrically oriented mental status evaluation particularly elicits distortion of thought: paranoia, ideas of thought control, grandiosity, etc. But none of this is specific to a particular cause, as any so-called psychiatric symptom can occur in a disease identifiable as neurologic. Conversely, so-called neurologic abnormalities are being increasingly recognized in some diseases currently categorized as psychiatric. References to psychiatrically oriented mental status and behavioral evaluation will be found at the end of this chapter.

Neuropsychologic testing

Just as the confrontation examination of visual fields may lead to formal perimetry, or the suspicion of papilledema to a computerized tomography scan, the bedside mental status examination may indicate the need for more extensive and better controlled evaluation of intellectual function. A great deal of work in this field has created sophisticated batteries of tests that help to identify abnormalities and to correlate them with focal cerebral dysfunction. Neuropsychologic batteries need to be skillfully administered and interpreted; they are time-consuming and, in many areas, a relatively scarce or absent resource, but they can provide important clarification (see Further reading section).

Summary of approach to general mental status assessment

Mental status assessment is not only aimed at detecting abnormalities that assist pathologic localization, but also at enhancing understanding of the whole patient, including the patient's ability to participate effectively in treatment and general health management. In evaluating mental status, you should observe the following points.

1 Draw upon your past experience and human insight in trying to understand the patient's emotions, behavior, and other factors affecting cognitive performance. Your ability to form a sympathetic relationship with the patient may be as important as any particular technique. You will learn much about the patient by taking an interest in him or her as a person.

2 Feel free to explore alternative and nonconventional ways of achieving the goals of mental status assessment, so long as these methods maintain appropriate respect for the patient. Adapting your means to a well-articulated goal works better than performing routine tests in a perfunctory fashion.

3 Try to establish both the best that the patient can do and the worst trouble that he or she is having. Peak performance informs you of a minimum capability – the nervous system has at the very least the structural integrity to achieve that level of performance. Delineation of a pattern of dysfunction (that may be temporary) can provide clues to localization.

4 Be alert to blocks in the process of evaluation – factors affecting the patient's performance, and factors affecting your ability to evaluate it. Impaired consciousness, inattention, aphasia, disruptive behavior, psychotic thought processes, etc., limit accession of a good data base. Your success will frequently depend upon your ability to work around these in an inventive and resourceful way. For your part, be alert to your own attitudes and responses: does your attitude convey a disinterest or impatience that may adversely affect the patient's performance? Do you seem judgmental? If you experience attitudes like these (as I sometimes do), adapt your interaction to minimize or circumvent their effect on the assessment.

5 Avoid unfounded assumptions and facile interpretations. Especially with memory testing, insist on positive evidence of the patient's best level of recall and new memory formation.

6 Utilize the patient's history and the observations of others to help set a standard of normal expectation for mental status testing.
7 Adapt the style of mental status assessment (formal, conversational and observational, neuropsychologic batteries) to the clinical context: the chief complaint, the concerns of others, the presence or absence of other neurologic or general medical dysfunction, the patient's functioning in daily life, etc.).
8 Draw upon the mental status observations of intimate care-givers and other contacts who can provide a much larger sample than you can encompass in the time that you have to spend with the patient.
9 Treat the mental status assessment as an ongoing endeavor, not a matter that can be definitively concluded in one session, or by one brief, scored test, such as the "mini mental status" examination. While such tests have their usefulness, they are very limited and should not ordinarily substitute for more individualized evaluations.

EVALUATION OF LANGUAGE AND SPEECH

Overview

Since language is a major vehicle of thought and our principal means of communication, language deficits both hinder and help evaluation of cerebral function. On the one hand, they limit our access to cognitive functions as well as history (see Case 1C), making mental status evaluation much more difficult. On the other hand, the pattern of language impairment greatly assists localization of cerebral dysfunction.

In the presence of language deficits, such as nonsensical speech or lack of response to the simplest commands, your first reaction may be to regard communication as almost hopeless. Yet examination of language performance yields frequent surprises and offers keys to diagnosis that are accessible to you if you are prepared to engage in some exploration: you may find that the patient who cannot state the place or year can, in fact, pick the correct answers from a multiple choice list. While you are analyzing language capacity, you will also discover that careful observation of manner of speech pays dividends in your understanding of affect and behavior.

Definitions

Aphasia, in a broad sense, is an acquired impairment of expression or comprehension of language. The term aphasia (or *dysphasia*) more specifically pertains to abnormalities of spoken language, but not of the articulation of speech (dysarthria) or the production of sound (dysphonia).

Alexia (dyslexia) refers to impairment or reading (and represents a subtype of aphasia).

Agraphia specifies a deficit in writing, again referring to language and not to penmanship.

Objective

Aphasia testing is designed to identify and characterize abnormalities of communication by language. As noted, disorders purely of producing sound (phonation) or enunciating words (articulation) that do not impair language as a symbolic method of communication are separable (see Chapter 5, section on CNs 9 and 10, and Chapter 8, section on speech). The goal of beginning language evaluation should be to gain confidence in a simple but systematic method of language analysis.

Testing

Begin your evaluation with a logical sequence of observations that does not depend upon any particular concept of language organization: listen to spontaneous speech and then empirically undertake trials of inputs and outputs. Determine for yourself what the patient can and cannot do in the uses of language that are fully familiar to you. Avoid the impulse to diagnose at the outset one classic type of aphasic syndrome or another.

At this introductory stage your examination should cover the following points.

Handedness

1 Ascertain handedness (see Chapter 4). (The left hemisphere is dominant for language in essentially all right-handers and a majority of left-handers.)

Spontaneous speech

2 Start by listening to the patient's spontaneous speech and any other phonation, if present. Think about the main features of ordinary speech, which include: (a) fluency of speech – the flow of words, phrases, and sentences: is it halting, labored, telegraphic, or smoothly flowing? (Quantity or amount of speech production is a separate variable: a patient may be fluent, but laconic.) (b) content – is speech coherent: does it make sense? Look especially for mistakes in words – does the patient substitute the wrong word (a verbal paraphasia such as pen for key).

Inputs and outputs

3 Try to define the inputs and outputs available for communication with the patient. If spontaneous speech is present, then verbal output exists, and you will already have gained some impression of its coherence and relevance. You can now try various inputs against this output, as in a question: "Please tell me your name." If the response is correct, you will have established that there is comprehension of a simple type of verbal input as evidenced by a correct answer. You might then extend this mode of communication to more complex questions requiring more involved answers, which stress comprehension and speech production more severely.

If there is little or no speech output, or if its output is not correctly responsive to the verbal input, then you will need to explore other inputs and outputs to see if communication can be established. Although inputs and outputs can be conveyed through any of the senses, we most often use some form of speech, writing, or signaling (see examples in Case 10B).

Nonverbal output

At times you will be able to infer at least partial comprehension of a verbal input from a nonverbal output. Clues come from social behavior and facial expression, such as a sudden alerting or smile when a specific name is mentioned.

The following case will illustrate the empirical use of inputs and outputs to establish language capabilities.

CASE 10B
An incoherent case

Leon Marston, a 71-year-old right-handed man, was brought to the emergency room because of incoherence and confusion. Neurologic physical examination was normal with the exception of a mild right upper motor neuron type of facial weakness and a right extensor plantar response. He spoke spontaneously in fluent phrases that were depleted of nouns and uttered many expressions like "Oh, you know" and "I guess so."

Various inputs and outputs were tested empirically; the results are shown in Table 10.1.

Summary of outputs

By this time the patient had shown the following outputs.

Motor: specific actions (sticking out tongue, closing eyes, holding pencil properly).

Behavioral: smiling, reaching out to his brother, showing irritation (swearing).

Verbal: spontaneous speech – occasional fluent phrases ("Oh, you know") and swearing; with cue, able to sing a line from "Jingle Bells."

Writing, reading, and graphics: he copied a circle and a large letter "T"; on

Table 10.1 Results of empirical input and output testing (Case 10B)

	Input	Output
Verbal	"Stick out your tongue"	Not done
	"Repeat: '10, 9, 8, 7' "	No response
	Examiner hummed tune of "Jingle Bells"	Patient sang one line recognizably
Written	"Is your name Leon?"	No response
	"Open your mouth"	Not done
	"C . . A . . T"	Did not read it aloud
	Examiner pointed to the letter T	Patient said "T" and occasionally named other letters, but not consistently
Visual (nonverbal)	Demonstration of eye closing and tongue protrusion	Actions mimicked
	Shown a tie	Did not name it
	Brother came into the room	Leon smiled and grasped his shoulder
Tactile	With his eyes covered, a pencil was put into his right hand	He felt it, held it appropriately and started to scribble aimlessly on his tray table
	Pencil was taken from him	Suddenly uttered, "Oh, damn it to hell."

one occasion he named the "T," but this was not regularly reproducible. He did not copy or read a sentence.

Course

Over the first few days of hospitalization he improved, demonstrating meaningful responses to the following additional inputs:

Verbal command: "Open your mouth" (response positive);

Written word: "CAT" (he read it aloud, but comprehension was not verified);

Progress in outputs: he could read words (as above) and spontaneous speech showed increased volume.

His speech gradually became more coherent, but he tended to repeat words or phrases over and over (perseveration) and made word or letter substitutions (paraphasias) such as "ink made" for "pen" or "ringer" for "finger." Repetition remained very difficult for him. He became angry with people who did not understand his speech and frequently swore. Rapid progress subsequently ensued in verbal and written comprehension and in forming longer, grammatical sentences, but frequent paraphasias and perseverations continued to intrude.

Diagnosis

From the pattern of his language difficulty, Mr Marston was diagnosed as having a predominantly posterior (fluent) aphasia with substantial resolution. His physician postulated a lesion in the left temporal lobe and attributed it to embolization of clot from a fibrillating left atrium.

Modality-specific results

The ability to respond correctly is often highly specific to the modality of testing. Sometimes a patient will not be able to say a word but can spell it, or can work with numbers but not the words for numbers. A patient may be unable to name an item, but succeeds in drawing a picture of it, or is perhaps able to choose the correct picture from multiple choices. Thus, if you think in terms of solving a systems problem, you may be able to find effective inputs and outputs that would not have seemed at all probable from the patient's apparent lack of speech and comprehension.

Definitions

Wernicke's

Wernicke's aphasia is one of the main types of aphasia (a "posterior" type) which is characterized principally by the capacity for fluent but error-filled or even nonsensical speech output and by poor comprehension, repetition, naming, reading, and writing. Note that speech production, especially acutely, may be greatly diminished even though it has fluent qualities when it does occur. The essential lesion is in the posterior part of the dominant hemisphere – the posterior superior temporal lobe. Other variations of posterior aphasia may involve adjacent temporoparietal areas.

Broca's

Broca's aphasia (motor, anterior) is characterized by nonfluent speech output, in contrast to very good to normal comprehension of speech and written material; there is poor repetition, writing, and naming. The responsible lesion includes Broca's area in the dominant posterior inferior frontal lobe, but is typically much larger. In a Broca's aphasia the cerebral organization of language output (both spoken and written) is disrupted. It is more than just dysarthria, although dysarthria usually coexists.

Global

Global aphasia can be thought of as a loss of all the language functions mentioned above – a combination of a severe anterior and a posterior aphasia (Broca's type and Wernicke's or other temporoparietal aphasias, respectively.) "Mixed aphasia" refers to the coexistence of partial deficits of both types.

Numerous other specific types of aphasia have been identified, representing loss of a particular function due to a focal lesion of a cortical or subcortical structure or connection. At this stage you will gain little from memorizing the characteristics of the many variations of aphasia. What you should be able to do, however, is to describe the abnormal features of language usage. You can then refer to text and tables that will help your localization, based upon these features (see Further reading section). Most of the cases of aphasia that you will see will not fit perfectly into one of the classic categories, although you will learn to categorize them broadly as more anterior or more posterior in type.

Summary

1 Listen to spontaneous speech, noting fluency, volume, and use of words, as well as sentence construction (syntax), melody and rhythm (prosody), etc. Distinguish errors or abnormalities of language from simple slurring of words (dysarthria).

2 By means of trying various inputs and outputs against each other, characterize speech and other verbal communication, including:

- (a) comprehension of spoken words, sentences;
- (b) naming letters, numbers, and objects;
- (c) repetition;
- (d) reading aloud and for comprehension;
- (e) writing.

3 Describe what you find; do not attach labels prematurely.

4 Correlate your language findings with other neurologic findings, such as the presence or absence of hemiparesis, sensory deficits, field cut, and nonverbal behavior.

5 One of the most common mistakes consists of accepting a function as normal on the basis of only very simple tasks: just because a patient can reply "yes" or "no" correctly, name a few objects, or produce a signature, does not mean that comprehension, naming, and writing are normal or almost normal.

6 Another common pitfall is to call an aphasia in which the patient has trouble with expression, an "expressive aphasia," and to equate this with a motor type of aphasia (anterior, Broca's type). Many patients with other types of aphasia have trouble expressing themselves (deficient word finding, paraphasic errors, or initial muteness). Before you postulate a Broca's type of aphasia, ascertain that comprehension is normal or nearly so in response to complex inputs.

OTHER HIGHER FUNCTIONS

Overview

Clearly, there are many important intellectual and perceptual functions of the human brain into which the basic mental status and language examinations offer only little insight. You can begin to think about the breadth and richness of human cortical function by reviewing the kinds of mental activities in which a person engages in ordinary life – running a household, working as a salesperson, planning a trip, hiking in the woods, designing a kitchen renovation, knitting a sweater, to name but a few. In addition to powers such as concentration, memory, language communication, etc., the person might need a sense of spatial relationships, ability to recognize and synthesize complex visual, tactile, and auditory data, and many other types of associations. Beyond these capacities are a multitude of talents, innovative and creative capabilities, and other human attributes that we witness in life.

The designation of some mental abilities as additional "higher functions" while others are typically included in the core, bedside mental status examination is quite arbitrary and subject to modification. Problems with visual recognition or spatial orientation, for example, can be just as disabling as certain language deficits. When is it particularly important to explore these other higher functions?

"Tip of the iceberg": you have discovered, either from history or examination, that one "cortical" function, such as language, is impaired. You wish to know whether this is an isolated deficit or whether it is part of a multifocal or diffuse cerebral disorder.

Deficit "denial": the patient is not functioning normally, but is unaware of any relevant symptoms – he or she lacks insight into the existence of a problem. You survey higher functions to determine whether there is a cerebral deficit that might be interfering with the patient's ability to recognize the existence of a problem (see Case 1D).

Lapsed performance: the patient is failing in a particular aspect of work or other activity and you wish to identify the responsible neurologic deficit (no explanation having been found on the basic examination). For example, a salesperson in a clothing store suddenly neglects familiar customers. Performance on survey of the usual mental status questions is good, but further exploration reveals an inability to recognize familiar faces or to appreciate the entirety of a picture apart from its details.

Further tests of "higher function"

Aspects of mental and behavioral function associated with the cerebral lobes of the right and left hemispheres are summarized in Chapter 13. In Chapter 14 the concepts of cerebral localization and dominance are briefly discussed. To pursue these subjects, consult the Further reading section at the end of these chapters and the present one. For now, it may be helpful to list some tests for "cortical functions" (aside from language) which go beyond simple observation and are commonly employed.

1 Accurate drawing or copying of complex diagrams or geometric figures (such as a cube) requires many abilities, including planning (frontal lobes) and visual–spatial synthesis and integration (parietal and occipital lobes, especially the right parietal). Drawing of daisies, clocks, etc., also emphasizes attention to both sides of space (neglect of the left side being a hallmark of large nondominant parietal lesions).

2 Calculations: the ability to perform arithmetic, is not a unitary function, but depends upon the way the material is presented and whether there are sequential operations. Thus, while dyscalculia is associated with the dominant parietal lobe, tasks of more than one step requiring planning or sequencing also depend upon anterior frontal lobe function. Similarly, calculations requiring particular spatial abilities (as when the numbers in a problem are displayed in a particular spatial array) may depend upon nondominant function to some degree. Do not test extremely rote calculations, such as simple items from the multiplication tables, as these draw upon remote memories and associations.

3 Right–left orientation can be tested by asking the patient to specify whether a designated object is on the right or left. The object can be located on the patient, in space, or on the examiner. Alternatively, ask the patient to show a right or left body part, such as holding up the right thumb. These right–left abilities are associated with the dominant parietal lobe, but again may require particular spatial abilities (as well as language function) in some instances.

4 Apraxia is defined as the inability to carry out a task despite all the necessary individual abilities seemingly being present. Of the various kinds of apraxia, one commonly tested is "left-hand apraxia" in which a command to wave, pretend to brush teeth, etc., with the left hand is not accomplished. The failure occurs despite evidence of language comprehension of the task (as evidenced by performance with the right hand) and lack of weakness or incoordination in the left hand. This type of apraxia is particularly associated with callosal disruption – the left sided temporoparietal language center is effectively disconnected from right cortical motor areas. Other, more complex types of apraxia relate more obviously to "higher function," but this example was offered because of its relative simplicity.

5 Difficulty in changing mental "set" (attention and orientation to a particular task or pattern of activity) is associated with frontal lobe dysfunction. A "card sort" test requires the patient to sort the cards into piles according to one criterion, such as suit. If then the task is shifted to sorting by odd or even numbers, for example, the patient may have trouble making this change. Clearly, this type of task that requires "switching gears" can be accomplished in many simple ways at the bedside or in the clinic.

SUMMARY OF ASSESSMENT OF HIGHER FUNCTIONS

There are various approaches to the evaluation of higher functions (apart from standard mental status and language testing).

1 Follow up clues from the history or other parts of the neurologic examination. For example, if a patient complains of trouble with eyesight, but you cannot find significant abnormalities of acuity, or fields, or eye movements, you should pursue tests of more complex visual comprehension and performance.

2 Look for deficits in functions that are known to be closely associated topographically with abnormalities that have already been identified. For example, if a patient has difficulty with writing (dysgraphia), you should be sure to include tests of calculation in your examination, since both of these are associated with the dominant parietal lobe. You can look up these clusterings of localized functions in standard medical and neurologic texts.

3 Start with a short list of mainly nonverbal "higher" functions:

(a) calculations;
(b) right–left distinction;
(c) spatial orientation;
(d) picture recognition;
(e) attention to left side of body and space;
(f) insight into deficit.

4 Use a textbook of neurology, behavioral neurology, or neuropsychology to conduct an in-depth and systematic survey of higher functions. This will probably seem tedious to you until your imagination is captured by an actual patient problem that confronts you or is vividly described (see Further reading section).

SUMMARY

Priorities

1 Attention: observe concentration and attentiveness generally and, if in doubt, test specifically (ability to register a memory task, digit span, serial subtractions, etc.). Unless attention is adequate, memory and cognitive tasks cannot be properly evaluated. Also, observe for particular kinds of inattention, such as neglect of the left side of space.

2 Recent memory: never assume it is present or intact unless you can cite incontrovertible evidence of retention and capacity for new learning. You may gain such evidence during the interview, but otherwise test it specifically.

3 Language: various forms of aphasia and confusional disorders often

mimic each other. If either language or thinking seems confused, test naming, repetition, following commands, reading, and writing.

Pitfalls

1 Mistaking an adequate fund of knowledge (reflecting remote memory) for normal recent memory.
2 Taking a poor mental status performance at face value rather than further analyzing its sources. These might include anxiety, depression, cultural differences, as well as retardation or dementia. Assess the ability to profit from clues, to improve with repetition and encouragement, to perform better when tasks are presented in alternative ways. Engage the patient affectively in the process of mental status testing. The goal is to determine how well the patient can do, not how badly.
3 Misinterpreting intermittent "memory lapses" as indicative of deteriorating memory capacity. Sporadic interference with registering or recalling information may be due to episodic events, such as seizure discharges, while memory performance is entirely normal at other times.
4 Divorcing the mental status examination from the patient's interests, background, and particular capabilities. Such attention helps to set reasonable expectations for normal cognitive performance or, at least, lack of deterioration.
5 Presuming that poor performance in the low-output patient reflects dementia, when actually there are insufficient data to judge. Beware of overlooking depressive pseudodementia.

PROBLEMS FOR SELF-STUDY

Problems

1 An elderly patient is thought by her family to be mentally normal, but on testing cannot perform the serial 7 test or name the Presidents back to Kennedy. Is the family missing something?
2 A middle-aged patient is brought in by his family because of the vague complaint that he is "not acting himself." He says nothing is wrong – he just wants "to live a little before I get too old." Formal mental status testing is within normal limits. Are you prepared to reassure the family?

Comments

1 No judgment should be made without assessing the patient's cultural and educational background, as well as her baseline cognitive status. Attention should be retested in a way that does not depend on calculations. Fund of knowledge should be assessed within a familiar context. If attention is adequate, test recent memory and other cognitive functions, with expectations adjusted to the patient's prior capabilities.
2 Recognizing that conventional bedside formal mental status testing is grossly inadequate to assess personality and behavioral changes,

such as disinhibition, consider the following points. (a) More detailed history from family and friends, emphasizing specific occurrences of altered behavior, perceived personality changes, or impaired judgment. (b) Additional interviewing to extend your personal observations of his behavior and to offer the patient a chance to "open up" about current interests, future plans, frustrations, reactions to events affecting his life, etc. (c) Further detailed physical neurologic examination, emphasizing items such as frontal release reflexes, as well as speech, comportment, and mental status. (d) Formal neuropsychologic testing. (e) Brain imaging, to rule out tumors and other lesions, especially in the anterior frontal lobes or temporal lobes that might be relatively "silent" on examination. (f) Other tests such as cerebrospinal fluid sampling for signs of inflammation and infection, electroencephalogram, etc., if warranted after imaging.

FURTHER READING

Alexander, M.P., Naeser, M.A., Palumbo, C. Broca's area aphasias: aphasia after lesions including the frontal operculum. *Neurology* 1990; 40:353–62. Evidence supporting an updated view and differentiation of aphasias commonly called "Broca's."

Cassem, E.H. Behavioral and emotional disturbances. In: Wilson, J.D., Braunwald, E., Isselbacher, K.J., *et al.* (eds) *Harrison's Principles of Internal Medicine*. 12th edn. McGraw-Hill, New York (NY), 1991. An introduction to the subject; includes the mini-mental status examination, which has drawbacks but has promoted standardized bedside testing.

Damasio, A.R. Aphasia. *New Engl J Med* 1992; 326:531–9. An authoritative, accessible, and concise review of the current understanding of aphasias, including the role of subcortical nuclei in the neural networks subserving language.

Glick, T.H. *The Process of Neurologic Care in Medical Practice*. Harvard University Press, Cambridge (MA), 1984. Interactions of patient and physician behaviors, and "integrated" mental status assessment (Chapter 6 and pp. 87–99).

Kirshner, H. *Behavioral Neurology: A Practical Approach*. Churchill Livingstone, Edinburgh, 1985. A readable, efficient survey of disorders of attention, cognition, language, and behavior.

Lazare, A. (ed.) *Outpatient Psychiatry: Diagnosis and Treatment*. 2nd edn. Williams and Wilkins, Baltimore (MD), 1989. Mental status and behavioral evaluation from a psychiatric point of view (discussed in Chapters 12–14, 16).

Margolin, D.I. Cognitive neuropsychology. Resolving enigmas about Wernicke's aphasia and other higher cortical disorders. *Arch Neurol* 1991; 48:751–65. Informative article on neuropsychology and cerebral localization, with special reference to posterior aphasias.

Mesulam, M-M. *Principles of Behavioral Neurology*. F.A. Davis, Philadelphia (PA), 1985. Leading text in the field, broad in scope and rich in detail: for the serious reader.

Mesulam, M-M. Large-scale neurocognitive networks and distributed processing for attention, language, and memory. *Ann Neurol* 1990; 28:597–613. Exposition of a modern reconciliation (distributed processing) of traditional arguments over discrete localization vs. diffuse substrates.

Nicholi, A.M. Jr (ed.) *New Harvard Guide to Psychiatry*. Harvard University Press, Cambridge (MA), 1988. The psychiatric history and mental status examination (Chapter 2) are discussed by Nicholi, and Mesulam writes on the neural substrates of behavior: the effects of brain lesions upon mental state (Chapter 5).

Simon, R.P., Aminoff, M.J., Greenberg, D.A. *Clinical Neurology*. Appleton and Lange, Norwalk (CT), 1989. An introduction to disorders of cognitive function: Chapter 1 (Approach to diagnosis) and 2 (Acute confusional states, and dementia).

Squire, L. *Memory and Brain*. Oxford University Press, New York (NY), 1987. In-depth reference on memory, its neuroanatomic substrate, and revealing examples of pathology.

Strub, R., Black, F. *The Mental Status Examination in Neurology*. 2nd edn. F.A. Davis, Philadelphia (PA), 1985. A good introduction to the subject for those who want to delve further into formal mental status testing.

Strub, R., Black, F. *Neurobehavioral Disorders: A Clinical Approach*. F.A. Davis, Philadelphia (PA), 1988. More on abnormal mental status and behavior, suitably pitched for the student or house officer.

Victor, M., Adams, R.D., Collins, G.H. *The Wernicke–Korsakoff Syndrome and Related Neurologic Disorders Due to Alcoholism and Malnutrition*. 2nd edn. F.A. Davis, Philadelphia (PA), 1989. The definitive text, based upon extensive, direct, clinical and pathologic study.

chapter 11

The Examination as a Whole: Overview and Write-up

A reprise

Having been introduced to all the major components of a neurologic examination, you are now in a position to "put it all together."

A number of issues, some of which have been touched upon in preceding chapters, should now be addressed directly.

1 Format and sequence of the neurologic examination:
(a) integration of the neurologic with the general physical examination; approaching the examination regionally or by neurologic system;
(b) the order of doing the neurologic examination;
(c) neurologic stress testing.

2 Measurement, grading, and observation:
(a) measurement of structure and function;
(b) grading systems;
(c) observing the whole: positive and negative features.

3 Recording the examination:
(a) a "long form";
(b) a "shorter form" and a "brief form";
(c) check lists.

4 Obstacles to a good neurologic examination.

5 Explaining the examination to the patient.
6 The neurologic examination and technology.

FORMAT AND SEQUENCE OF THE NEUROLOGIC EXAMINATION

The format of the neurologic examination should promote the following goals:
1 to facilitate important comparisons (and make differences more memorable);
2 to help avoid unintended omissions;
3 to promote efficiency by minimizing repetition and change of directions to the patient.

In performing the examination, neurologists tend to proceed system by system rather than region by region: they test motor functions throughout the limbs and subsequently reflexes throughout the limbs, rather than testing arm strength, reflexes, pulse, blood pressure, etc., and then going on to another part of the body. The system by system approach facilitates the comparison of strength, for example, between the two arms and between arms and legs. Efficiency is at stake also: when you give directions for resistive strength testing, most patients quickly catch on to the idea and do not need to be told to pull or resist for each new muscle group tested. If you move from testing strength, to sensation, to pulses, and on to joint examinations, your directions must frequently change and the whole process must be repeated for the next limb.

In contrast to a systematic examination, you will recognize certain problems, for example, low back and leg pain, that require a focused, regional approach at least initially: motor, sensory, reflex, vascular, and musculoskeletal examinations would be performed on the involved extremity, before deciding whether to survey these functions elsewhere (see Chapter 19).

INTEGRATION OF THE NEUROLOGIC EXAMINATION WITH THE GENERAL PHYSICAL EXAMINATION

In patients without neurologic complaints (as will be discussed in Chapter 19), simple observation in the course of the general examination will provide many of the neurologic data that you need; the few other specific tests required can be done in the course of the general examination of the head and neck, trunk, and limbs.

For patients who require a more thorough neurologic examination, I suggest that you start by maintaining formal neurologic testing as a more or less separate part of the overall examination. Once you have become adept and comfortable with the comprehensive neurologic assessment, adapt your method to the occasion and to the format that works best for you. Clearly, to do a thorough, system by system neurologic examination on many general medical, surgical, or obstetric patients would be like "the tail wagging the dog." But premature fragmentation of the examination will risk serious errors of omission in patients who deserve a thorough evaluation.

Order of examination

When you need to work-up a patient with a major neurologic problem, the following approach should be considered.

1 Obtain your initial mental status and behavioral data as you greet the patient and take a history. Observe the kinds, quantity, and appropriateness of mental and physical output. Look not only for structural and behavioral details, but try to capture a sense of the patient as a whole.

2 Include the cervical vascular examination, the funduscopic, and inspection of the tongue and throat with your general examination of the head and neck.

3 Otherwise, examine cranial nerve functions in order, as part of the neurologic examination proper.

4 For motor assessment, test limb and neck tone (resistance to passive movement) and resistive strength. Inspection of the musculature and observation for involuntary limb movements, muscle twitches, etc., can be done as various parts of the body are exposed throughout the examination as a whole.

5 Sensory testing should be done systematically, except that facial sensation is usually included with cranial nerve functions. The Romberg test (while stressing proprioception) can be accomplished at the same time as testing of stance and gait.

6 Part of the coordination examination can be fulfilled by observing stance, gait, speech, and spontaneous movements of the limbs throughout the history and general examination. However, specific tasks of limb coordination (such as finger–nose, finger-tapping, rapid alternating hand movements, heel–shin, heel-tapping, and tandem gait) benefit from immediate comparison of performance of right vs. left, arms vs. legs.

7 Deep tendon (stretch) reflexes are best tested in sequence, moving back and forth from one side to the other. Depending on the case, these are followed by the "pathologic reflexes" – always check the plantar responses – and corticobulbar reflexes. The superficial abdominal reflexes, if tested, are best checked before abdominal palpation. If anal reflexes or sensation are to be tested, these are done at the time of the rectal examination. The corneal and palatal (gag) reflexes can be examined with the other cranial nerve functions.

8 Having obtained initial, informal mental status and behavioral information earlier, now complete this evaluation, employing more formal and detailed testing as indicated (see Chapter 10).

Modifications

This basic order offers a systematic approach that will facilitate comparisons and minimize omissions. However, any tests that may seem stressful, painful, or embarrassing to the patient, should ordinarily be performed at the end of the examination. Be prepared to modify your regular order in particular patients; do not leave key components of the examination until the patient is overtired, irritated, or otherwise less cooperative. This applies particularly to ill or hospitalized patients and to aspects of the examination that require attentive participation. For example, if a patient complains primarily of abnormal sensory symptoms, consider testing sensation before becoming involved in arduous motor testing.

NEUROLOGIC STRESS TESTING

Testing a neurologic function can be approached from opposite directions: from easy to hard or from hard to easy. To test balance you can begin with the simplest tasks, such as standing and walking, and then progress to more demanding maneuvers, such as walking heel-to-toe (tandem gait) or standing on one foot with eyes closed. Success with easier tests demonstrates only that some functions exist, but not that they are normal. Success with difficult tasks quickly confirms very good, and probably intact, function, unless a history of subtle decline suggests otherwise.

Stress tests

Challenging the higher ranges of neurologic function (in an examination situation) might be called "neurologic stress testing." In order to stress the system sufficiently, you may need to simulate real-life activities, such as comprehending the substance of a difficult paragraph, as opposed to simply reading and remembering a test sentence or two. Even so, more demanding tests will not necessarily address the mental qualities needed by a physicist or the coordinated finesse of a fast typist. The stress is relative: what challenges one patient may bore another.

In practice, stress tests are efficient if the patient succeeds, but inefficient if the patient fails. Your elderly patient has difficulty walking heel-to-toe (tandem gait): does poor eyesight, leg weakness, balance, or anxiety play a role? What part of the test system accounts for the difficulty? You will need to go back to simpler tasks to clarify the reason for impaired performance. Overwhelming a patient's capacities at the outset may result in undermining his or her confidence, which will need to be restored in order to make the most of further testing.

Facilitation

As you develop competence in neurologic examination, you will probably find it best to proceed from easier tests to harder ones in order to build confidence and not complicate interpretation. In taking this approach you will run the risk of initially requiring tests that seem too simple or even silly, but a brief explanation will usually suffice: "These are routine tests designed to check how well your body is working. I hope you will bear with them." Then, as the difficulty of the tests increases, the patient will come to recognize the challenge involved and you will be able to observe at what point and in what way performance falls short of the mark.

MEASUREMENT, GRADING, AND OBSERVATION

Structure and function

You have already encountered semiquantitative measurements in the examination of pulses, reflexes, and resistive strength. In some areas of assessment more precise measurements can be made (especially with technologic assistance); in others your ingenuity will be taxed even to fashion a verbal description of what you observe. While structure and function are integrally related, our main access to the nervous system is through performance. In contrast to the skin, for example, the neuromuscular system reveals itself more by how it works than by how it looks or feels, and we measure responses more than structures themselves. An acutely "weak muscle" is not shrunken. Similarly, a patient may become acutely blind from optic nerve disease without the optic discs showing any signs.

Quantitation

In general, the degree of attempted quantitation at the bedside should be appropriate to the accuracy and precision of observation: there would be little point in grading the briskness of reflex responses on a 1–10 scale if the observer can reproducibly distinguish only trace, low, moderate, and high levels of reaction. For tests requiring active patient participation, variable or incomplete effort may obscure subtle intrinsic differences. Strength testing obviously depends on the will to exert. Rather precise measurement of certain sensory perceptions, such as the duration of a vibratory stimulus, can be made at the bedside, but the result is only as good as the patient's attention and communication ability: slow or unreliable reporting stultifies precise quantitation of perception. Pain, or guarding against anticipated pain, also influences output, often in an erratic way. If a patient fears that sudden exertion (as in testing arm strength) may precipitate a painful spasm, guarding will be excessive and output reduced. The most that can then be documented by grading is the peak level actually observed; the patient can perform up to that level, but might do even better under different circumstances, for example, when less tired, in less pain, and better motivated.

To recapitulate, the observations and tests that you wish to document may run a gamut from changes in fixed structures to the most complex human functions. At each level you should continually explore ways to make your observations more accurate and measurements more precise.

Measuring structures

Some external structures that can be directly measured are listed below:

1 circumference of the head;

2 degrees of lateral curvature of the spine (scoliosis);

3 circumference of a limb (such as the lower leg, mainly reflecting the bulk of the calf muscles);

4 diameter of the pupil (variable).

Measuring output

Tests of function can be graded, utilizing variables such as the following:

1 duration (length of perception of a vibrating stimulus);
2 intensity of stimulus – threshold of perception (amplitude of sound);
3 linear distance (width of base in stance or gait, or length of stride);
4 frequency (oscillations in tremor).

Most grading done at the bedside is not highly precise, but even a crude semiquantitation often serves better than mere qualitative impressions. With technical assistance, precise measurements of almost any function can be made (see Further reading section), but other sources of variability, such as motivation, need also to be taken into account. Since we are ultimately interested in whether a patient functions normally in ordinary human activities and reactions, consider the kinds of observation you can make. These include the following:

Assessing function

1 spontaneous activities:
   (a) volitional motor activity (standing up and walking);
   (b) semivoluntary activity (fidgeting);
   (c) autonomic activity (natural breathing).
2 responses to ordinary external stimuli:
   (a) startle to sudden, loud sound;
   (b) verbal and nonverbal responses when spoken to;
   (c) glancing towards movement in the visual periphery.
3 practical operational capabilities:
   (a) activities of daily living (climbing a flight of stairs, brushing one's teeth, or putting on a coat);
   (b) ability to divide attention; doing two or more things simultaneously (note the colloquial deprecation, "He can't walk and chew gum at the same time").

You will encounter most difficulty in assessing higher aspects of human performance, for example:

1 ability to show initiative;
2 creativity;
3 ability to operate under stress;
4 capacity to deal with novel situations.

Such expressions of human performance and potential become significant issues in assessment of early dementia and in other insidious deteriorations.

Grading systems: a summary

The three most common grading systems apply to tendon reflexes, strength, and pulses, and are set out in Table 11.1. As noted, tendon jerks are usually graded on a 0–4 scale. The response is often documented at the appropriate joint on a stick figure with ++, for example, and the translation therefore becomes 2+ (two plusses). The plus does not signify "greater than 2," but rather just 2. Similarly, pulses (such as the carotids) are often described as 2+, again meaning 2 on a scale of 0–4.

Table 11.1 Grading systems applicable to reflexes, pulses, and strength

Tendon reflexes (see Chapter 9)	Arterial pulses (see Chapter 4)	Strength (see Chapter 6)
0–4	0–4	0–5
(0, 1+, 2+, 3+, 4+)	(0, 1+, 2+, 3+, 4+)	(0, 1, 2, 3, 4−, 4, 4+, 5)

In contrast, however, resistive muscle strength is most often graded on a 0–5 scale. In this system, 3/5 indicates ability to resist gravity only, whole 4/5 signifies strength against active resistance. However, 4/5 covers such a wide range, from feeble resistance to almost normal, that it is advisable to qualify 4/5 further. This can be accomplished by interpolating plusses or minuses. Thus 4+/5 means greater than straight 4 (not simply 4, as would be the case with reflexes or pulses). This problem can be obviated by using a wider scale, a decimal (4.5/5), or some other transitional notation (4–5/5). Do not confuse 4/5 (4 on a scale of 5) with a left/right comparison, such as 3/4 (3L/4R).

POSITIVE AND NEGATIVE SIGNS

As you think about the entirety of the neurologic examination – observing and testing structure and function in physical and mental respects – you will recognize that some abnormal signs literally jump out at you, and others represent an absence of normal activity. The clonic jerks of a limb during a focal seizure typify one type of positive sign, while the momentary lapses in speech that occur in an absence seizure are negative. (Similarly, vertigo is a positive symptom and low energy a negative one.) Some positive signs are active, occurring spontaneously (for example, a resting tremor). Others need to be elicited (like a Babinski sign). To pick up negative signs you need to be actively on the lookout for them: is something missing?

CASE 11A
Slowing down

A 71-year-old retired professor was referred for neurologic evaluation because of "failure to thrive." Successful treatment of an arthritic condition did not seem to be combating the general slowing down that his wife had noticed. Observation revealed an unusually soft voice, a paucity of facial expression, and a slow gait, with diminished arm swing.

These signs were all negative. They were picked up as important neurologic signs only because observers "stood back" far enough to gain an overall impression – to see what was missing as well as what was there. The pattern of signs suggested a diagnosis of Parkinson's disease. A negative sign, like the unblinking countenance of a parkinsonian patient, may "stare you in the face," but still taxes your powers of observation (see also Case 8A).

CASE 11A *(continued)*

On further specific testing, cogwheel rigidity in both arms was demonstrated, and subsequently a slight resting tremor in the hands appeared. (No weakness, excessive fatigue, cerebellar type of ataxia, thyroid or other metabolic derangement, or depression was evident.)

Of the positive signs, the cogwheel rigidity must be elicited, whereas a resting tremor is evident across the room. For the patient, tremor usually proves less disabling than the negative phenomenon of akinesia, a decrease or slowness of motor activity, coupled with difficulty initiating movements. In general, diminished or absent function takes more of a toll on activities of daily living than signs that are overtly displayed. A slow reduction in activity is frequently not even recognized by the family or clinician as a manifestation of disease. In retrospect, the professor and his wife agreed that the onset of his slowing down could be dated back at least 2 years. Thus, Parkinson's disease, a treatable condition, often escapes medical attention until disability is quite far advanced or positive signs supervene.

Paradoxically, the clinical concept of positive and negative signs does not necessarily correspond to the underlying mechanism. What might seem to be positive clinically may, in fact, turn out to be negative physiologically. For example, asterixis, or so-called liver flap (seen mainly in metabolic encephalopathies), is a positive sign that can be elicited: the dorsiflexed, outstretched hands show quick, downward jerk-like movements or flaps. These are not actually positive muscle contractions, but rather electromyographically silent: they are momentary lapses of the previously assumed posture (with an acute corrective phase after the lapse). Whatever the mechanism, a lapse is as important as a jerk. Slowing down is as noteworthy as speeding up – which is, in fact, what some parkinsonian patients experience: they may "freeze" in their tracks on one occasion, while on another they may rush forward (festinate), as if to catch up with their center of gravity.

RECORDING THE NEUROLOGIC EXAMINATION: LONG AND SHORT FORMS

Like the examination itself, documentation in the record has specific goals, but no particular style is infallible. Recording the examination ensures the following:

1 communication with other care-givers;
2 you will be able to remember findings with sufficient accuracy and detail in the future;
3 imposing a form of quality control on your examination: remind yourself of omissions, stimulate clearer observations, and make better connections between one part of the examination and another;
4 provide a record for legal and administrative purposes.

In theory, all observations made are worth recording, either as positives or negatives. In practice, for the sake of efficiency, we usually describe in detail only the abnormal findings and those that are useful to quantitate as baseline data. However, it is important to indicate specifically what tests have been done, and not use self-serving but vague terms such as "neurologic (examination) physiologic" or "nonfocal." Impressions should not substitute for description in recording the examination: specify what the patient did and did not do in practical terms. Do not describe the findings of the language examination as an "expressive aphasia" or the difficulty with walking as a "cerebellar gait."

You may recall the very first case illustration presented in this book (Case 1A), in which a 19-year-old college sophomore experienced a seizure. She described feeling a contortion in her face and witnessed her left arm shaking uncontrollably, while mentally feeling momentarily overwhelmed by some ineffable force. While under evaluation she developed left face and arm twitching which progressed to a generalized tonic–clonic convulsion. Her complete examination was not documented then, but will be presented here, as an illustration of a thorough write-up. Some neurology clerkships require this level of detail. Residents often provide such detail selectively, in areas of special concern. Following this "long form," a "shorter form" and "brief" record will demonstrate practical compromises between comprehensive documentation and inadequate detail.

"Long form" examination write-up (Case 1A)

Objective

On neurologic examination (9.15 am) the patient appeared alert and very articulate, but severely anxious.

Head

No abnormalities of shape; no palpable defects or tenderness. Blowing, moderately high-pitched bruit lasting through most of systole, heard over the right orbit and less well over the right temple. Superficial temporal pulses 2+ symmetric. Normal funduscopic bilaterally with spontaneous venous pulsations; no papilledema, hemorrhages, abnormal vessels, or optic pallor.

Neck

Full range of motion without tenderness. Carotid pulses 2+ bilaterally. No bruit on left. Right: a continuous low-pitched rushing sound heard over the right anterolateral neck from the clavicle to the angle of the jaw; increased with inspiration and markedly diminished with moderate pressure over the anterolateral neck, at the angle of the jaw – not obliterating the carotid pulse.

Cranial nerves

1 Identified smell of cloves with each nostril.

2 Visual acuity: "20/20" (corrected) with pocket screening card, o.u. (both eyes). Visual fields: normal in each eye to finger confrontation and to a 5 mm white test object. No extinction on double simultaneous stimulation.

3, 4, 6 Pupils 5 mm equal and briskly reactive to light and accommodation. Extraocular movements full horizontally and vertically; no nystagmus, no ptosis.

5 Motor: firm masseter and temporalis contractions and no jaw deviation on forced opening. Sensory: normal touch, pin, and cold in upper, mid, and lower face bilaterally. Corneal: brisk, direct, and consensual reactions bilaterally.

7 Forehead wrinkling full and symmetric. On forced eye closure, eyelashes buried less fully on the left; with eyes open, left palpebral fissure slightly wider than right. Left nasolabial fold slightly flattened; upon showing teeth left side of the mouth moved less well than the right; no droop at rest or with spontaneous smiling. Taste not tested.

8 Auditory acuity normal to 512 Hz tuning fork. Air conduction greater than bone conduction bilaterally; Weber midline.

9, 10 Brisk bilateral and symmetric gag and palate elevation. Phonation and swallowing normal.

11 Forced head turning to right and left and head flexion, all full strength. Shoulder shrug strong and symmetric.

12 Tongue protruded in the midline and

outpouched well in both cheeks. No fasciculations or atrophy.

Motor system (patient right-handed)

Muscle bulk: normal throughout
Muscle tone: normal throughout
Adventitious movements: no fasciculations, tremor, flap, etc.
Strength: resistive strength entirely normal on the right and in the left leg; slight weakness in the left upper extremity.

		(Scale 1–5)
Arm:	abduction	4+
	extension	4+
	external rotation	4+
	internal rotation	5
Forearm:	flexion	4+
	extension	4
	pronation	4+
	supination	4+
Hand:	dorsiflexion at wrist	4
	abduction of the fingers	4
	flexion at wrist	4+
	opposition of the thumb	4+
	flexion of distal phalanges	4+

Sensory system

Light touch: normal threshold and subjective feeling to cotton wisp on distal and proximal extremities bilaterally.
Pin: normal threshold in upper and lower extremities bilaterally.
Temperature (cold): subjectively normal and symmetric on right and left limbs.
Joint position sense: normal to fine movements in thumbs and toes.
Vibratory sense: normal threshold in fingers and toes bilaterally.
Discriminative ("cortical") modalities: normal graphesthesia and stereognosis (coins) in both hands. Normal touch localization and symmetric two-point discrimination on palms.
Romberg test: normal.

Coordination

Finger–nose test: normal.
Finger-tapping movements in the left hand slower than expected for handedness (right). Rapid supination/pronation slower

	on left, but ?consistent with handedness (right). Heel–shin and heel-tapping tests: normal. Gait: normal including tandem. Speech: normal rhythm and articulation.
Reflexes (can also be shown on a stick figure)	Deep tendon reflexes — *Right* / *Left* Brachioradialis 1+ 2+ Biceps 2+ 3+ Triceps 2+ 3+ Knee jerks 2+ 2+ Ankle jerks 2+ 2+ Others: the right plantar response flexor, left neutral. Superficial abdominal reflexes present in all quadrants. Chvostek negative. No snout, jaw jerk, or grasp reflex.
Back	Spine: straight, full range of motion, no tenderness
Mental status (2 hours after witnessed seizure)	Mental status appeared entirely normal with appropriate affect and a very responsive, perceptive, and verbal manner; fully oriented; normal concentration and attention; answered with precision and showed an excellent recall for previous items of our conversation and history; recalled a four-line story perfectly after 5 minutes; calculations (such as total value of one of each type of coin) done quickly and accurately; no left–right confusion; proverbs quickly and appropriately abstracted; read a complex test paragraph aloud and with excellent comprehension; complex three-step commands involving right and left done correctly; no paraphasic errors in speech; naming and repetition normal; writing to dictation grammatic and handwriting legible (example saved); accurate description of items in a picture; drawings (clock face and cube) done very well (drawings saved).

"Shorter form" write-up

The examination in Case 1A can also be presented in summary form, still documenting the positive findings and the most important pertinent negatives. Economy is achieved by omitting much of the detail and extent of the normal findings. This is more like the examination note that a senior neurology resident or an attending might write. As you gain experience you will be better able to judge the degree of documentation that is really useful.

Objective

Examination (9.15 am): patient alert, but severely anxious.

Head	Right orbit and temple: blowing, moderately high-pitched bruit, nearly pansystolic. Superficial temporal pulses 2+ symmetric. Normal funduscopic bilaterally with spontaneous venous pulsations.
Neck	Carotid pulses 2+ bilaterally. Left: no bruit. Right: continuous low-pitched rushing sound over the right anterolateral neck from clavicle to angle of jaw. Increased with inspiration, markedly diminished with moderate pressure over the anterolateral neck, at the angle of the jaw – not obliterating the carotid pulse.
Cranial nerves	CN 2–12 within normal limits (WNL) except on left side of face: decreased eyelash burying, nasolabial fold, mouth movement with grimace; slightly increased palpebral fissure; forehead symmetric. Pupils 5 mm, briskly reactive bilaterally.
Motor system (patient right-handed)	Strength: normal on right and in the left leg. Slight weakness in the left upper extremity: 4+/5 at all groups except 4/5 extension at elbow, dorsiflexion at wrist, finger spreading; 5/5 internal rotation of arm.
Sensory system	Normal primary and discriminative modalities.
Coordination	Normal limb coordination except finger-tapping movements on left hand slower than expected for handedness. Stance, Romberg, gait including tandem within normal limits.
Reflexes (can also be shown on a stick figure)	Deep tendon reflexes: Brachioradialis 2+ left, 1+ right; biceps, triceps 3+ left, 2+ right; knee and ankle jerks 2+; right plantar response flexor, left neutral.
Mental status (2 hours after witnessed seizure)	Mental status appeared entirely normal with appropriate affect. Fully oriented. Normal concentration, attention, and recent memory. Speech conversationally normal. Drawings (clock, cube) normal.

"Brief form" write-up

Anyone familiar with medical records will be fully aware that even more condensed write-ups are the rule. Even when patients on a medical service have neurologic problems, the format is apt to resemble the following (examination of a different patient):

Alert oriented ×3 (person, place, and time).
Carotids: no bruits; neck supple; *discs* sharp.
CN 2–12: within normal limits (WNL).
Motor: WNL.
Sensory: WNL.
Coordination: finger–nose WNL; heel–shin: side-to-side tremor (bilateral); ataxic, wide-based gait; Romberg normal.
Reflexes: 2+ (shown with stick figure). Toes: ↓↓ (plantar responses flexor).

This is adequate in many respects, although more detail (JPS, ataxia, etc.) would be desirable. As will be discussed in Chapter 19, some additional specification (e.g. pupillary size and reactivity) is valuable as baseline information.

Examination check lists

Preprinted examination check lists are very helpful for assisting good documentation of the examination, if used thoughtfully. Such forms will remind you of omissions and can encourage specification of what tests have been done. For now, use whatever forms or formats are provided or specified. Later, in practice, you may wish to adopt a preprinted form that suits you.

OBSTACLES TO A GOOD NEUROLOGIC EXAMINATION

Blocks to an effective examination result from both patient-based and clinician-based factors. Some problems arise from specific alterations in the patient's level of consciousness, responsiveness, communicative abilities, and behavior. Despite major obstacles, some very useful observations can be made, even in the presence of coma. Patients should never be written off as "unexaminable." How to obtain a data base from "difficult to examine" patients is discussed in Chapter 18.

Pressures on the examiner

Your own pressures and stresses also affect the examination. Just as the patient may display various forms of negativism, you will find yourself at times feeling negative about having to examine a certain patient. Excessive time pressure is a major obstacle to a good neurologic examination, especially when mental status and behavioral issues are at stake or sensation needs to be examined in detail. By the same token, severe fatigue can quickly erode your thoroughness. When examining under the duress of time pressure or fatigue, realities that cannot be easily altered, try to diagnose yourself and find constructive means of compensation: seek direct assistance from others and ask for help in establishing priorities (see Chapter 12, section on rapid emergency formulation). Specify any important omission in your problem list (this enables you to finish the examination at a later stage, if the patient's condition permits delay). Most importantly, guard against fabricating any findings.

Perfunctory performance

Finally, the greatest hindrance to a good examination may be narrow-minded thinking. If you force your approach to the examination into a rigid format, losing sight of the real goals of assessment and the special situation of each individual patient, you will miss much of value. A perfunctory examination, directed more towards avoiding criticism than successful problem solving, will neither help the patient nor satisfy you.

EXPLAINING THE EXAMINATION TO THE PATIENT

Overview examination

As a rule, the patient who understands the purpose of the neurologic examination will participate in it more effectively. The process of examination can also benefit the patient in terms of better informed self-observation and self-testing. For you, learning to describe the examination in lay terms will increase your efficiency.

Patients can relate quickly to the purpose of some parts of the examination, such as strength testing. However, many patients are not aware that by testing muscular strength you are also testing connections that run all the way from the front half of the brain through the spinal cord and out through nerves to the muscles. With this knowledge the patient can understand the rationale for testing parts of the body that may be remote from the focus of symptoms, such as headaches.

Some parts of the examination may stimulate the patient's interest and curiosity. The funduscopic examination serves to illustrate this point: the idea that the back of the eye is so revealing – that you can actually see a bit of the central nervous system (the optic nerve head), as well as many details of arteries and veins – fascinates many patients.

On the other hand, certain test procedures strike patients as intimidating, embarrassing, silly, or weird. Some patients will bring to your examination the burden of prior, off-putting experiences with particular aspects of testing. The prospect of pin testing may provoke anxiety unless you offer explanation and reassurance. The perineal sensory and reflex examination (see Chapter 19) is awkward, at best; certainly, perineal testing may produce discomfort if not accomplished with care, but even more important is the sense of humiliation or resentment that may linger if the purpose of the particular procedure is not understood. A patient with urinary incontinence will more readily appreciate the need for a thorough perineal examination if you explain the reason: a neurologic abnormality that results in loss of urinary control can also cause numbness in the genital and anal areas ("the nerves run together").

Whether, when, and how much to explain

Remember that most people never have had a thorough neurologic examination: they are likely to be familiar with knee jerk reflex testing and parts of the eye examination, but little more. The neurologic examination is not only quite unfamiliar, but much longer than any other part of the physical examination. Patients often express surprise at so many strange tests and thus appreciate some items of explanation.

The extent and timing of any explanatory comments should ideally be individualized, that is, based upon your assessment of the patient through the preceding parts of the encounter or from past interactions. Moreover, you will need to experiment with different styles of commentary until you find a mode that is congenial and adaptable. For starting purposes, imagine the questions that would arise in the mind of a (nonmedical) member of your family, if subjected to a neurologic examination. Try (within limits of time) to comment briefly on those tests that you think might arouse the greatest concern.

Preferably, offer any comments to the patient before you do the test or just as you are starting rather than after completion. But if a patient is stimulated to ask you a subsequent question ("I noticed that my reflexes are low – does that explain why I was never good at athletics?") you should, of course, respond. You might say, "There is a great deal of normal variation in reflexes. Your reflexes are normal. Brisker reflexes are not better; the reflexes I am testing now do not measure your coordination."

Ordinarily you will probably prefer to discuss the results of your examination after all parts of it are completed. This does not mean, however, that as you proceed you cannot occasionally mention that a test is normal. Especially if your examination is lengthy, as it might be in looking at the fundi, a brief word is reassuring. When you have finished, it will usually be appropriate to provide feedback on your findings, for example, "Your examination is mostly normal, but there are a few points I want your eye doctor to check further." Or yet again, "You told me that your feet feel numb, and I find that you don't feel touch and vibration as well as expected. This helps me to understand your symptoms better, and we can now plan some tests to help get to the bottom of the problem."

THE NEUROLOGIC EXAMINATION AND TECHNOLOGY

Over the years, attempts have been made to achieve greater quantification of neurologic testing, at least in part through the application of technology. For sensory testing there have been hairs calibrated for stiffness so as to provide a quantifiable and reproducible touch stimulus; electric current can produce precisely graded noxious stimuli; strength is assessed with dynamometers and other devices. These have had little appeal to generalists; nor do most neurologists utilize such techniques in daily practice.

In fact, what seems to have happened in large measure is that technologic advances have been accepted more for localizing lesions and elucidating pathology and pathogenesis than for quantification of the examination. Technology has largely leapfrogged over the primary clinical data base towards the definition of the disease process itself. To be sure, in certain areas, technologic methods have exploited improved sensitivity and quantification to achieve better data for localization. For example, in the complex world of nystagmus, the use of electronystagmograms, often combined with quantitative caloric testing, produces superior localizing data. Videotaping has enhanced the study of movement disorders, but, even more, the prolonged video monitoring of suspected epilepsy patients, combined with ongoing electroencephalogram recording, allows for a much higher level of correct seizure diagnosis in difficult cases. Similarly, physiologic sleep monitoring (polysomnography) couples actual observation with quantitative recording of eye movements and electromyography. This enables specific diagnoses that the physician could only suspect from the history, but rarely would have the chance to observe.

Computer-based techniques for analysis of muscular performance or of balance and gait, have established a growing niche in rehabilitative medicine. Restorative programs can be planned in a quantitative fashion and progress plotted by means of detailed feedback on the parameters of motor output.

There is rather little presently to recommend to students, residents, generalists, or even neurologists in the way of new technologic aids for routine use in bedside examination. However, once the history, examination, and preliminary formulation have pointed the way, valuable new technologic resources are being made available to characterize the disease process itself. Imaging and additional selected neurodiagnostic methods will be outlined in Chapter 15. Reference to quantification in the neurologic examination will be found in the Further reading section.

SUMMARY

1 Technology is on the march, but do not wait for it to render the neurologic examination obsolete. Neuroimaging is liberating both the patient and the physician from anxiety over lurking lesions, such as brain tumors in headache cases. Ideally, this should leave you more time for the whole patient and for disease and injury prevention.
2 As time goes by you will find your own preferred way of integrating the neurologic examination with the general physical examination. I think it is helpful to preserve enough continuity in neurologic testing so that you can readily make comparisons (such as upper vs. lower extremities), minimize changes of position, and avoid repeating instructions (as in testing strength, tone, coordination, and sensation in upper and lower extremities).

3 Despite the fact that conventional neurologic grading systems for strength, reflexes, and pulses are clumsy and confusing, score and document key findings, especially abnormal ones. Doing so will make you a better observer and will facilitate communication with other care-givers. In general, you can combine efficiency with specificity by using an examination check list that allows for detailing important baseline and abnormal findings.
4 Pay attention to negative as well as positive signs and symptoms. Like white spaces in a work of art or rests in a musical score, neurologic performance is judged by what does not happen, as well as what does.
5 Without overdoing it, some ongoing explanation of the examination, while it is in progress, can reassure and educate the patient; also, offer encouragement frequently – neurologic assessment is a strange and intimidating process for many patients.

PROBLEMS FOR SELF-STUDY

Problems

1 A 27-year-old housewife presents with fatigue, which is most noticeable when she climbs up- and downstairs, walks substantial distances, and when she carries out her daily activities, especially later in the day. On examination she "appears sad, sort of down in the mouth." Her grips are strong and she is able to stand on heels and toes. What further aspects of her examination would you wish to emphasize?
2 A 77-year-old man is noted by his family to be growing increasingly subdued and isolated. He takes part much less in dinner table conversations and appears bored, often drowsing off into brief naps. No cardiovascular or other systemic problems are identified and he seems to be strong, have normal tone, and a normal gait for his age, as he is observed coming in and out of the consulting room. How would you analyze this presenting picture?

Comments

1 Fatigue and weakness, as negative symptoms, are often more disabling than positive symptoms and signs. In her case it would be important to grade proximal strength and functional motor performance (climbing stairs), and to do so late in the day at the peak of her symptoms. While evaluating for neuromuscular disorders such as myasthenia gravis, also consider depression, including metabolic causes.
2 This elderly man is also developing negative neurologic signs of diminishing output. More information from the family about his actual level of intellectual and physical function would be essential. How is he "at his best"? You should observe and elicit symptoms and signs of depression, but at the same time assess his mental status for evidence of coexistent dementia. Normal tone and gait make parkinsonism unlikely, but this possibility should be monitored in

later encounters. A thorough systemic, neurologic, and possibly psychiatric work-up is needed.

FURTHER READING

Koller, W.C. When does Parkinson's disease begin? *Neurology*, 1992; 42(Suppl. 4): 27–31. The negative signs of parkinsonism, such as "slowing down," may be difficult to recognize early, but they exemplify the need to consider the full dimensions of neurologic assessment in order to see the patient as a whole. This whole article considers biologic as well as clinical markers.

Munsat, T.L. *Quantification of Neurologic Deficits*. Butterworths, Boston (MA), 1989. For those curious about methods presently used only in specialized situations, but perhaps harbingers of future techniques.

Potvin, A.R., Tourtellotte, W.W. *Quantitative Examination of Neurologic Functions*. Vols I and II. CRC Press, Boca Raton (FL), 1985. More on quantification.

part 3

Systematic Formulation in Neurologic Diagnosis

chapter 12

Principles of Diagnostic Formulation

Introduction to Part 3

Finally, diagnosis! Clinical formulation caps your construction of a data base. As previewed in Chapter 1, Table 1.1, a comprehensive formulation of a neurologic problem has four parts:

1 anatomic (topographic localization);
2 pathologic (the disease or reaction of tissue);
3 pathogenetic (the mechanism of disease);
4 etiologic (the root causes).

Up to this point you have been urged not to shortcircuit data gathering because of interpretations that may be starting to gel in your mind. Premature formulation should not truncate basic data collection. However, you inevitably start to form impressions as you elicit the history and perform the examination. Every piece of history, every finding, will increasingly stimulate associations with your growing fund of substantive knowledge of the field. These interpretations develop into a so-called "running formulation" – an assessment that builds from each new clue. Your running formulation will in turn suggest direction and emphasis in your history taking and examination. In this way, the process of formulation benefits the data collection process.

Running formulation

With experience this interaction will become almost second nature. For now, practice a systematic method, as will be outlined in this chapter.

Clinical–anatomic study guide

Chapters 13 and 14 contain brief summaries of the most commonly used facts, rules, and constructs that help in topographic localization in the central nervous system. It is important to remember that the conventional clinical–anatomic constructs oversimplify neuroanatomy for the purpose of forming some practical principles that are memorable and useful in a clinical context. Although they bypass much of the richness and subtlety of actual neurologic function, such constructs have conventionally served this purpose well. Utilize them as a starting point in your diagnostic formulation, not as an end to your thinking. If you prefer, you may read Chapters 13 and 14 before reading the more general approach to formulation presented here.

Clinical constructs

Laboratory data

Up to this point laboratory and imaging data have not been folded into the data base. Your preliminary formulation should ordinarily guide the choice of ancillary tests. Moreover, for numerous important pathologic processes, neuroimages or electrophysiologic tests do not reveal abnormalities: you still need to be able to reason clinically. Chapter 15 offers an introductory approach to the role of imaging and other neurodiagnostic tests.

Relevance of imaged abnormalities

An increasingly important facet of neurologic formulation might be celled "retrodiagnosis" or the "diagnosis of relevance." Is the imaged abnormality (or anatomic variation) pertinent to the symptoms and signs? Some of your patients will come to you already bearing a neuroimage or electrophysiologic test which has been interpreted as abnormal. The "lesion" seen on this test (which may have been ordered by another caregiver) has now assumed the status of a chief complaint, often dwarfing the original symptoms. Your most pressing diagnostic challenge may be to set the clinical formulation and the laboratory "abnormality" in proper relationship to one another – to diagnose relevance or irrelevance.

THE PROCESS OF FORMULATION

A systematic method

The foremost pitfall in diagnostic formulation consists of a tendency to jump prematurely or haphazardly from symptoms and signs to particular diagnoses with which you may happen to be familiar. Instead, use a bridge of logic to cross from data base to interpretive formulation. The hardest part is getting started.

Summarize the data base

A helpful first step is to summarize the hard core of the data base – those symptoms and signs that you believe to be most significant and reliable. As you proceed with your formulation, you may realize the significance of data that you had initially put aside.

To illustrate, consider again the case of Susan Squires, the 19-year-old right-handed college sophomore whose history is briefly presented in Chapter 1 and whose neurologic examination is recorded in detail in Chapter 11. Her history and findings might be summarized as follows.

Case 1A: Summary of history and examination

This young woman presented with the abrupt onset of left arm shaking and a sense of losing control. Prior history was negative except for several "blackouts" in the past 2 years and a very high current level of stress. Her neurologic examination (following recovery from an observed convulsion) showed only mild left facial weakness (forehead sparing) and mild proximal and distal left upper extremity weakness, a left plantar response that was neutral (versus flexor on the right), and a loud vascular sound over the right orbit and right side of the neck (the latter obliterated by jugular venous compression).

This concise listing of the ostensibly most significant ingredients of the data base sets the case in front of you: it is in a form that you can start to digest.

ANATOMIC LOCALIZATION

Either symptoms or examination findings can indicate the topographic localization of a disorder (Fig. 12.1). In the present case, the motor events and findings provide the most concrete clues to localization. Where in the extent of the motor pathways, from frontal cortex to face and limb muscles, could the dysfunction be? The primary object here is not so much to pinpoint an exact location as to define the range of possibilities based upon the data at hand. Since Susan Squires experienced contortion of the left face and shaking of the left arm, and since weakness was found in these same areas, localization must take into account both of these features: the lesion responsible for left arm weakness must be on the right side in the brain (above the pyramidal decussation); moreover, because of the facial involvement, the lesion must be in or above the pons – the level of segmental brainstem outflow to the muscles of facial expression. Thus, the motor system must be involved at or between the cortex and the pons.

Arm weakness

Facial weakness

But consider the matter of the left facial weakness in more detail: is the left facial weakness due to a segmental, lower motor neuron (LMN) type of dysfunction? Or is it due to a lesion of an upper motor neuron (UMN) (suprasegmental) pathway from the right motor cortex to the left CN 7 nucleus? (If you are unfamiliar with these terms and concepts see discussion of segmental and suprasegmental links in Chapter 5, and for a more comprehensive coverage see Chapter 14.)

There are two reasons for implicating the suprasegmental, UMN (corticobulbar) pathway: first, the facial weakness spared the forehead,

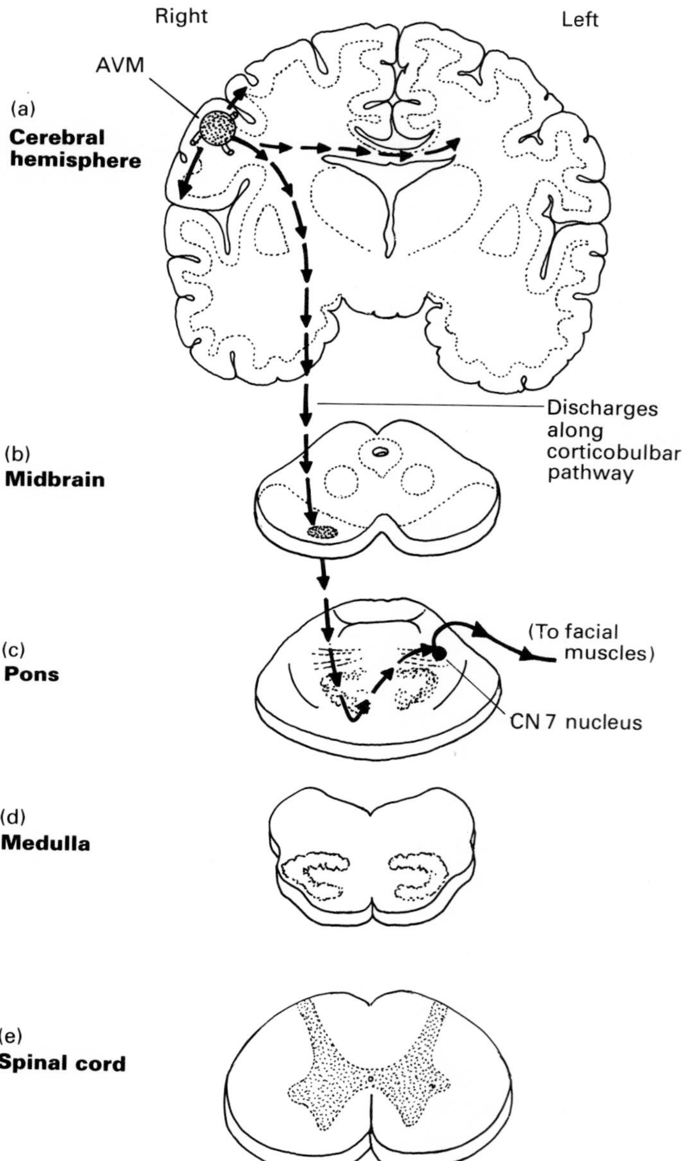

Fig. 12.1 A template for central nervous system long tract localization applied to Case 1A. (a) The cerebral hemispheres in coronal section (not in scale to the brainstem and spinal cord) show the right-sided, subcortical location of the arteriovenous malformation (AVM) in Case 1A. The arrows descending along the path of the corticobulbar tract in (a), (b), and (c), are meant to suggest intermittent (clonic) seizure discharges causing the initial left facial twitching. Later, the discharges spread to adjacent areas of cortex and then across the corpus collosum to the left hemisphere.

suggesting the UMN type of facial weakness (see Chapter 5, section on CN 7). Second, to account for the left facial weakness by means of a left pontine (or peripheral) lesion would be incompatible with a single anatomic focus: we have already established that a lesion at or above the pons, accounting for the left arm weakness, would have to be on the right side. (In addition, recall the finding of an abnormal vascular sound on the right side of the head and neck.)

Right cortical lesion

Thus, a single responsible lesion would have to involve the right motor cortex or the descending corticobulbar and corticospinal fibers on their route to the brainstem and cervical spinal cord, respectively. But can we further narrow the range? The only clue comes from the occurrence of shaking. If this is to be interpreted as epileptic seizure activity, then we could learn from a textbook that motor seizures with focal onset are thought virtually always to be cortical phenomena. So we might surmise that the epileptic discharge arose in or spread to the right frontal (motor) cortex, involving the areas somatotopically representing face and arm (Fig. 13.6). Short of laboratory tests, such as neuroimaging techniques, this localization cannot be substantially refined or validated.

PATHOLOGIC FORMULATION

As you already know, the pathology of a lesion is defined as the type of abnormal tissue or tissue reaction. In place of normal brain tissue, is there scarring, tumor, infection, blood clot, tissue devitalized by circulatory failure, etc.? In addition to tissue changes that can be seen under the light microscope, it is increasingly important to think about "biochemical pathologies" that affect tissue function without visible changes, or with change only apparent to ultrastructural examination. At this level the distinction between structure and function, between structural pathology and abnormal physiology, blurs increasingly.

You might think that a pathologic diagnosis would have to come from pathologic examination, and ultimately this is true. However, the clinical method can certainly narrow the range of probable pathologic processes and sometimes even suggest a particular one that is likely. Neuroimaging can also narrow the differential diagnosis and even define certain types of pathology, such as a fresh blood clot (hematoma), but beware of inferring too much! A brain abscess and a malignant tumor might look very much alike in certain cases (see Table 15.2).

Temporal profile

Our first approximation comes from the temporal profile of the history: what was the nature of onset of the symptoms, the ups and downs (if any) and tempo of the course? Were the symptoms and signs abrupt or gradual in onset, transitory, episodic, relentlessly progressive, or resolving? A stroke (an infarction or hemorrhage) comes suddenly, as the term implies, although there may be prior warnings or subsequent progression. The symptoms and signs of tumors usually progress gradually, although at an uneven pace, and occasionally the course is punctuated by sudden changes.

Case 1A, formulation (continued)

What can be said from our data base about the pathologic diagnosis in the case of Susan Squires? The abrupt onset of acute symptoms and signs indicates an acute dysfunction, but not necessarily an underlying lesion of recent development. The additional history of prior nocturnal episodes over 2 years, which were suggestive of seizures, indicates a relative chronicity of the underlying pathology. The occurrence of a focal seizure would account for the new symptoms, but would not distinguish among any of the types of lesions that might constitute a seizure focus in the cerebral cortex.

Examination findings

In the examination only the abnormal vascular signs, the bruit-like sounds over the right orbit and neck, would suggest that blood vessels might be involved in the pathology. Assuming a unitary explanation, the pathologic focus would not be simply a small scar, but rather a vascular lesion, perhaps a very vascular tumor or (as you might learn from a textbook) more likely yet an arteriovenous malformation (AVM). (The fact that the sounds in the neck can be damped or obliterated by compression of the jugular vein does provide a clue that their source is not an arterial stenosis.)

Neuroimaging

In this case the neuroimaging technique (contrast-enhanced computerized tomography (CT) scan) provided not only excellent localizing data but demonstrated the major pathology – an AVM – as well. This lesion was in the right frontal lobe, near the motor strip areas for face and arm. The AVM presumably caused changes in neurons and glia to constitute an epileptogenic focus.

EEG

An electroencephalogram (EEG) demonstrated paroxysmal activity and slow waves (see Chapter 15) in the right frontoparietal region.

PATHOGENETIC FORMULATION

The pathogenesis is the mechanism or process of production of the pathology. A given type of pathology, such as infarction, can result from several different mechanisms, each of which produces identical or highly similar structural changes: brain infarction may be due to an *in situ* thrombosis of a cerebral blood vessel, an embolic occlusion of a vessel, or much less commonly a spasm or compression of a blood vessel – all of which deprive a part of the brain of nutrient blood flow.

Case 1A, formulation (continued)

In the Squires case, the pathology is the AVM and the associated neuronal–glial changes. Relatively little is known about the detailed pathogenesis of a seizure focus or of vascular malformations. The latter appear to be developmental in nature, stemming from an anomaly of embryogenesis and/or fetal development. In this case it seems likely that the epileptogenic focus was created by ischemia (due to arteriovenous shunting of blood), by other local metabolic effects, or by compression of surrounding tissue by the AVM. There was no evidence of recent hemorrhage on CT scan. More common processes resulting in epileptogenic foci include traumatic brain injury, embolic infarction, and metastatic tumor growth, to name just a few examples.

Use of temporal profile

The source of your first inferences about pathogenesis will usually come from the history, just as for the pathology. If a patient suffered a cerebral infarction, the detailed mode of onset and progression of the symptoms and signs would suggest whether embolism or thrombosis would be more likely. In the former instance, the onset is typically very sudden and the extent of the deficit is usually maximal at or within minutes of the onset. In contrast, a thrombotic process may be heralded by stereotypic warning symptoms (transient ischemic attacks), and the deficit may develop in a stepwise or stuttering fashion, as the occlusion is completed. Such profiles are by no means foolproof, but offer some help.

Use of risk factors

A second type of historical information relevant to the pathogenesis derives from your data on risk factors (see Table 2.1) obtained in the past medical history. A positive history of hypertension does not discriminate very well among the common causes of stroke, but the absence of hypertension diminishes the likelihood of intracerebral hemorrhage.

ETIOLOGIC FORMULATION

The etiology, or root cause, of a pathologic process cannot always be clearly distinguished from the pathogenesis. Nonetheless, efforts to identify the true origins of disease states are important epidemiologically, and sometimes for the individual patient as well. In the case of a patient with a history of heavy smoking presenting with a seizure, the pathology and pathogenesis may be metastatic spread of bronchogenic carcinoma to the brain, but the ultimate cause is mainly the carcinogenic toxicity of cigarette smoke. Obviously, in many instances there will be several interactive causes, involving both exogenous and endogenous factors. In the case of Susan Squires' AVM, the etiology is no more clear than the pathogenesis, but the possibility of a teratogenic factor in pregnancy cannot be excluded.

Thus, your information bearing upon etiology often comes, at least in part, from a knowledge of risk factors that you can identify in the patient's history. These may be mainly individual, such as cigarette smoking, or represent group risk factors that the patient is not always able to control, such as environmental toxins. In some instances, the presumptive etiology will be immediately and decisively evident – as when a patient is rendered paraplegic in a single vehicular accident, the patient having been driving at excessive speed while severely inebriated. In the Squires case we can then outline the formulation as follows.

Case 1A summary

1 Anatomic localization: from clinical analysis of symptoms and signs we can say that the site of dysfunction involved the right frontal cortex, including the motor strip and, more specifically, face and arm areas of cortical representation. From neuroimaging we know that the lesion is indeed centered in that area.

2 Pathology: AVM with presumed associated glial reaction and possible ischemic changes, but no evidence of hemorrhage. The temporal profile of the history only indicated some chronicity punctuated by recurrent acute symptoms. This was a case in which the neuroimages established a specific gross pathologic diagnosis because of the pathognomonic correspondence of CT findings and pathologic characteristics.

3 Pathogenesis: we presume that the seizures originated from the AVM or its vicinity, but no direct data in the case bear upon the questions of how the seizures in this instance were generated or how the AVM developed. We would need to extrapolate from a general neuroscience knowledge base.

4 Etiology: again, no direct data from the case.

THE DIAGNOSTIC FORMULATION AS A WHOLE

For present purposes, the anatomic (topographic) and pathologic parts of the formulation deserve more of your attention than do the pathogenetic and etiologic assessments. These latter aspects depend on a pathophysiologic understanding of the origin and mechanisms of neurologic disease, which will concern you increasingly as you enlarge your knowledge base in neurosciences and neurology. For now, while improving your techniques of information gathering by history and physical examination, you need to be very clear about how your data enter into the diagnostic process – and how far you can go with them. The main uses of the history and examination are summarized below.

1 *History.*

(a) The chief complaint opens the door to the present illness and focuses attention on the main symptoms to use for localization.

(b) The temporal profile of the present illness often provides clues to the category of pathologic (and pathogenetic) process – acute vs. chronic, episodic vs. persistent, progressive vs. resolving, etc. The site and distribution of symptoms helps anatomic localization, often as much or more than physical signs.

(c) The past personal, family, social, occupational, and environmental histories are important sources of data on risk factors which help suggest possibilities and probabilities of pathology, pathogenesis, and etiology. Such information usually does not confirm a diagnosis, but points laboratory investigation in productive directions.

(d) The review of neurologic symptoms is a safety net, designed to catch important pieces of the history that did not emerge in the present illness. These symptoms may help to localize or identify the disease.

2 *Neurologic examination*: findings primarily assist with anatomic localization (such as loss of visual acuity in one eye implicating the retina or the optic nerve). Sometimes the character of the finding (such as an isolated dense homonymous hemianopia) suggests the likely pathologic and pathogenetic diagnosis. In this instance, embolic infarction of the contralateral visual cortex appears to be the most likely cause, because other localizations or pathologic processes are usually accompanied by additional findings (see Case 5A).

SYNDROME DIAGNOSIS

Based upon your history and examination, you will increasingly be able to discern a pattern in the clinical picture – a sense that the elements of the data base are starting to hang together, to cohere as an entity. These symptoms and signs, organized in the context of a temporal profile, form a characteristic clinical expression, a syndrome. As you gain more experience, you will often be able to recognize that you have encountered such an entity, even if you cannot yet put a label on it.

Stroke syndrome

To illustrate a common neurologic syndrome: a 73-year-old right-handed woman slumps over in her chair. You find a hemiparesis and sensory deficit, homonymous hemianopsia, hyperreflexia, and an extensor plantar reflex, all on the right. She is mute and does not show comprehension of simple commands. This clinical event has the stamp of a stroke syndrome – an acute, seemingly spontaneous event with deficits localizable to the left cerebral hemisphere. You would not be able to tell definitely from this information whether the pathology is infarction or hemorrhage, or whether the pathogenesis (if this be an infarct) is thrombotic or embolic. From the standpoint of vascular territories, an infarct would be in the carotid/middle cerebral artery distribution. The absolutely sudden onset, without preliminary symptoms, suggests that an infarct would most likely have had an embolic pathogenesis.

This vignette reveals a pattern of historical events and findings that clinicians have come to recognize in case after case. Syndromes have a clinical (and often mechanistic) coherence. There is not necessarily a unitary cause for a clinical syndrome; in fact, a syndrome typically has alternative causes, and thus differs from a specific disease entity. While recognition of clinical syndromes will be helpful to you as your knowledge base grows, your emphasis at this stage should be on the process of logical formulation based upon the data at hand.

Acting on partial data and incomplete formulation

In practice, clinical data gathering, formulation, diagnostic testing, reformulation, and therapeutic intervention do not proceed entirely in serial fashion, but often partly in parallel. History alone should prompt certain laboratory tests or initial therapies even before a full differential diagnosis is articulated or a best diagnosis hypothesized.

1 History (chief complaint): "I just had a little seizure – I'm taking Dilantin." Question of inadequate anticonvulsant level. Possible need for supplementation. Order phenytoin (Dilantin) serum level.

2 History (risk factor): a patient who is known to be anticoagulated on Coumadin complains of an increasing headache after bumping his head. Question of intracranial hematoma. Possible need for neurosurgery. Order a prothrombin time (and alert staff to the need for a cranial CT scan).

3 History (risk factor and initial observation): "Mr Crowe, my neighbor, is an alcoholic. He hadn't been seen in weeks, so the police broke in and brought him right to the hospital. He's very confused." Possible Wernicke–Korsakoff syndrome, and/or hypoglycemia. Treat with intravenous thiamine and glucose while proceeding with work-up.

Most cases that require a tentative working diagnosis and plan of management, despite only scanty information, are not emergencies. It is in the emergency arena, however, that a systematic approach to initial formulation based on partial data ranks highest in priority.

RAPID EMERGENCY FORMULATION

Concurrent examination and formulation

In an emergency situation, the concept of a "running formulation" takes on literal meaning. Whereas in nonemergency work-ups we emphasize an orderly, systematic history and examination, an emergency imposes a need for rapid prioritization. Instead of allowing interpretation of data to develop more slowly, so as not to truncate data gathering, the "quick and dirty" emergency formulation dominates the choice and sequence of history taking, examination, and laboratory tests.

Compressed sequence of diagnosis and management

The order of progression suggested below cannot be applied to all cases and situations. You should modify and build upon this scheme as you acquire specific knowledge of particular diseases or injuries and their modes of presentation. The path of assessment is based upon the steps that an experienced neurologist might take if called for a neurologic emergency evaluation. What cannot be adequately conveyed in print is the degree to which several of these activities proceed simultaneously: the vital signs and level of consciousness have been evaluated by the time the neurologist arrives. Blood tests are being drawn and an intravenous line inserted while the initial history is being obtained. The emergency physician will probably be relating the gist of the known history as the neurologist looks at the breathing pattern and eyes. A call for neuroimaging may well be initiated at that point, while more of an examination is being carried out. Ideally, another physician or nurse will be obtaining additional history from emergency medical technicians (EMTs), family, or other witnesses, while additional items of neurologic function are being assessed.

Table 12.1 Emergency formulation: diagnostic and therapeutic issues

1 Vital signs and temperature	Is the patient perfusing? (Adequate pulse and blood pressure)	If not, further immediate attention to cardiovascular factors, urine output, blood loss, etc.; ?Shock
	Is respiration adequate? (a) ?Respiratory drive	Assure patent airway, oxygenation of blood ?Medullary or cervical lesions; ?Arterial O_2, CO_2, pH; ?Opioid or other drug effect. Give antagonist
	(b) ?Ventilatory mechanics	?Cervical cord, phrenic nerve, thoracic cord, intercostal nerve dysfunction; ?Primary muscular or neuromuscular junction dysfunction; ?Chest injury
	Is temperature normal?	?Fever ?Stiff neck, other meningeal signs; evidence of other infection, heat stroke; Obtain stains, cultures, etc.; ?Cool patient
2 Level of consciousness	?Awake and alert	Obtain further history
	?Lethargic, stuporous, comatose	?Evidence of head injury (safeguard spine), ?Other space-occupying lesion; ?Stroke (especially brainstem). Correlate with eye signs, pattern of weakness, posturing, plantar responses, etc. (see Chapter 18); ?Toxic, metabolic problem. Draw blood studies. Give glucose, thiamine, opioid antagonist
3 Eye signs	?Abnormal pupillary size, reactivity	?Enlarging or nonreactive pupil(s) ?Transtentorial herniation; drug effect (see Chapter 13)
	Eye movements: gaze deviation, ocular palsy	?CN 3 palsy; ?hemispheric or posterior fossa lesion (see Chapter 17)
	Funduscopic examination ?Hemorrhages, papilledema	?Acute or chronic increase in intracranial pressure (see Chapter 4); ?Subarachnoid hemorrhage; ?Hypertensive encephalopathy
4 Plantar responses (and deep tendon reflexes)	?Babinski signs, hyperreflexia	Correlate with eye findings and weakness, sensory loss
	?Areflexia	?Acute polyneuropathy; spinal shock
5 Motor, coordination	Hemiparesis, pariparesis, quadriparesis	Correlate with level of consciousness; eye signs (Table 17.1); breathing pattern; reflexes, tone, posturing, sensory level, if present
	?Proximal or distal pattern of weakness	
	?Ataxia	?Cerebellar hemorrhage, brainstem or cerebellar infarct
	Swallowing, cough failure	?Acute neuromuscular, brainstem dysfunction
6 Sensory loss	?Sensory level, trunk or neck	Correlate with evidence of spinal injury or disease; (see Chapter 14)
7 Thought processes, affect, behavior	?Irrational, violent, mute, etc.	?Confusion (delirium); ?psychosis, etc.

Meanwhile the neurologist's thinking process might be characterized by the questions listed in Table 12.1, each leading to some further neurologic (or non-neurologic) action.

Rapid neurologic formulation is a hodge-podge from the standpoint of analytic process. As you can see, some thinking is driven by certain prescribed rules, for example: (a) ''tend first'' to vital cardiopulmonary and systemic functions, including body temperature extremes, that will cause or compound neurologic damage or lead to shock and arrest; (b) ''don't miss'' certain conditions that are highly treatable, such as hypoglycemia, bacterial meningitis, opioid overdose; (c) ''start the ball rolling'' to get a patient with a herniation mass lesion onto measures to lower intracranial pressure and then into surgery.

Tend first

Don't miss

Start the ball rolling

Other thinking is driven by a recognition that localization within the nervous system is required for diagnosis and treatment: there can be no rule of action until the location and nature of the problem are defined. Is the problem in the brain or spinal cord or peripheral nervous system? In what specific part? And to what pathologic process are these parts subject? For example, what is the level of consciousness? Is the coma due to bihemispheric cortical dysfunction? Is it metabolic?

The logic of rapid formulation and initial management is not, therefore, in its clarity of process, but in its adherence to the principle of time-dependent treatability: what are the disorders that can be treated acutely and for which is time of the essence?

Time-dependent treatability

SUMMARY OF DIAGNOSTIC FORMULATION

1 Form the data base:

Subjective data	Symptoms	History
	Self-observation Third party observation Past records	
	Sensory Mental status Motor (cranial nerves) Coordination Reflexes Head and neck, spine,	Examination
Objective data	Other general examination	

2 Summarize the data base: identify the main parts that will be used initially in formulation.

3 Formulate the diagnosis (based on symptoms and signs):

(a) anatomic/topographic – localization;

(b) pathologic – type of tissue change;
(c) pathogenetic – mechanism of pathologic change, steps leading to deranged structure/function;
(d) etiologic – root cause, initiating factor.

4 Laboratory/imaging data added: often diagnostic tests are begun after only partial data collection and formulation.

5 Reformulation (after incorporation of laboratory, imaging data, and further observation of course of illness) leads to:
(a) further primary data collection (history, physical, laboratory tests);
(b) accessing resource data to clarify the diagnosis (texts, articles, more experienced or knowledgeable colleagues/supervisors, etc.);
(c) modification of differential diagnosis; prioritization of further work-up, diagnostic observation; diagnostic/therapeutic trial;
(d) definitive therapy/symptomatic therapy;
(e) management and further observation of therapeutic course.

PROBLEMS FOR SELF-STUDY

How far can you proceed with formulation based upon the data supplied in the following case summaries? Consider anatomic localization (topography), pathology, pathophysiologic mechanism, and etiology.

1 A 54-year-old right-handed woman presents with a history of acute onset of double vision and left frontotemporal headache. She is not diabetic and has not experienced recent trauma. On examination, she has mild left ptosis, an enlarged left pupil with decreased reactivity, and an abducted left eye with decreased adduction, elevation and depression. Her neck is not stiff and there is no fever. *Problems*

2 A 72-year-old woman with a history of rheumatoid arthritis fell 3 days ago and has noted increasing difficulty with gait since that time. She has also been feeling sore "all over". Examination reveals a thin, wasted woman who displays poor effort on strength testing but definite weakness of the right arm and leg. There is right greater than left hyperreflexia, a right extensor plantar response, and an equivocal response on the left. Moderate vibratory loss is noted in both feet. No cranial nerve abnormalities are found except for an asymmetry at the mouth with a tendency to smile more out of the left side of the mouth than the right and a shoulder shrug which is slightly weaker on the right than the left. No jaw jerk, snout or grasp reflex is present.

3 The husband of a 60-year-old right-handed woman reports that she suddenly developed "ragtime" speech this morning. She does not follow commands nor can she name objects, read, repeat, or write grammatically. A partial right superior quadrantanopia is present. No motor, sensory, coordination, or reflex abnormalities are detected.

4 A 43-year-old man complains of chronic, insidious development

of unsteadiness of gait, intermittent vertigo, and impaired hearing (noted when using the telephone). Examination reveals a mild left facial droop and decreased ability to wrinkle up the forehead on the left. Hearing is markedly decreased on that side. Gait is slightly wide-based and ataxic.

Comments

1 Localization: the headache suggests a problem in the left anterior quadrant of the head, but the pain could be referred. Assuming the double vision is binocular, then the neuromuscular systems controlling eye movements could be affected anywhere from the posterior fossa (brainstem) to the eye muscles themselves. The concurrence of ptosis, an enlarged and less reactive pupil and the specified oculomotor deficits implicates left CN 3, including its parasympathetic fibers (as discussed in Chapter 5), but does not specify just where the lesion is located.

Pathology and pathogenesis: a cranial nerve (or nucleus) can be affected by compression (mechanical or ischemic damage), inflammation, hemorrhage, infarction, tumor, etc. From the temporal profile, the sudden onset makes intrinsic tumor unlikely, but does not exclude compression from sudden expansion of a cerebral aneurysm (which turned out to be the pathogenesis in this case). (Aneurysms of the Circle of Willis that involve CN 3 are located at the junction of the internal carotid and posterior communicating arteries, where CN 3 is affected peripherally.) There are no symptoms of bleeding, but this would need to be confirmed by neuroimaging and, if indicated, by lumbar puncture. Analysis of risk factors is helpful in that diabetes is not known to be present. (Diabetes can cause cranial nerve infarction which typically spares any major pupillary dysfunction.) The etiology of arterial defects that lead to berry aneurysm formation is thought to be congenital, but is poorly understood.

2 Localization: UMN signs in the right shoulder, arm, and leg indicate a corticospinal tract lesion in the upper cervical cord on the right or in the brain on the left. The key point of ambiguity is whether the slight asymmetry of her smile is relevant. If so, then the lesion must be in the left upper pons or higher (e.g. internal capsule, cerebral white matter, or motor cortex). Uncertainty also exists regarding the hint of bilateral corticospinal involvement, as deep tendon reflexes and the plantar response on the left may possibly be abnormal. Bilateral involvement from a single lesion usually implicates the spinal cord or brainstem (as will be further discussed in Chapter 14).

Pathology and pathogenesis: the progressive course raises the question of an expanding mass lesion, but could also be inflammatory, etc. Of help here is the known rheumatoid arthritis, a risk factor for several types of neurologic problems. A review of known complications would identify the occurrence of atlantoaxial (C1–C2) dislocation and fracture of the odontoid process of C2, often after only moderate trauma. While other possibilities should not be ignored, progressive high cervical cord trauma from an unstable spine at C1–C2 should be ruled out promptly. In this case, neuroimaging confirmed this anatomic diagnosis, from which intermittent compressive pathology (swelling, contusion, or necrosis) in the cord could be inferred. Treatment with high-dose corticosteroids for spinal cord swelling and stabilization of the cervical spine was instituted.

3 Localization: language disorder in a right-handed patient implicates the left hemisphere. The fluent, noncomprehending character of the aphasia suggests a "posterior" (temporoparietal) localization, but even if this knowledge were not available to you, the right superior quadrantanopia localizes to the left temporal white matter or the left occipital cortex (inferior bank of the calcarine fissure). Other postchiasmal locations are much less likely (see Fig. 13.17).

Pathology and pathogenesis: the sudden onset strongly favors a stroke. In the temporal lobe, infarction is much more likely than hemorrhage, in the absence of trauma or a blood coagulation disorder. However, playing these odds would not be sufficient; neuroimaging by CT or magnetic resonance imaging (MRI) should be done to rule out hemorrhage, especially since anticoagulant therapy might be indicated. As it turned out, her infarct, like most focal infarcts in this region, was embolic in pathogenesis.

4 Localization: while gait difficulty in itself does not localize, its association with vertigo (a vestibular symptom) and impaired hearing all point to the posterior fossa – the brainstem, cranial nerves, and cerebellum. These symptoms are common enough that they might be unrelated to the gait difficulty, but the LMN type of facial weakness (forehead involved) points to the region of the cerebellopontine angle on the left. Here, CN 7 and the acoustic and vestibular divisions of CN 8 are all in close proximity to each other, the pons, and the cerebellum.

Pathology and pathogenesis: in the temporal profile of symptoms, the insidious development suggests the likelihood of a mass lesion, such as a tumor. While other possibilities would need to be considered if appropriately selected neuroimaging were negative, an MRI (or contrast-enhanced CT) should be the first step. In this case, an "acoustic neuroma" (Schwann-cell tumor of CN 8) was indeed found and surgically removed, relieving the symptoms caused by compression. Aside from some families with a genetic predisposition to this tumor (a type of neurofibromatosis or Von Recklinghausen's disease), the etiologic basis is not understood.

FURTHER READING

Chimowitz, M.I., Logigian, E.L., Caplan, L.R. The accuracy of bedside neurologic diagnoses. *Ann Neurol* 1990; 28:78–85. This comparison and categorization of diagnostic accuracy by neurologic residents and staff attendings offers insights into sources of error. A background discussion of methods of diagnostic formulation is included.

Glick, T.H. *The Process of Neurologic Care in Medical Practice.* Harvard University Press, Cambridge (MA), 1984. Patterns of diagnostic mistakes and ways of thinking that will help avoid them (Chapter 5).

Kassirer, J.P. Diagnostic reasoning. *Ann Int Med* 1989; 110:893–900. A broad analysis of how physicians generate and validate diagnostic hypotheses.

Landau, W.L. Strategy, tactics, and accuracy in neurological evaluation. (editorial) *Ann Neurol* 1990; 28:86–7. Editorial comment on the Chimowitz *et al.* article (above) with a listing of recommended methods.

Mumenthaler, M. *Neurologic Differential Diagnosis.* 2nd edn. Georg Thieme Verlag, Stuttgart, New York (NY), 1992. An introduction to syndrome diagnosis (Chapter 1).

Weiner, W.J. (ed.) *Emergent and Urgent Neurology.* Lippincott, Philadelphia (PA), 1992. The STAT situations that require rapid formulation and action.

chapter 13

Priority Anatomy: A Clinical–Anatomic Study Guide

Introduction

Data collection from the patient can proceed to a point without neuroanatomic knowledge, but localization requires an understanding of some anatomic facts and relationships. The compendium that follows will highlight the information that you will need most for getting started. Necessarily, this high priority information is condensed to make it clinically functional. In Chapter 14, simplified clinical constructs used in everyday practice are further articulated and briefly contrasted with the underlying anatomy.

GLOSSARY OF SELECTED TERMS

Segmental: in functional neuroanatomy this refers to a cross-sectional slice of the brainstem or spinal cord containing the input or output structures for communication with the periphery; it also designates the roots and nerves at that level and the muscles innervated by that central nervous system (CNS) segment (see Fig. 9.2).

Suprasegmental: neurons and tracts from a higher level of the CNS that influence segmental neurons by synapsing on them or on interneurons. Also, sensory long tracts projecting higher in the neuraxis. Any CNS structures in the cerebral hemispheres, cerebellum, or otherwise nonsegmental (see Fig. 5.1).

Supranuclear: used synonymously with suprasegmental when referring to the brainstem (where segmental neurons are organized in cranial nerve nuclei).

Corticospinal tract: a white-matter tract which includes myelinated fibers (axons) of neurons in the primary motor cortex (and other nearby cortical areas), some of which are destined to synapse on anterior horn cells (see Fig. 6.1).

Corticobulbar tract: same as above, but destined for brainstem motor nuclei. (Strictly speaking, bulbar refers to the medulla, but is widely used, in this context, to refer to the brainstem generally, see Fig. 5.1.)

Upper motor neuron: a neuron of the motor cortex (most typically) whose axon is a fiber of the corticospinal or corticobulbar tracts; a suprasegmental motor neuron (see Fig. 6.1).

Lower motor neuron: a segmental motor neuron; an anterior horn cell (by which we usually mean an α motor neuron) at spinal levels or a neuron of a brainstem motor nucleus (see Fig. 9.2).

Final common pathway: a term for segmental motor outflow, such as the anterior horn cell and its axon that contributes to an anterior root and motor nerve. Whatever the multiple inputs to anterior horn cells, they are the only motor access to muscle (analogous situation in the brainstem).

Neurons, 1st, 2nd, 3rd order: this is the designation of connecting sensory neurons, starting from the periphery. The 1st order neuron (1st neuron, primary afferent neuron) has its cell body in a dorsal root ganglion (or cranial nerve sensory ganglion); its central process (axon) synapses with a 2nd order neuron (2nd neuron) located at some level of the spinal cord or brainstem. This neuron in turn synapses with a 3rd order neuron (3rd neuron), that in the simplest scheme of a three-neuron chain is located in the thalamus and projects to the sensory cortex.

BRAIN AND SKULL: INTRACRANIAL COMPARTMENTS

Volume expansion

The brain vitrually fills the intracranial cavity formed by the bony skull, which is rigid and unyielding after infancy. Volume expansion results from space-occupying lesions inside the brain or overlying it, swelling of brain substance (edema), active increase in the ventricular volume (hydrocephalus), or changes in intravascular volumes. The effects depend upon the degree, location, and time course of the expansion. For example, tumors can grow to remarkably large size with few neurologic symptoms if the enlargement progresses very gradually and without compromise of key structures. Therapeutic intervention capitalizes upon the interdependence of these tissue compartments. Neurosurgeons can remove a tumor or blood clot or shunt the cerebrospinal fluid (CSF) from a hydrocephalic ventricular system; controlled hyperventilation constricts cerebral blood vessels, decreasing the size of the vascular compartment. (Do not confuse the widely distributed tissue compartments, referred to here, with the fixed divisions or compartments of the skull and dura, to be described next and illustrated in Fig. 13.1.)

Compartments

The supratentorial compartment comprises all intracranial space above the tentorium cerebelli, the dural "tent" over the cerebellum (Fig. 13.1). The midbrain is the neural connection between the cerebral hemispheres of the supratentorial space and the remainder of the brainstem, and the cerebellum in the infratentorial compartment (posterior fossa). Any communication from one compartment to another constitutes a potential site for brain herniation (bulging through an opening). This occurs when the pressure in one compartment rises sufficiently to squeeze part of its contents toward or into an adjacent, lower-pressure compartment (Fig. 13.2). In the case of the tentorial notch, the process is called transtentorial herniation – either downward ("central") or downward and horizontal. A medially directed as well as downward force vector, from a lateral mass, causes the medial temporal lobe to bulge through the tentorial notch: temporal lobe herniation. Transtentorial herniation impacts the midbrain, the CNs 3, and the posterior cerebral arteries on the side of the herniation and/or the opposite side, as the midbrain is shifted against the rigid edge of the tentorium (Fig. 13.2).

Tentorial herniation

Subfalcial herniation (shift)

A major division within the supratentorial compartment is produced by the fold of dura in the sagittal plane (falx cerebri) that partially separates the right and left cerebral hemispheres. Expansive pressure from a lesion in one hemisphere may cause herniation of brain tissue (cingulate gyrus) under the free edge of the falx and displacement of the ventricles (see Fig. 13.2a) to compress the opposite hemisphere in a right to left, or left to right shift. An expansive mass effect does not necessarily imply a shift, especially in that bilateral mass effects may balance each other, side to side.

Tonsillar herniation

A third and much rarer type of herniation, usually from cerebellar mass lesions, causes bulging of the most caudal cerebellar tissue ("tonsils") into the foramen magnum. The medullary distortion occurring with tonsillar herniation (cerebellar pressure cone) threatens respiratory drive and other essential life functions. The cerebellum can also herniate upward into the tentorial notch.

The pathophysiology of herniation syndromes is not understood in fine detail, despite their apparent physical simplicity. You can see that herniating tissue would itself be distorted, the tissue that it compresses or displaces might be damaged, arterial and venous circulation compromised, CSF flow obstructed, etc. – depending upon the degree and rapidity of displacement, force vectors, and the response of critical structures to distortion (see Further reading section).

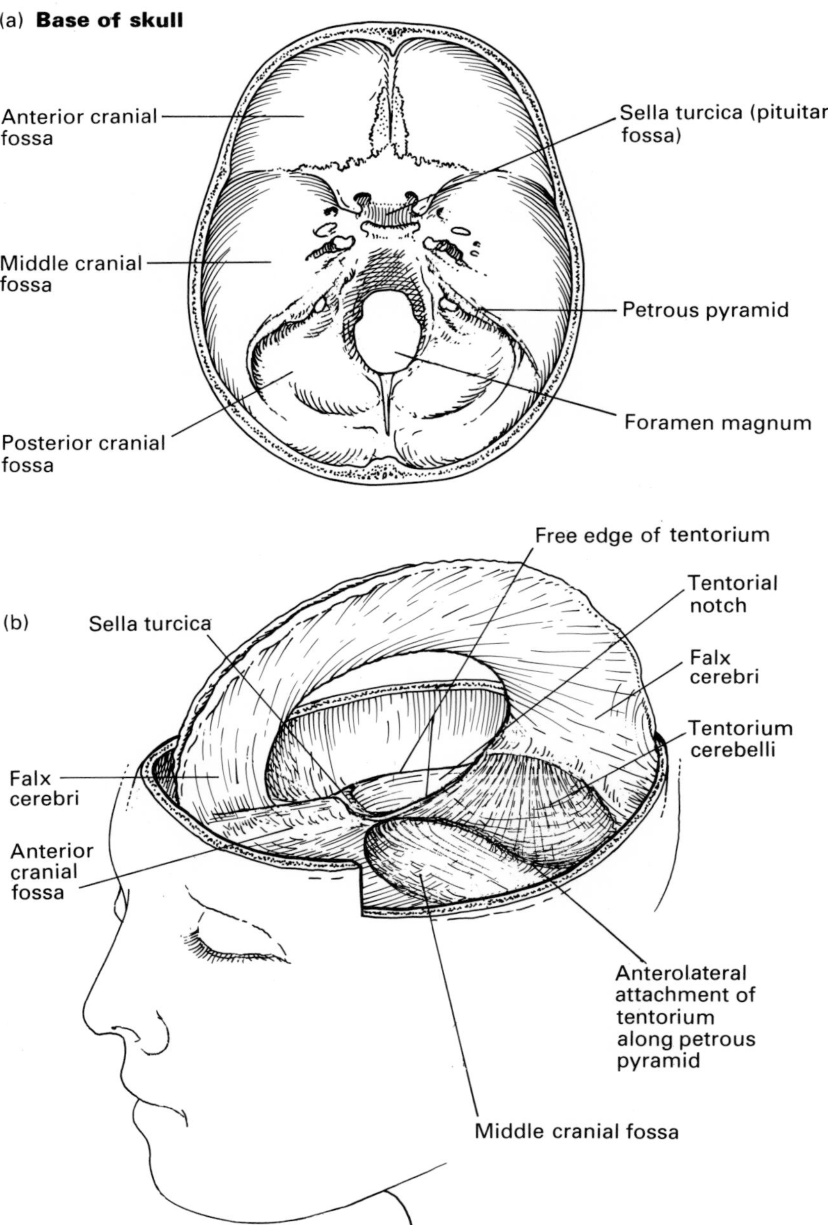

Fig. 13.1 Bony and dural compartments of the skull. (a) In the base of the skull on each side are the anterior cranial fossa (for the base of the frontal lobe), the middle fossa (temporal lobe), and the posterior fossa (brainstem and cerebellum). (b) View of the falx cerebri and tentorium cerebelli in place. The falx merges posteriorly in the midline with the peak of the tentorium cerebelli (tent over the cerebellum). The sloping leaf of the tentorium is shown on the near side. The tentorium attaches anterolaterally along the petrous pyramid and anteromedially the free edge forms the tentorial notch and borders the sella turcica (before terminating at the anterior clinoid process).

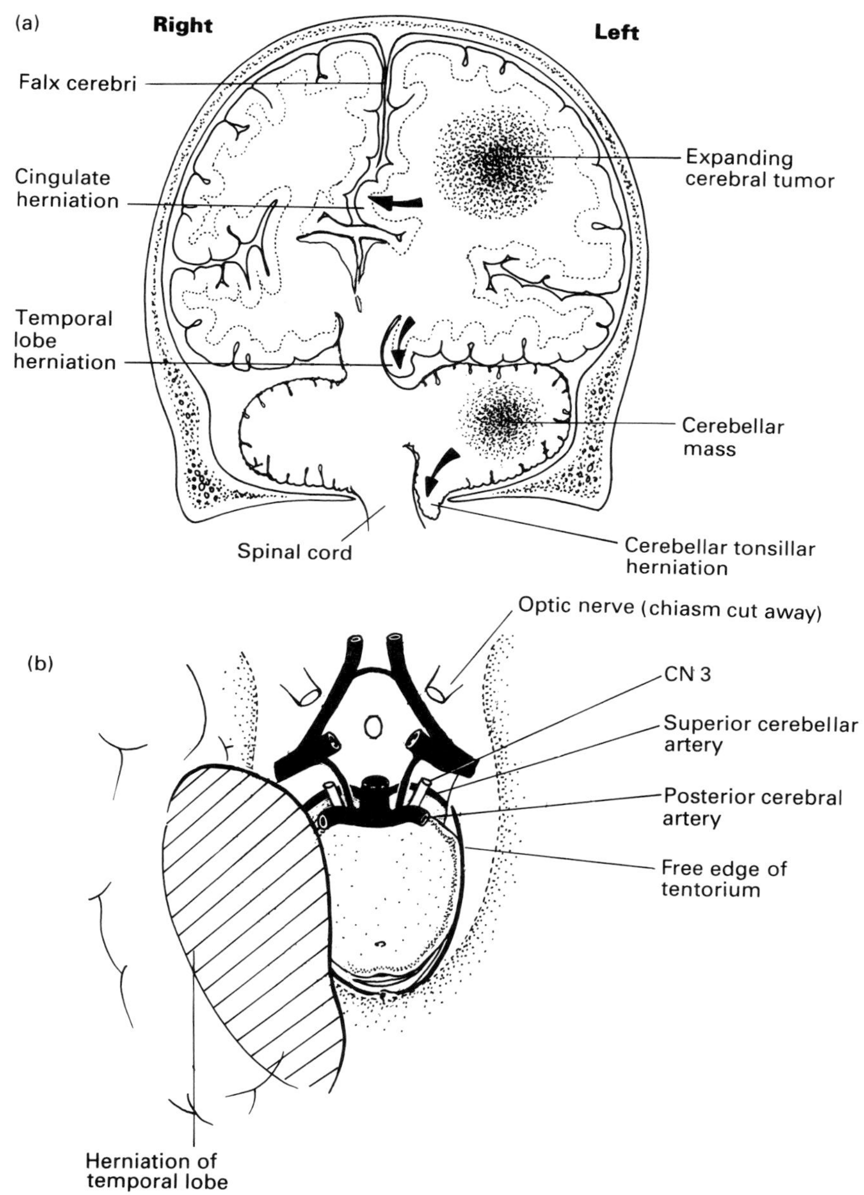

Fig. 13.2 Brain herniations. (a) Three types of herniation are shown schematically: the mass lesion in the left hemisphere causes a left to right shift with subfalcial (cingulate) herniation, in which the cingulate gyrus is forced under the free edge of the falx cerebri. Temporal lobe, transtentorial herniation (so-called uncal herniation, after the uncus of the medial temporal lobe). In tonsillar herniation (cerebellar pressure cone), a left cerebellar mass displaces the cerebellar tonsil(s) downward into the foramen magnum, with distortion of the caudal medulla. (b) View (from above) of the tentorial notch in a transtentorial (temporal lobe) herniation, with compression of the ipsilateral midbrain, forcing it against the contralateral tentorial free edge.

VASCULAR ANATOMY: AORTOCRANIAL AND INTRACRANIAL CIRCULATIONS

The main aortocranial arterial trunks are shown in Fig. 13.3 and the superficial territories of the three major cerebral arteries on each side are depicted in Figs 13.4 and 13.5. The major brain arteries and their larger branches are located in the subarachnoid space: they are surface vessels (except for fine penetrating branches arising from their initial portions or "stems"). Eventually their most distal branches penetrate the cortex.

Characteristic vascular lesions

Characteristic pathologic changes can be categorized by location in the vascular tree. The extracranial vessels and their large-caliber intracranial branches are subject to atherosclerosis (see Fig. 13.3). The Circle of Willis constitutes the site of most saccular (berry) aneurysms (see Fig. 15.2). The small, penetrating vessels, originating as side branches from the major intracranial trunks, plunge as end-arteries deep into the substance of the brain and bear the brunt of direct hypertensive changes, leading to intracerebral hemorrhage and small, deep infarcts (lacunes). The small, superficial cortical branches terminate the surface arborization and represent the lodging sites for most small emboli.

As a generalization, isolated occlusions of a common carotid, innominate, or subclavian artery (the parent vessels of arterial supply to the brain) do not cause stroke, because of collateral routes to the internal carotid and vertebrobasilar systems.

Aortocranial vessels

The internal carotid artery (ICA) rises into the skull without any branches to enable collateral flow prior to its first intracranial branch, the ophthalmic artery. Since the ICA supplies much of the perfusion to the ipsilateral retina and hemisphere, carotid occlusion may cause a telltale pattern: episodes of ipsilateral, monocular visual loss and contralateral motor, sensory, and other cerebral deficits. (See subsequent section on crossing of long motor and sensory tracts and refer back to Case 4A.) Occlusion of an internal carotid artery does not necessarily result in any cerebral infarction because of possible collateral flow to its intracranial branches, the larger being the middle and anterior cerebral arteries.

The vertebral arteries do have cervical branches which permit anastomotic reconstitution of flow in case of occlusion of the vertebral artery at its origin. Occasionally, vertebral blood flows in retrograde fashion if pressure relationships are reversed by proximal subclavian occlusion (see Fig. 13.3).

Major intracranial arteries

Middle cerebral artery

The middle cerebral artery (MCA) is the largest of the three main intracranial arteries on each side and represents a continuation of the internal

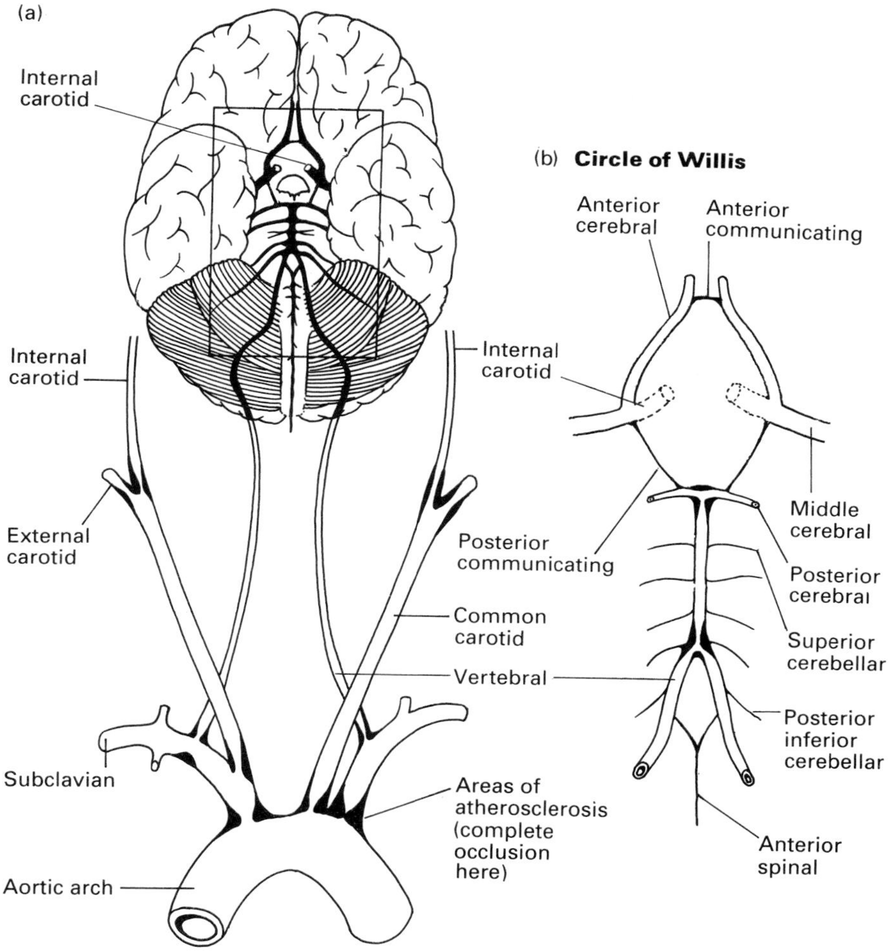

Fig. 13.3 Aortocranial circulation. (a) Schematic of the "great vessels" (arteries) of the upper chest and neck and of the arteries at the base of the brain. The internal carotid arteries supply the "anterior circulation" of the brain (mainly the anterior and middle cerebral arteries); the vertebral arteries supply the "posterior circulation" (vertebrobasilar system, including the posterior cerebral arteries). Typical areas of atherosclerosis at major vascular bifurcations and junctions are depicted. (b) The Circle of Willis is the anastomotic ring joining the anterior and posterior circulations and the right and left sides. There are two posterior communicating arteries connecting the anterior and posterior circulations (internal carotid to posterior cerebral arteries), but just one anterior communicating artery between the right and left anterior cerebral arteries. Anatomic variations of the Circle are common.

carotid artery. The MCA irrigates virtually the entire lateral aspect (convexity) of the hemisphere (see Fig. 13.4). Thus, the middle cerebral artery is not medial. Many of the deep structures of the cerebrum, including much of the basal ganglia and cerebral white matter, and part

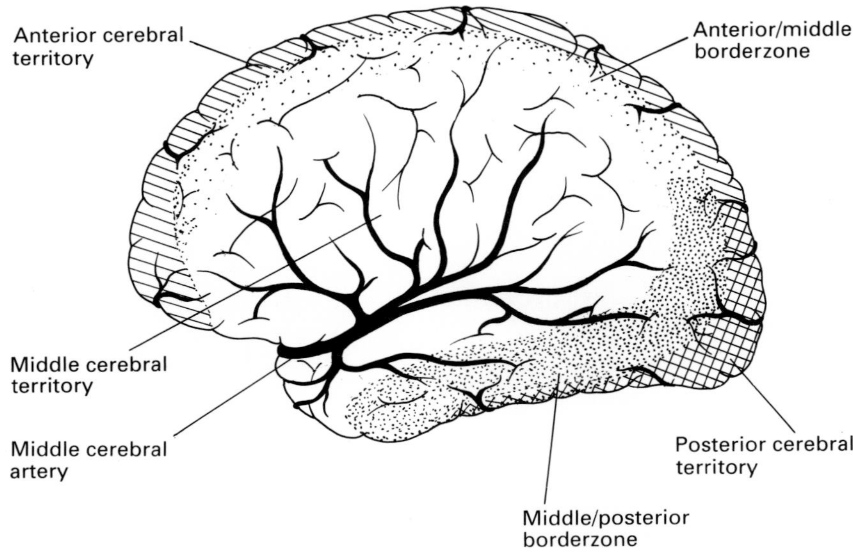

Fig. 13.4 Middle cerebral artery (MCA), surface distribution. The MCA ramifies over the lateral surface (convexity) of the brain. Superiorly and anteriorly the adjacent terminal branches and territory of the anterior cerebral artery (ACA) are depicted. Inferiorly and posteriorly the adjacent branches and territory of the posterior cerebral artery (PCA) are shown. The light and darker stippled areas indicate the cortical borderzones between the MCA–ACA and between the MCA–PCA, respectively. (The deep territory of the MCA is not depicted here – see Fig. 13.6.)

of the internal capsule, also lie within the MCA territory (Table 13.1).

Anterior cerebral artery

The anterior cerebral artery (ACA) provides circulation to much of the medial aspect of the hemisphere, not only anteriorly but back to the posterior parietal lobe (see Fig. 13.5). The medial occipital lobe (including the primary visual cortex) and the posterior–medial–inferior parts of the temporal lobe are mainly supplied by the posterior cerebral artery (PCA).

Posterior cerebral artery

The proximal PCA also irrigates parts of the midbrain, thalamus, and variably a small part of the internal capsule.

Internal capsule

The pattern of perfusion of the internal capsule is confusing: blood flow is derived from the deep penetrating branches of the MCA and from the anterior choroidal branch of the ICA. The PCA and posterior communicating arteries contribute slightly and variably.

Borderzone territories

The arterial "borderzones" (or "watersheds") are at the juncture of major arterial territories – for example, where the MCA territory meets the ACA territory (see Fig. 13.4). Potential or actual cross-circulation may occur between these distal fields, through small anastomoses. If a middle cerebral artery is occluded, its borderzone may well be effectively collateralized through the borderzone of the adjacent arterial system. In the case of general circulatory failure, however, with low pressure in all cerebral arteries, the perfusion failure is maximal in the borderzone

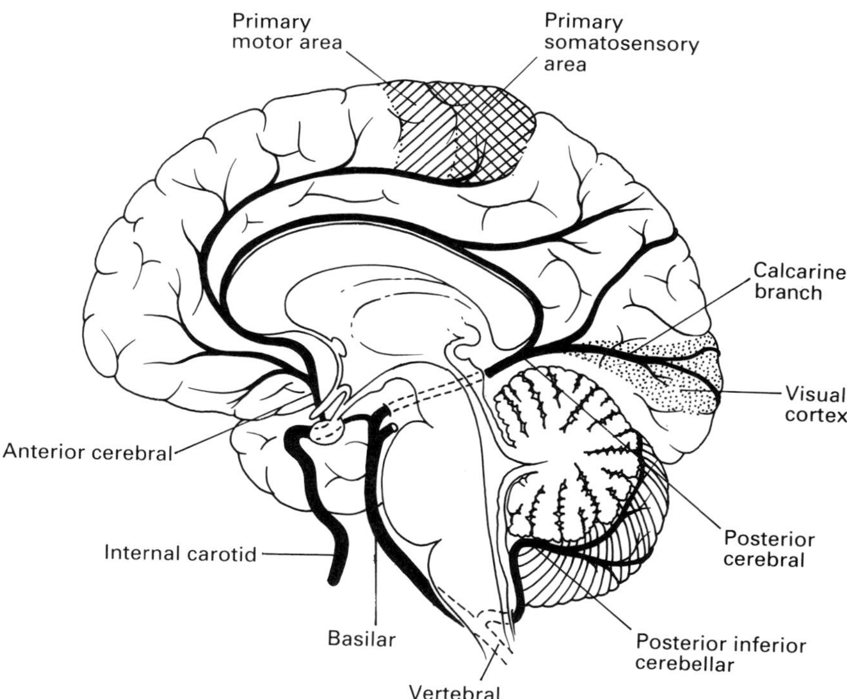

Fig. 13.5 Anterior cerebral artery (ACA) branches on the medial surface of the brain. The cortical territory of the ACA includes the leg, foot, and genital areas of the primary motor and primary somatosensory cortex (see Fig. 13.6). Among the branches of the posterior cerebral artery (PCA) the calcarine branch, supplying visual areas, is emphasized in this drawing. Not shown are the PCA branches to the medial and inferior parts of the occipital and temporal lobes and the thalamus. Also depicted in this selective rendition is the origin and cerebellar branching of the posterior inferior cerebellar artery from the vertebral artery. The medullary branches (see Fig. 14.5) are not shown.

areas: neither artery can supply its own distal territory or collateralize any adjacent territory. Infarction in the MCA–ACA borderzone high on the convexity of the frontal and parietal cortex affects proximal arms, trunk, and thighs (see Fig. 13.6 and the discussion of somatotopic representation in Chapter 14).

Vertebrobasilar system

Each of the two vertebral arteries supplies much of the medulla and inferior parts of the cerebellar hemisphere, on the same side; each contributes to the formation of the anterior and posterior spinal arteries (see Fig. 14.8 and the section on spinal column, cord, and nerve roots, below). The vertebral arteries join to form the basilar artery (a unique anatomic occurrence of two smaller arteries merging into one larger trunk!). Branches of the basilar artery irrigate much of the remaining brainstem and most of the cerebellum. The consequence of a single large midline

Table 13.1 Vascular territories: main arterial trunks and selected branches

	Trunk vessels	Major branches and divisions	Territory
Anterior circulation	Internal carotid arteries (no internal carotid branches in neck)		
		Ophthalmic arteries (other small intracranial branches)	Retina
		Anterior cerebral arteries (ACAs)	Medial hemispheric surface (leg areas of primary motor and sensory homunculus)
		Middle cerebral arteries (MCAs)	Lateral hemispheric surface. Deep territory: parts of central white matter, internal capsule, basal ganglia
		superior (anterior) division of MCA	Primary motor and sensory cortex; Broca's area, etc.
		inferior (posterior) division of MCA	Temporoparietal language areas (including Wernicke's); optic radiations, etc.
Posterior circulation	Vertebral arteries (right and left)		Medulla (most), cerebellum (posterior inferior parts)
		Anterior, posterior spinal arteries	Spinal cord
	Basilar artery (unpaired)		Pons; midbrain (most parts); cerebellum (anterior inferior, superior)
		Posterior cerebral arteries (PCAs) right and left	Visual cortex, medial occipital; hippocampus, posterior–inferior–medial temporal lobe; thalamus (including sensory nuclei); midbrain (small parts)

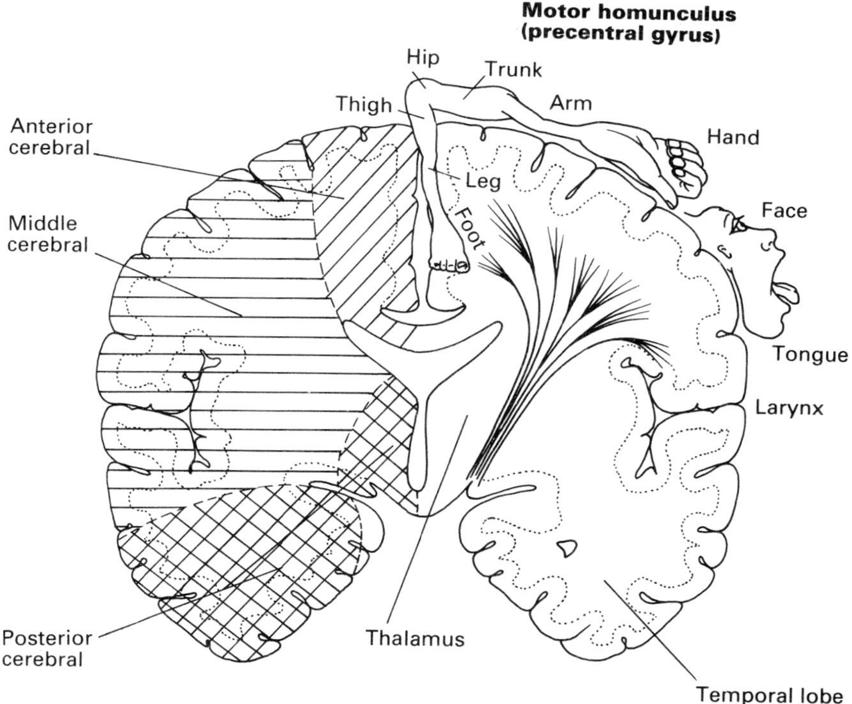

Fig. 13.6 Cortical motor homunculus in relation to vascular territories. Traditional somatotopic representation of the parts of the human body on the primary motor cortex. The cortical and deep territories of the anterior, middle, and posterior cerebral arteries are schematically depicted in this coronal section. Also shown are the consolidation of fibers from the cortical areas into a more compact bundle of corticospinal and corticobulbar fibers running through the posterior limb of the internal capsule. The vascular supply to the posterior limb of the internal capsule comes mainly from deep middle cerebral artery branches and/or the anterior choroidal artery, (not shown), and sometimes small contributions from the posterior cerebral and posterior communicating arteries. (Homunculus adapted from: Penfield, W., Rasmussen, H. *The Cerebral Cortex of Man*. Macmillan, New York (NY), 1950.)

arterial trunk is that impaired perfusion affects tissues of the brainstem and cerebellum bilaterally, and sometimes the territories of both PCAs, as well (see Fig. 14.8). Since each of the two PCAs is typically smaller in caliber than the parent basilar artery, an embolus that enters the basilar may not be able to exit. Occlusion of the "top of the basilar" often produces devastating infarction in the midbrain and in the PCA territories beyond.

Anatomy of intracranial hemorrhage

Every hemorrhage, whether from a cerebral artery within the brain or a saccular aneurysm in the subarachnoid space, erupts from a vessel that has a territory of normal perfusion. However, the extent of the hemorrhage does not respect the boundaries of that territory. Hemorrhages expand along lines of least resistance, often along white matter cleavage planes or even into the ventricular system. Thus, the anatomic distribution of a clot should be described not in vascular territorial terms, but in terms of the particular cerebral lobes or other specific structures

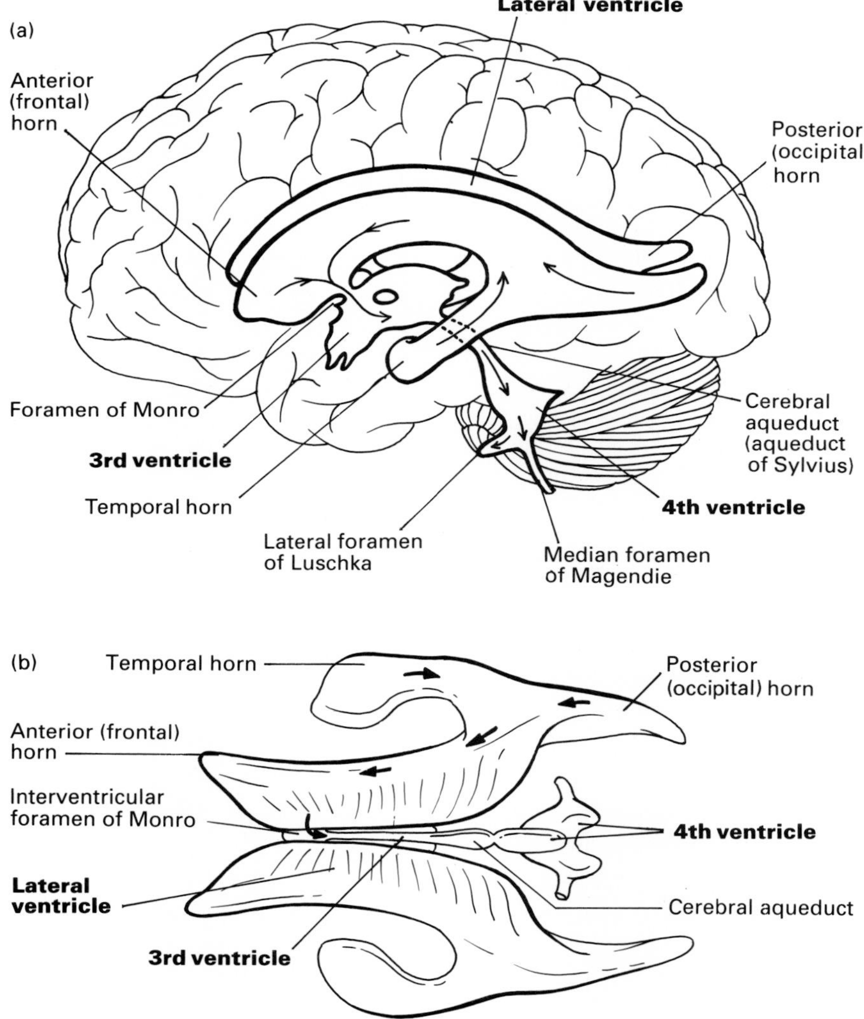

Fig. 13.7 The ventricular system. (a) Profile of ventricular system, superimposed upon a lateral view of the brain. The arrows show the general direction of net movement of cerebrospinal fluid (CSF) through the ventricular system. CSF is formed in all ventricles, but primarily in the lateral ventricles. (b) A view of the ventricular system from above, again showing the direction of net movement of CSF.

(basal ganglia, thalamus, etc.) involved. Hypertensive brain hemorrhages occur in four characteristic sites: the lateral basal ganglia (including the putamen), the thalamus, the cerebellum, and the pons. Other, "atypical," locations are associated with intracerebral hemorrhages in the context of coagulopathies, trauma, vascular malformations, etc.

Middle meningeal artery

The external carotid arteries and some of their palpable branches were described in Chapter 4 (see Fig. 4.2). The middle meningeal artery, coursing within the dura on the inner surface of the skull, is particularly vulnerable to trauma where it is applied to the thin, squamous portion of the temporal bone. A skull fracture in this temporal area often crosses the middle meningeal groove, lacerating the artery and leading to an epidural hematoma, which often produces transtentorial, temporal lobe herniation, if not promptly treated surgically.

CEREBROSPINAL FLUID PATHWAYS

CSF is produced by the choroid plexuses in the ventricular system (Figs 13.7 and 13.8), mainly in the lateral ventricles, and net flow is then out of the ventricular system, into the subarachnoid space around the brain and spinal cord, and finally to absorption into the venous system, mainly via the superior sagittal sinus. Figs 13.7 and 13.8 show the CSF pathways from the lateral ventricles through the paired foramina of Monro to the 3rd ventricle and via the aqueduct of Sylvius to the 4th ventricle, then out three small foramina into the subarachnoid space.

Hydrocephalus

Obstruction anywhere along these CSF pathways produces a "back-up" dilatation of upstream ventricles. If obstruction occurs at the aqueduct, for example, the 3rd and lateral ventricles expand and ventricular CSF does not communicate with the subarachnoid space, including the spinal subarachnoid space. This is a noncommunicating form of obstructive hydrocephalus (ventricular enlargement). If the block to CSF flow is outside the ventricular system (e.g. in a scarred-down subarachnoid space around the upper brainstem) then the hydrocephalus affects all the ventricles to some extent. It is termed communicating, since ventricular CSF can circulate to the spinal subarachnoid space. Here it can be tapped by lumbar puncture (under appropriate circumstances) and the CSF pressure will reflect changes in ventricular pressure. Passive ventricular dilatation, due to surrounding tissue loss, is called hydrocephalus *ex vacuo*.

SPINAL COLUMN, CORD, AND NERVE ROOTS

The major anatomic relationships of the bony spinal column, the spinal cord, and roots are directly relevant to numerous clinical situations, such as performing a lumbar puncture, analyzing back pain, and dealing with possible spinal cord compression, including one of the most preventable types of neurologic disorder, spinal trauma.

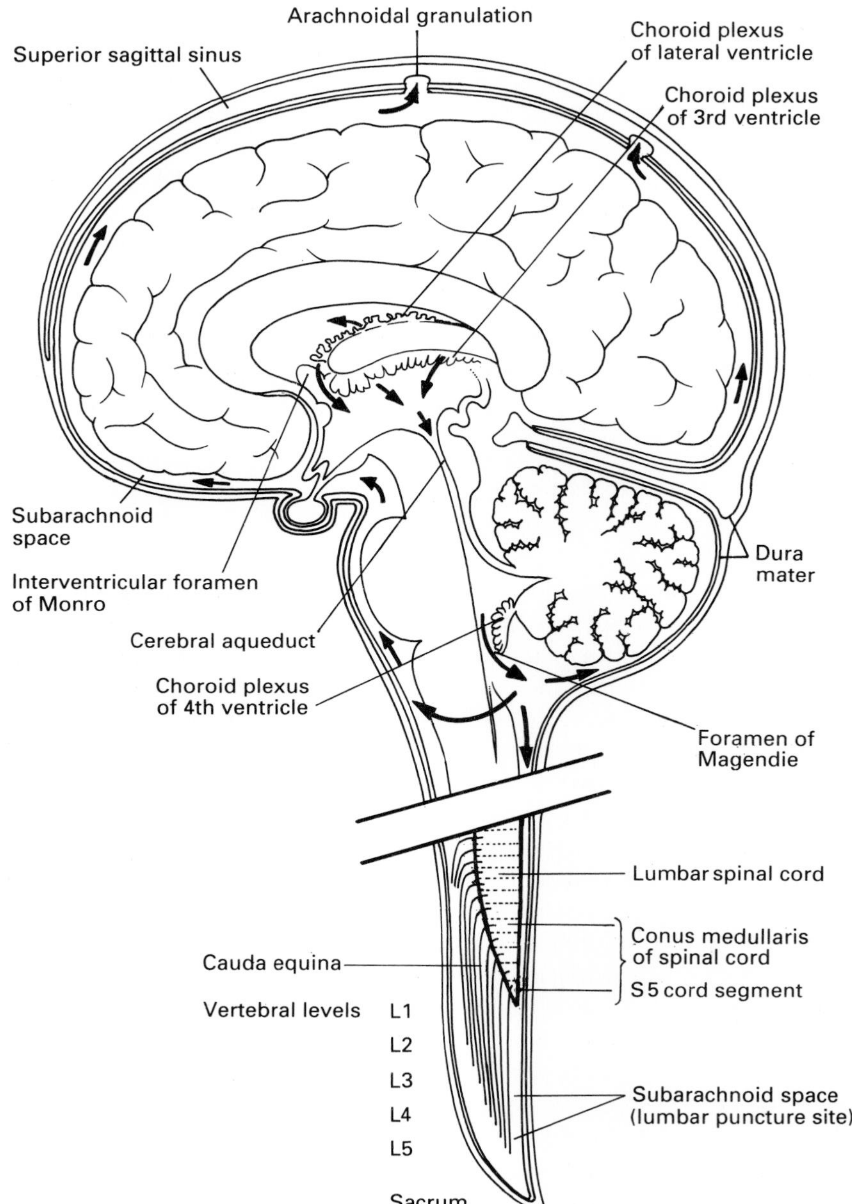

Fig. 13.8 Circulation of the cerebrospinal fluid (CSF): ventricular and subarachnoid pathways, represented in a midsagittal plane. Only the upper cervical and lumbosacral levels of the spinal canal are included. The end of the spinal cord and the cauda equina are shown in a simplified, schematic version to emphasize the surrounding subarachnoid (CSF) space and safe levels for lumbar puncture. Some CSF absorption occurs at spinal levels as well as at the principal site, the superior sagittal sinus.

Spinal cord/spinal column disproportion

The disproportion between the length of the spinal cord and the length of the bony spinal column (Fig. 13.9) is a central fact of spinal neurology below the cervical region. In the adult, the spinal cord itself ends at approximately the L1 vertebral level, but the spinal roots hang down in a "horse's tail" (cauda equina) to exit at the appropriate intervertebral foramina; for example, the L4 anterior root emerges from the 4th lumbar cord segment opposite vertebral level T12, but exits between the L4 and L5 vertebrae.

Risk of cord compression

Any pathologic process that is known to be below the L1 vertebral level will not ordinarily impinge upon the spinal cord. A potentially compressive lesion at vertebral level L4 does not carry the extreme degree of urgency that a similar lesion at T4 would entail. This is not to say that compression of a spinal root or the whole cauda equina would not be potentially serious, but the emergency is not so grave as when the spinal cord itself is threatened. The most common diseases that cause low back pain strike below the L1 vertebral level; protrusion of an intervertebral disc preferentially involves the L4–L5, L5–S1, and L3–L4 levels. By the same token, lumbar puncture in the adult at the L4–L5, L3–L4, or even (though not recommended) the L2–L3 levels, does not risk puncture damage to the spinal cord itself.

Lumbar puncture level

Root exit level

The level of exit of a spinal root, with respect to the vertebra of the same number, differs from the cervical to lower regions (see Fig. 13.9). The C1–C7 roots pass above their respective vertebral bodies, because the C1 root exits between the skull and C1. The C8 root is "extra" (as there is no C8 vertebra); it is located between C7 and T1. From there on down, starting with the T1 root, the remaining roots pass below the vertebra of the same number.

Herniated disc

At the lumbar level the root affected by a herniated intervertebral disc often is the next lower one, however. For example, an L4–L5 disc typically impinges on the L5 root, which is vulnerable as it descends across the L4–L5 disc space to exit at L5–S1. Note that the sacral segments are fused, so that there are no discs between S1 and S2, etc. (see Chapter 19, selective examination for low back/leg pain).

Spinal trauma

The segmented column is especially vulnerable to trauma at its intervertebral joints, resulting in displacement of one vertebral body and posterior arch relative to an adjacent one, above or below. In the absence of underlying bone or joint pathology, this occurs only with major trauma (in which head injury may divert attention from coexistent spinal injury).

Within the spinal canal, combinations of pathologic processes may conspire to produce compressive cord injury. For example, it is not uncommon for a cervical or thoracic intervertebral disc or bony spur to mildly indent the subarachnoid space and even the cord without apparent

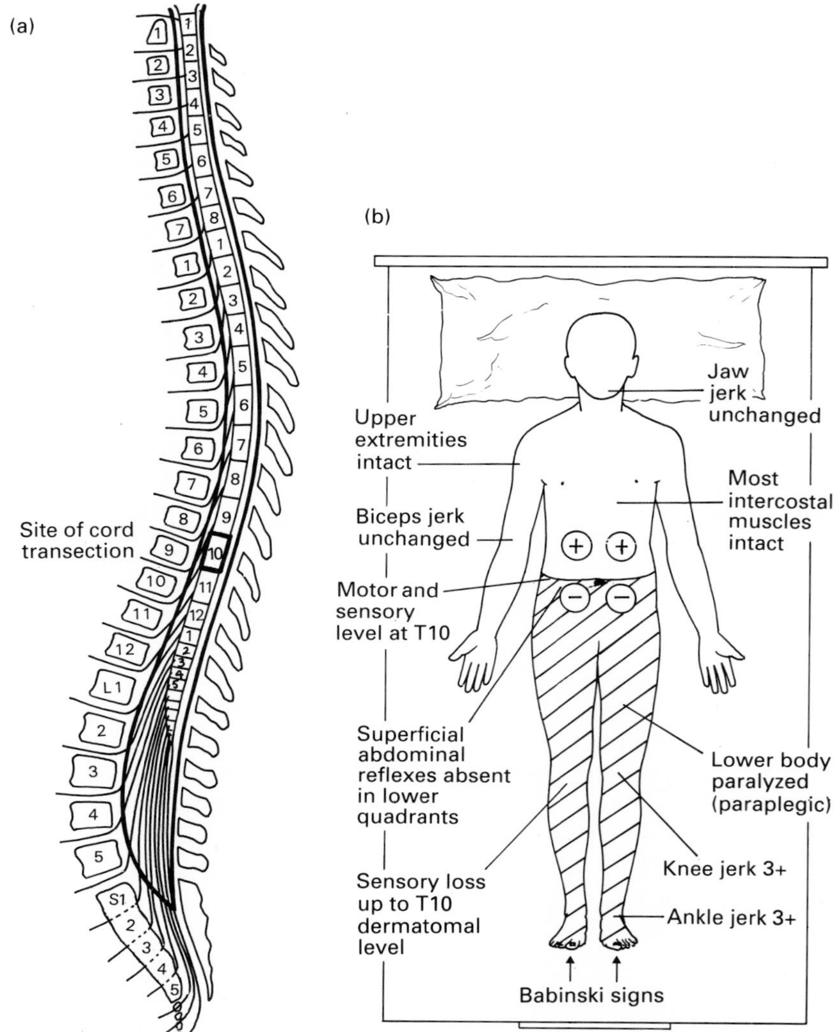

Fig. 13.9 Spinal cord, vertebral, and clinical levels. (a) Note the disproportion between the spinal cord and spinal column: below the cervical region the cord segments are progressively rostral to the vertebral segments. This cord ends at approximately L1–L2 (usually T12–L2). The site of a lesion transecting the spinal cord is shown at cord segment T10. Note that sacral vertebral segments are fused; the roots exit via foramina, not interspaces. (b) A clinical level at T10 with motor, sensory, and reflex markers indicated. After initial spinal shock, deep tendon reflexes in the legs are hyperactive and extensor plantar signs (Babinski signs) present. Superficial abdominal reflexes are present in the two upper quadrants (above T10, marked by the umbilicus), but absent in the two lower quadrants. Descending sympathetic and parasympathetic pathways in the cord (not shown) are also disrupted (but descending sympathetic fibers leaving the cord above T10 to enter the sympathetic chain are preserved).

clinical effect. Since the spinal cord is housed in relatively tight quarters in the spinal canal, superimposed trauma might then cause more damage than would otherwise be expected. The cord is tethered within the spinal meninges, with only a rather thin layer of CSF in the subarachnoid space, a potential subdural space, and a small epidural space.

Compressive lesions

Any mass, whether tumor, abscess, hematoma, bony spur, or protruding intervertebral disc, at a vertebral level from C1 to L1, carries a high potential for cord compression and irreversible neuronal injury. The vertebrae, intervertebral disc spaces, and the intraspinal plexus of draining veins are common sites for the growth and spread of metastatic tumors and abscesses that progressively impinge on cord and roots.

Arterial circulation to the spinal cord

The arterial supply to the cord (see Figs 13.3, 14.3, and 14.8) seems surprisingly tenuous for such a crucial structure, but arterial occlusion is quite unusual. Two small posterior spinal arteries (from the vertebrals) perfuse the posterior third of the cord. The anterolateral two-thirds of the cord depends on the anterior spinal artery, which arises rostrally from a branch from each vertebral artery and is collateralized at intervals by branches from the segmental intercostal arteries from the aorta. (There is usually one especially large intercostal feeder.) Most threats to the spinal blood supply (aside from damage in trauma or spinal surgery) come from the aorta in the form of vascular operations, dissections, or atherosclerotic/embolic processes that occlude one or more intercostal branches. In Chapter 14 the anterior spinal artery syndrome is used to exemplify one pattern of spinal cord topographic diagnosis.

GENERAL FEATURES OF BRAINSTEM TOPOGRAPHY

Divisions

The three main rostrocaudal divisions of the brainstem are the midbrain, pons, and medulla (Table 13.2). Cranial nerve nuclei 3–12 are arrayed down the brainstem, revealing its overall segmental character (though less regular than in the spinal cord).

Strata of the brainstem

In a ventrodorsal plane two major layers, the basal (ventral) stratum and the dorsal stratum (tegmentum) are evident (Fig. 13.10). The long fiber tracts from the cerebral hemispheres to the spinal cord tend to run in the ventral stratum (although the ascending sensory tracts move dorsally as they proceed rostrally and approach the thalamus). Generally, the long tracts remain ventral to the cranial nerve nuclei which are concentrated in the tegmentum. Because of this separation, focal lesions such as small strokes can damage tracts while sparing nuclei, or vice versa. In the midbrain a third stratum, the tectum or roof, which is dorsal to the aqueduct, contains the paired superior and inferior colliculi that are involved in the visual and auditory systems, respectively.

Table 13.2 Brainstem localization: midbrain, pons, medulla

	Midbrain	Pons	Medulla
Principal cranial nerve nuclei	CN 3 oculomotor, CN 4 trochlear	CN 5 Trigeminal (main sensory, motor); CN 6 abducens; CN 7 facial	CN 8 acoustic, vestibular; CN 9 glossopharyngeal; CN 10 vagus; (CN 11 cranial portion); CN 12 hypoglossal
Role in conjugate eye movement control	Vertical gaze (midbrain/pretectal area)	Horizontal gaze (pontine center, see Chapter 17)	(Vestibular inputs to pontine, midbrain centers)
Role in pupillary size and reactions (see text)	Edinger–Westphal/CN 3 complex: parasympathetic outflow; passage of descending sympathetic tracts	Passage of descending sympathetic tracts	Continued passage of descending sympathetic tracts
Role in consciousness/ alertness	Midbrain portion of reticular system		
Best-known neurotransmitter/ neuromodulator sources	Dopaminergic (substantia nigra, ventral tegmental area, etc.); enkephalinergic (periaqueductal gray); seratonergic (raphe nuclei)	Noradrenergic (locus coeruleus); seratonergic (raphe nuclei)	Seratonergic raphe nuclei (nucleus raphe magnus, etc.)
Position of long tracts			
Corticospinal tract	Cerebral peduncles (basis pedunculi)	Base of the pons	Medullary pyramids
Dorsal column/medial lemniscal sensory system	Dorsal lateral tegmentum (approaching ventral posterior nuclei of thalamus)	Medial lemnisci	2nd order neurons in dorsal column nuclei; internal arcuate fibers form medial lemnisci
Spinothalamic fibers (2nd order neurons)	Dorsal lateral tegmentum – blending with lemniscal fibers	Lateral	Lateral
Relationship to cerebellar peduncles	Superior peduncles (cross in midbrain tegmentum)	Middle peduncles	Inferior peduncles
Arterial supply	Top of the basilar artery; small branches from proximal posterior cerebral and posterior communicating arteries	Basilar artery branches (incl. anterior inferior cerebellar artery branches to pons)	Vertebral arteries and branches, (incl. posterior inferior cerebellar artery branches to lateral medulla)
Characteristic vascular pathology	Embolic infarctions (top of basilar or posterior cerebrals); thrombotic infarction of proximal posterior cerebrals	Thrombotic infarction (basilar artery and small branches); hypertensive hemorrhage	Infarction: thrombotic (or embolic) occlusion of vertebral artery or posterior inferior cerebellar artery ("PICA")

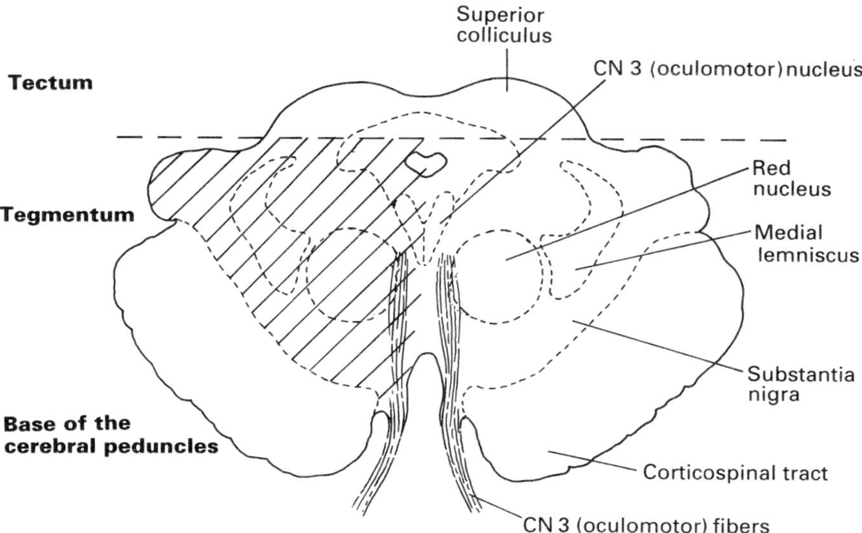

Fig. 13.10 Strata of the midbrain. The tectum (only in the midbrain) is dorsal to the aqueduct and includes the colliculi. The tegmentum (diagonal hatching, shown on one side only) comprises all of the area ventral to the tectum and dorsal to the base of the cerebral peduncles. Cranial nerve nuclei are located in the tegmentum, and the corticospinal and corticobulbar tracts run in the base. Several classic vascular syndromes result from combined involvement of the motor tracts in the base, the exiting CN 3, and/or tegmental structures.

Cranial nerves

The cranial nerves do not cross (with the exception of CN 4 and those fibers from CN 3 nuclei that are destined for the superior rectus and some fibers to the levator palpebrae muscles). Crossed function is achieved by decussation of the descending (or ascending) long suprasegmental tracts, such as the corticobulbar tracts which are the upper motor neuron (UMN) tracts synapsing on the cranial nerve motor nuclei.

Long tract crossing

Two of the long tract systems of greatest diagnostic importance (see pp. 266–71) cross in the brainstem: the corticobulbar/corticospinal tracts and the dorsal column/medial lemniscal system for vibration, conscious joint position sense, and fine touch. (Fibers of the third major tract, the lateral spinothalamic tract, cross at successive levels of the spinal cord, as will be described later.) Like the afferents entering at a spinal level, virtually all afferents entering the brainstem are 1st order neurons with their cell bodies outside the CNS in ganglia corresponding to the spinal dorsal root ganglia. The 2nd order neurons cross in the brainstem on their way to the contralateral thalamus.

CRANIAL NERVE CONTROL OF EYE MOVEMENTS

In keeping with the general pattern of uncrossed cranial and spinal nerves innervating ipsilateral structures, the cranial nerves controlling eye movements are uncrossed (with the clinically minor exceptions noted earlier). CN 3 (oculomotor) mediates vertical, horizontal (adduction), and rotatory movements. CN 4 (trochlear) also acts both vertically and in rotation; these actions of CNs 3 and 4 must be analyzed in relationship to the position of the eye, which determines the result of muscle traction on it (see Fig. 5.6). CN 6 (abducens) is instrumental only in horizontal movements (see Figs 5.6 and 5.7), since it innervates only the lateral rectus muscle, which abducts the eye.

Muscle actions dependent on position

Neural control on the right and left side is closely integrated: the two eyes must move exactly together in order to maintain binocular fusion and avoid double vision. Since turning the eyes towards the right involves abduction of the right eye and adduction of the left eye, the function of CN 6 (pons) on the right and CN 3 (midbrain) on the left must be coupled or "yoked" to produce this conjugate movement. The crossing of a connecting pathway in the brainstem, the medial longitudinal fasciculus (MLF), accomplishes this hook-up, as well as connections with the trochlear and vestibular nuclei. You can remember that the MLF fibers connecting CN nuclei 6 and 3 must be crossed, since CN 6 on one side works in concert with CN 3 on the other side. A lesion in the MLF preventing the horizontal gaze message from reaching CN 3 (the adducting eye), results in double vision caused by the syndrome of internuclear ophthalmoplegia (INO) (see Fig. 5.7). As a neat proof that this typical form of INO is related to horizontal gaze and does not merely reflect a medial rectus palsy, consider convergence: both eyes adduct in response to a visual or mental stimulus to converge (mediated bilaterally at a midbrain level). In the INO syndrome, both eyes adduct normally in convergence.

Internuclear connections

MLF

An overall schema for control of conjugate eye movements, or gaze, is contained in Chapter 17. Note that the brainstem control of horizontal gaze is situated in a "pontine gaze center" in the same area as the abducens (CN 6) nucleus: both act in horizontal eye movements – a fact that may help as a mnemonic.

CONTROL OF PUPILLARY FUNCTION

The intrinsic mechanism for control of the size and reactivity of the pupils balances two major forces, the parasympathetic and sympathetic systems. The parasympathetic fibers join the 3rd nerve and act to constrict the pupil. A parasympathetic lesion causing dilatation and loss of reactivity must occur at some point along the intracranial or orbital course of the 3rd nerve itself, or in the midbrain where the parasympathetic fibers arise in the Edinger–Westphal/CN 3 nuclear complex. Most cases

Parasympathetic lesion

of an enlarging pupil with decreasing reactivity result from compression of the peripheral CN3 in its course outside the brainstem.

The sympathetic fibers to the eye do not run with a cranial nerve (except terminally, at the eye), but travel by a circuitous route: they pass from the hypothalamus down the brainstem to spinal cord segments T1 and T2, then to the sympathetic chain of ganglia, and finally upward with the carotid and ophthalmic arteries to the eye (Fig. 13.11). This sympathetic input di-

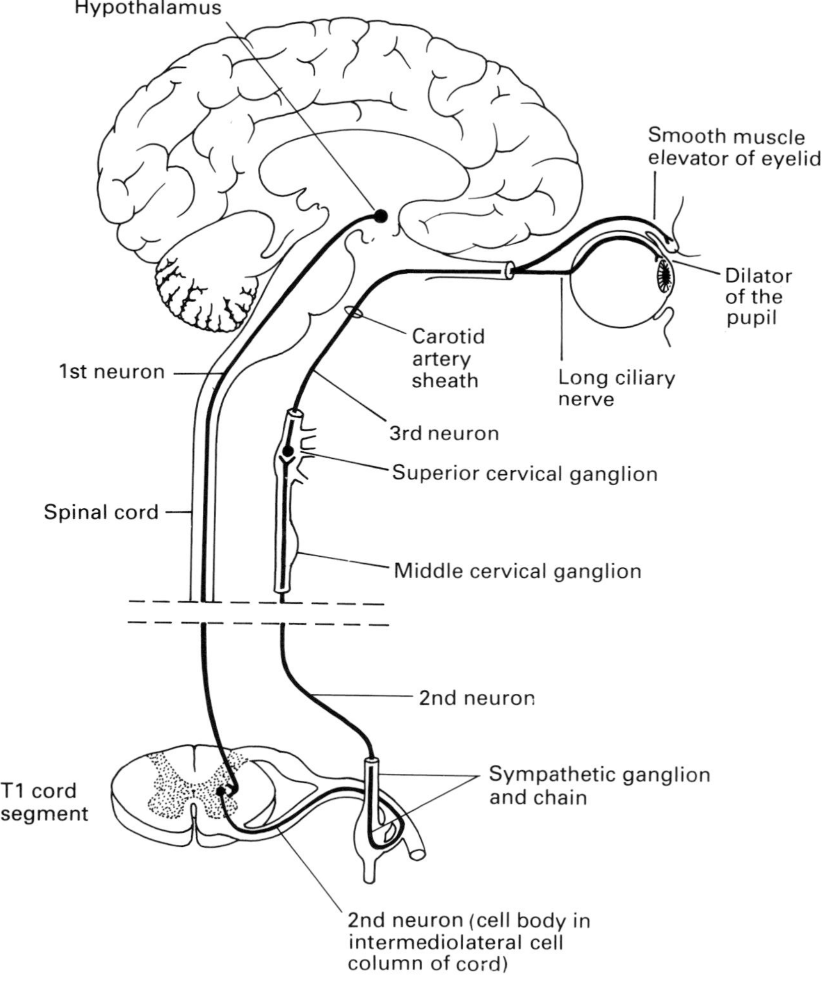

Fig. 13.11 Sympathetic pathway to the eye. In simplified form, this pathway consists of a three neuron chain. The 1st neuron is in the hypothalamus, projecting caudally to the intermediolateral cell column of gray matter at spinal cord segment T1. The 2nd neuron enters and runs up the sympathetic chain of ganglia (outside the vertebral column) to synapse in the superior cervical ganglion. The 3rd neuron ascends with the internal carotid artery into the intracranial vault, then forward into the orbit to innervate the dilator muscle of the pupil and the (smooth muscle) elevator of the upper eyelid.

Sympathetic lesion, Horner's syndrome

lates the pupil; a lesion of these fibers thus causes a smaller pupil (miosis) but does not obliterate reflex constriction (although this reaction may be hard to see because of the already small pupil). As a result of the long course of the nerves that comprise this schematic "three-neuron" sympathetic pathway, the site of a sympathetic lesion causing pupillary constriction may be located in the brain, spine, chest, neck, or orbit. The full Horner's syndrome also comprises lid droop (ptosis) and, depending on the site of the interruption, decreased facial sweating ipsilateral to the lesion.

Clues to brainstem level

In trying to localize a lesion within the brainstem, pupillary findings play an important role (see Table 13.2). Assuming a lesion within the brainstem: an enlarged pupil with decreased or absent reactivity indicates a midbrain level; an extremely small ("pinpoint") pupil suggests a pontine or medullary level of involvement, since the descending sympathetic tract could be affected in the pons or medulla, thus causing pupillary constriction, without affecting the parasympathetic output from the midbrain at all. Obviously a sufficiently extensive midbrain lesion could affect both the sympathetic and parasympathetic systems; the pupils might therefore be midsize, but nonreactive, as is often the case in advanced stages of damage to the midbrain (or caudal diencephalon).

For the correlation of pupillary changes with lesions of the afferent and efferent fibers, see Tables 5.5 and 5.6. Also, refer to the section on visual pathways later in this chapter.

OTHER AUTONOMIC FUNCTIONS

The autonomic control of bladder, bowel, and sexual function will be exemplified by the major neural connections to and from the urinary bladder.

Sympathetic supply to bladder

The spinal sympathetic and parasympathetic pathways that control bladder function are depicted schematically in Fig. 13.12. Sympathetic control, as always, begins in the hypothalamus, which is influenced by limbic and other cortical inputs. Descending sympathetic fibers (relevant to pelvic function) synapse in the intermediolateral column of the upper lumbar spinal cord, where the "2nd neurons" pass through the lower sympathetic ganglia and lumbar splanchnic nerves to the more peripheral (inferior mesenteric) sympathetic ganglion. From there, shorter postganglionic fibers innervate smooth muscles of the bladder. (This is the typical pattern for abdominal and pelvic viscera, whereas the ganglionic synapse elsewhere is usually in the sympathetic chain.)

Parasympathetic supply to bladder

The higher parasympathetic control from the hypothalamus is not as well defined as the descending sympathetic tracts. The segmental outflow from the sacral spinal cord to the bladder and other pelvic viscera originates from segments S2–S4, passes through the pelvic splanchnic nerves, and then synapses in peripheral ganglia in or near the organ involved. Short postganglionic fibers innervate visceral smooth muscle.

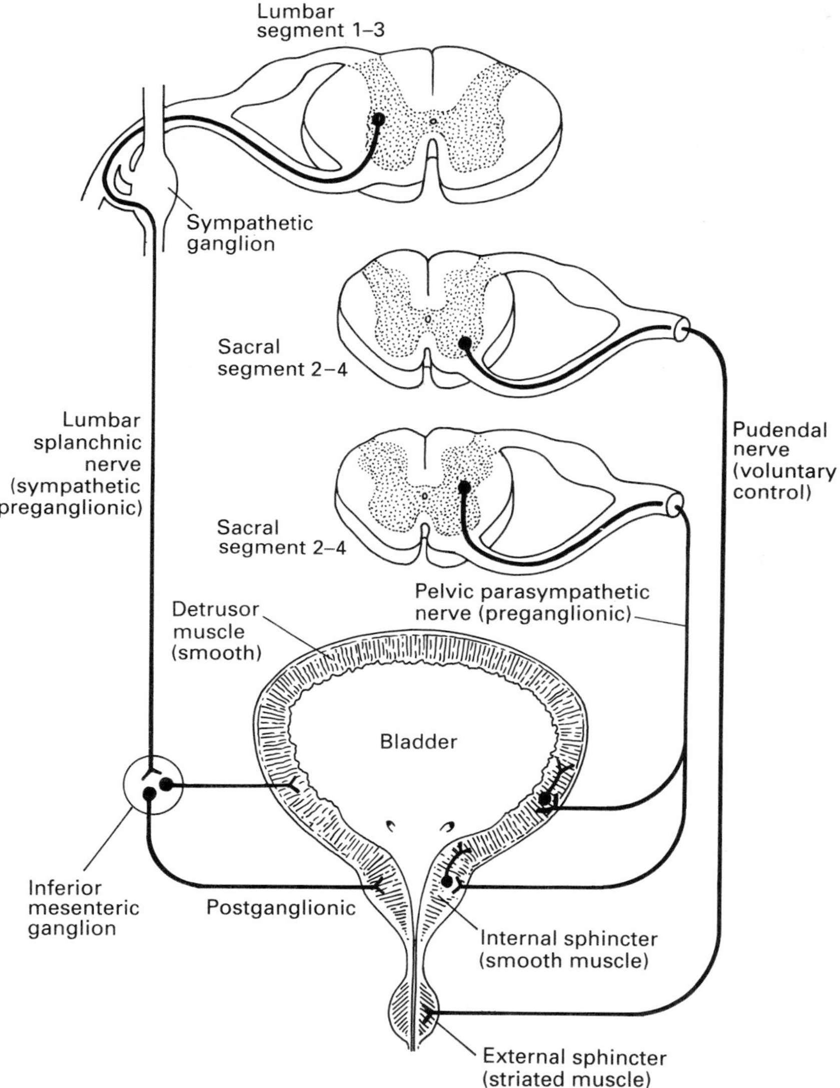

Fig. 13.12 Urinary bladder, efferent control. The parasympathetic supply from the sacral spinal cord (S2–S4) to the smooth muscle of the bladder provides the main autonomic control. Note the synapse of the preganglionic parasympathetic neuron with the postganglionic neuron in the bladder wall. The role of the sympathetic supply from the lumbar splanchnic nerves (approximately L1–L3) is less clear. There is also voluntary control of the external sphincter. (The afferents from the bladder are not shown.)

Autonomic afferents

When the sacral spinal cord is cut off from higher control, reflex emptying of the bladder can occur. This depends, in part, on visceral afferents. (As the afferents approach the spinal column they diverge from the autonomic efferents, since their cell bodies are in the dorsal root ganglia, like other afferents.)

Balance of inputs

Autonomic function of the urinary bladder, sexual organs, and lower gastrointestinal tract thus depends upon a balance between sympathetic and parasympathetic mechanisms and upon a delicate relationship with limited voluntary motor control. Autonomic control of urination is predominantly parasympathetic; erection depends upon parasympathetic input, whereas ejaculation has a sympathetic component.

Suprasegmental control

The role of cortical and other suprasegmental control of urination is much more complicated than is evident from the rule that UMN problems cause a spastic bladder, while lower motor and afferent disorders result in a flaccid bladder. Nonetheless, this is a useful first approximation. The typical effect of bilateral upper motor dysfunction (as in upper spinal cord demyelination in multiple sclerosis) is the development of a spastic bladder. This is a small bladder that reacts excessively to relatively small filling volumes and pressures. The patient experiences frequency, but voids only small amounts, leaving some residual urine. The suprasegmental motor tract dysfunction must be bilateral, because of peripheral merging of the right and left autonomic inputs to the bladder and other midline organs.

Lesions in segmental pathways

Bilateral destruction of the spinal cord autonomic outflow to the bladder (especially the sacral parasympathetic system), as well as loss of afferent input, results in a decreased or absent response to bladder filling. The bladder then enlarges and eventually overflows, causing a dribbling incontinence or sometimes a flood. What actually happens in the individual patient cannot be definitely predicted from this formula, as there may be different balances of the several factors noted. Moreover, the occurrence of bladder infection alters bladder responsivity and size.

Clinical approach

In summary, when you encounter a patient with apparent neurogenic bladder, bowel, or sexual dysfunction, consider the following factors, based upon a "systems" approach and relevant anatomy and physiology:

1 non-neurologic problems, such as anatomic obstruction and infection;

2 the level of a suprasegmental lesion in the neuraxis: (a) status of brain function, including frontal lobe behavioral control, such as inhibition; affective factors, such as the role of depression in cases of impotence; (b) neuroendocrine disorders, especially at a hypothalamic–pituitary level; for example, a prolactin-secreting pituitary tumor causing impotence; (c) a spinal cord lesion above the sympathetic output to the pelvic viscera (see Further reading section);

3 the level of the lesion with respect to key structures at a segmental level, such as the parasympathetic output of the sacral cord;

4 involvement of neural structures outside the spinal cord and column, such as peripheral nerves, like the pudendal (see Fig. 13.12);
5 whether the lesion is bilateral;
6 involvement of afferent pathways, affecting sensory perception;
7 whether sympathetic or parasympathetic function is solely or predominantly affected (this depends upon the anatomic location of the lesion, pathologic selectivity of particular diseases, and any pharmacologic effects, either from agonist or antagonist drugs; see Further reading section).

GLOSSARY OF SYNONYMOUS AND EASILY CONFUSED TERMS

Dermatome: a dermatome (such as the right 4th lumbar) is the skin area innervated by afferent fibers that will meet their cell bodies in one dorsal root ganglion (right L4). The central processes of these neurons form the right L4 dorsal root that enters the spinal canal at the L4–L5 vertebral interspace and joins the spinal cord at the L4 cord level. Some of these fibers synapse in the dorsal horn; some others ascend in the dorsal column.

Dorsal horn/posterior horn: dorsal (posterior) part of spinal central gray matter (cell bodies of sensory neurons etc.). Distinguish dorsal horn (gray matter) from dorsal column (white matter).

Dorsal root/posterior root: central process (axon) of dorsal root ganglion cell, as well as its peripheral process (axon) up to the point of joining the anterior root to form a mixed peripheral nerve.

Dorsal root ganglion (DRG): cluster of cell bodies of 1st order sensory neurons, located approximately at the intervertebral foramen.

Dorsal columns/posterior columns: white matter tracts in posterior part of spinal cord – transmit vibration, fine touch, and some position sense. A group of tracts, as in the dorsal columns, may be called a fasciculus, as in fasciculus gracilis and fasciculus cuneatus, the two major components of the dorsal columns (see *Tract*).

Dorsal column nuclei: nuclei gracilis and cuneatus in the caudal medulla. These contain cell bodies of 2nd order neurons in dorsal column system.

Nucleus dorsalis: cell bodies of 2nd order neurons in the unconscious proprioceptive (spinocerebellar) pathway. Nucleus dorsalis is also known as Clarke's column of gray matter. Do not confuse it with the dorsal columns of white matter or with a dorsal column nucleus.

Tract: a group of anatomically and functionally related CNS fibers with a common origin and destination. Different tracts may run in an anatomically distinct group that is sometimes called a fasciculus. Multiple fasciculi may be located in a distinct sector of the spinal cord white matter called a funiculus. The dorsal funiculi are also known as the dorsal columns.

Ventral horn/anterior horn: anterior (ventral) part of spinal central gray matter – cell bodies of "anterior horn cells" including the α motor neurons (lower motor neurons).

Ventral root/anterior root: axons of anterior horn cells up to the point that they join the posterior root to form a spinal nerve or mixed peripheral nerve; still the same axons after that, but no longer called roots.

Ventral columns/anterior columns: white matter tracts in the ventral part of the cord, including the anterior corticospinal tract and the reticulospinal tract of the "ventromedial" group of descending tracts. The spinothalamic tracts comprise the "anterolateral" system of ascending pathways.

NEURAL PATHWAYS: THE MAJOR LONG TRACTS

The long fiber tracts are the heart of the clinical neuroanatomy of the CNS: the visual system, the two main somatosensory systems (pain–temperature and fine touch–vibration–position), and the fine motor control system (corticospinal–corticobulbar). Of course, many other neural systems – including the limbic system, autonomic tracts, memory centers and circuits, and the whole expanding field of neurochemical projection – are essential for human function, but not of first priority in diagnostic localization.

Crossed control

Long tracts typically cross over to the opposite side of the CNS, enabling one cerebral hemisphere to relate primarily to the opposite side of the body and visual space. As will be noted in the next chapter on clinical constructs, this generalization applies to fine motor activity, to the two major sensory systems, and, in effect, to visual reception. However, multisynaptic uncrossed pathways also contribute to motor and sensory function in ways that are not reflected in the simple model provided here.

Descending motor tracts

Corticospinal tracts

The corticospinal tracts run from the cerebral cortex – mainly from the motor cortex of the posterior frontal lobe – to segments of the spinal cord where some fibers synapse with anterior horn cells that send their axons to muscles. The decussation of the predominant lateral corticospinal tract is in the caudal medulla (see Fig. 6.1). The corticobulbar tracts are analogous to the corticospinal tract in that these are cortical neuronal fibers that are destined for brainstem motor nuclei (see Fig. 5.1). The term "bulbar" is loosely used to refer to brainstem (rather than strictly referring just to the medulla). Thus, corticobulbar means linkage from cortex to brainstem, just as corticospinal relates cortex to spinal cord. Those corticobulbar tract fibers destined to decussate in the brainstem do so just rostral to their intended cranial nerve nuclei. (Motor tracts will be emphasized in the section on constructs of suprasegmental control in Chapter 14.)

Ascending sensory tracts

Two great sensory systems account for the transmission of most conscious, somatosensory information to the brain. One of these consists of the spinothalamic pathways (anterolateral system) of which the important part diagnostically is the lateral spinothalamic tract, conveying pain and temperature information (Fig. 13.13). The other system is the dorsal column–lemniscal group of pathways (Fig. 13.14) responsible for the sense of vibration and some aspects of conscious joint position, and fine tactile sense. (The term "lemniscal" refers to the medial lemniscus, which is the name assigned to this pathway after it has crossed in the brainstem.)

Features of the simplest general model of sensory transmission include the following.

Segmental sensory structures

1 The minimum segmental sensory apparatus comprises the peripheral sensory receptor (or free nerve ending), the peripheral nerve fiber with its cell body in the dorsal root ganglion, the central axon (of that same nerve cell) that forms the proximal dorsal root, and the synapse of some of these fibers with neurons in the dorsal horn gray matter of the spinal cord (Fig. 13.15).

Some 1st order neuron fibers enter CNS tracts

2 Once within the spinal cord, the incoming axons are designated as CNS fibers, with different supporting cells. The segmental organization of peripheral input to the spinal cord gives way to a much more complex pattern within the spinal cord: some 1st order neuron fibers synapse immediately; others ascend or descend from one to several segments before synapsing in a dorsal horn; still others ascend the length of the spinal cord before synapsing, as will be described.

1st order neurons do not cross

3 No matter what the pattern of ascent or descent, or the modality served, the fibers of the 1st order neurons never cross sides. Thus, the segmental sensory input to the spinal cord (like the segmental motor output) is ipsilateral.

Key 2nd order neurons cross

4 The neurons with which these 1st order sensory fibers synapse are designated 2nd order sensory neurons, wherever they are located in the spinal cord or in the brainstem. Not all ascending sensory tracts cross or cross completely, but those that hold most importance for clinical diagnosis do decussate. In any sensory system in which fiber crossing does occur, it is an axon of the 2nd order sensory neuron that crosses.

3rd order neurons do not cross

5 Continuing with the simplest, most direct model of sensory pathways, the 2nd order neuron synapses in the thalamus. From there a 3rd order neuron projects to the ipsilateral primary somatosensory cortex.

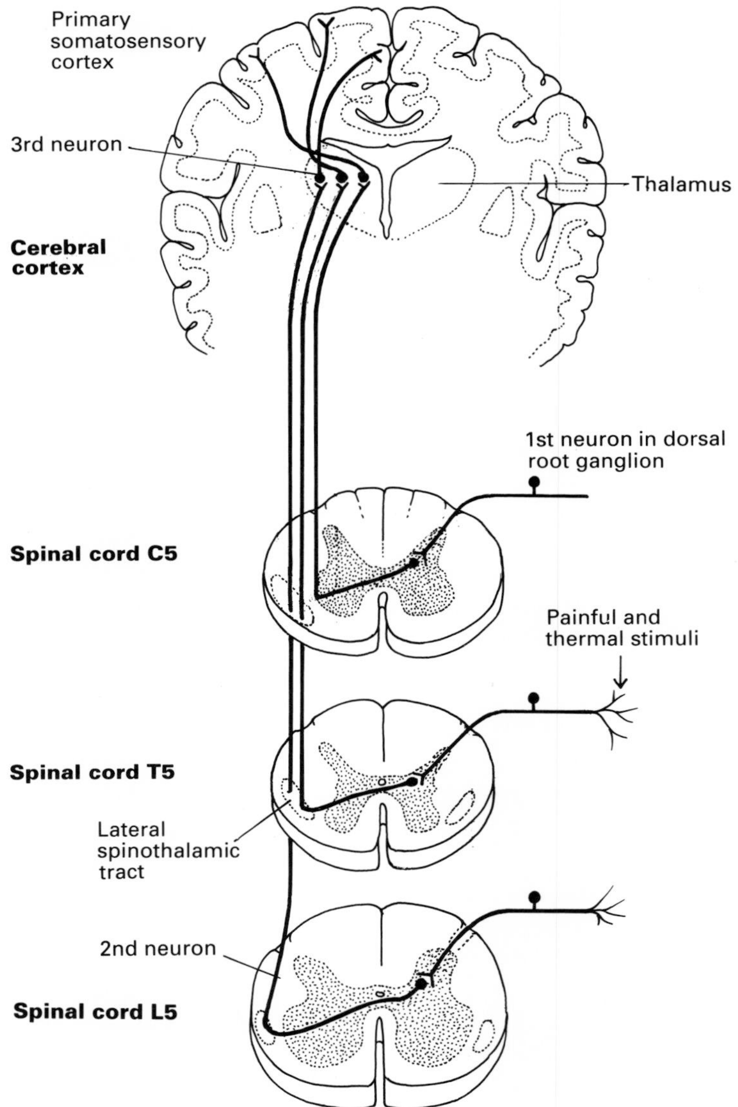

Fig. 13.13 Pain–temperature pathway. This very simplified pain–temperature pathway is schematically shown in terms of a three neuron chain. The 1st order neuron with its cell body in the dorsal root ganglion sends its central process to synapse in the dorsal horn of the spinal cord. The 2nd order fiber crosses the midline (usually during ascent of one or two segments) to join the lateral spinothalamic tract. The 3rd order neuron in the thalamus projects to the cortex. (This model does not reflect the complex collateralization and intermediate synapses of most fibers. The laminar localization of the dorsal horn synapse is not represented here.)

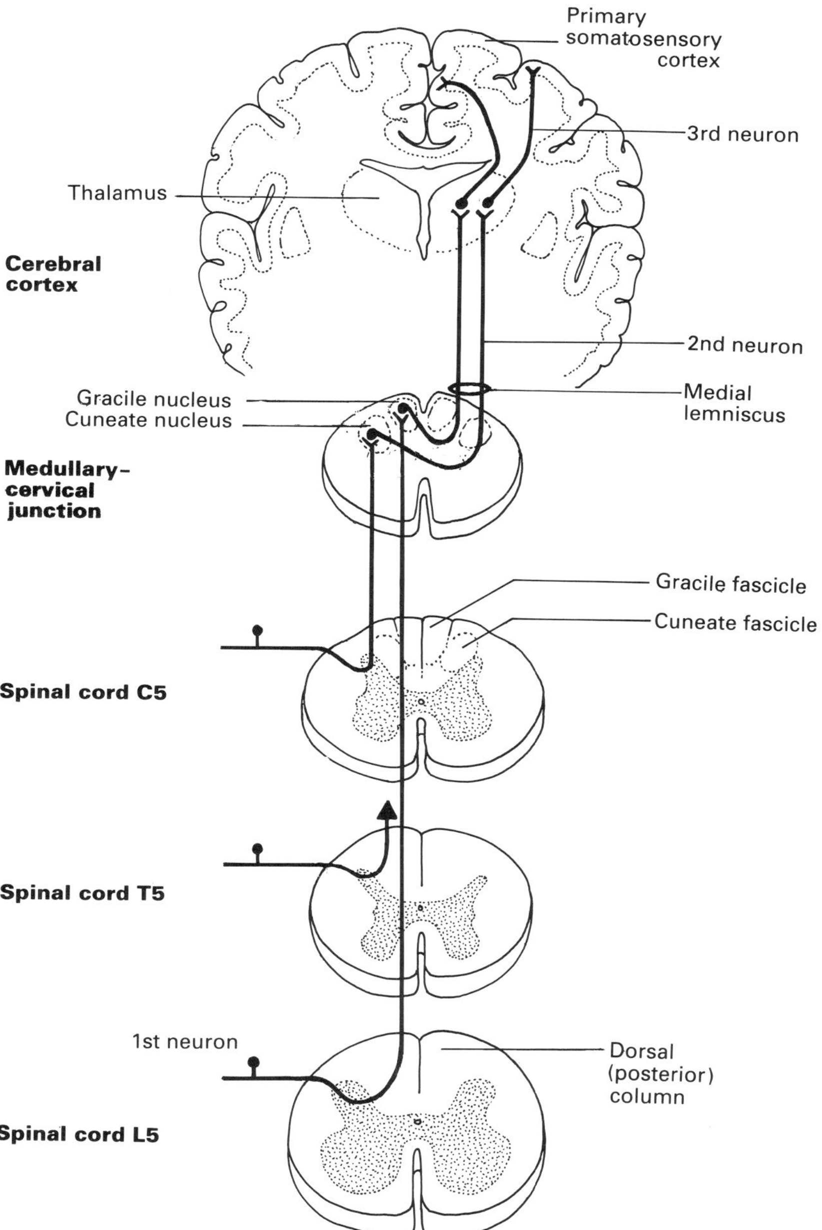

Fig. 13.14 Dorsal column–lemniscal pathways. These pathways are associated with vibration, high spatial resolution touch, and certain aspects of joint position sense. The 1st order (primary afferent) neurons have their cell bodies in the dorsal root ganglia; their central processes enter the spinal cord and (in this construct) rise ipsilaterally in the dorsal columns to synapse with the 2nd (order) neurons in the dorsal column nuclei (gracile and cuneate nuclei) of the caudal medulla, near the medullary–cervical junction. These 2nd order neurons send their axons across midline to enter the medial lemniscus of the opposite side and then ascend to the thalamus to synapse with the 3rd order neurons which project to the sensory cortex. This schema represents only the simplest, fastest pathway and does not account for collateral branching, the more widely distributed pathways for touch, or for joint position sense fibers that are more dorsolaterally placed.

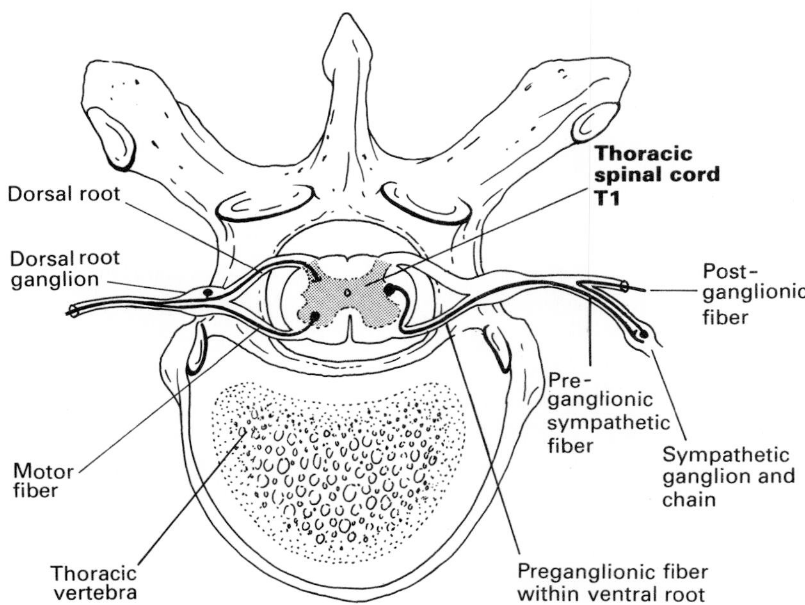

Fig. 13.15 Spinal segment (thoracic). The afferent and efferent fibers of a spinal cord segment are seen in relationship to the anatomy of the vertebra. Note the position of the dorsal root ganglion, with a dorsal root fiber and ganglion cell (shown only on the left) and the sympathetic ganglion with pre- and postganglionic fibers (illustrated only on the right). (Visceral afferents are not specifically depicted.)

Spinothalamic tract (anterolateral system)

The lateral spinothalamic tract (see Fig. 13.13) is one of the two key tract systems for clinical diagnosis. Even so, we utilize for this purpose only a small amount of the information conveyed by this pathway – the messages transmitted by those fibers in the so-called "neospinothalamic" system that form a direct link to the thalamus and thence to the sensory cortex. (Many other fibers or their branches synapse on reticular or other neurons of the spinal cord, brainstem, and thalamus.) The fibers of the 1st order neurons coming in from the periphery synapse with the 2nd order neurons of the dorsal horn gray matter at the level of entry, or branch, and ascend or descend before synapse. The fibers of the 2nd order neurons then ascend a few segments as they cross to the other side of the spinal cord to assume their position in the lateral spinothalamic tract of the other side. On reaching the thalamus they synapse with the 3rd order neuron (which may enter a local circuit or project to the cortex).

Successive levels of crossing

Thus, a lesion interrupting this ascending lateral spinothalamic tract will cause a loss of pain and temperature sensation below the level of the lesion, but on the other side of the body. (The pain–temperature sensory level is typically 1–2 segments below, but cannot be above, the numbered segmental level of cord lesion.) The spinothalamic tract does not cross as a whole, at one level, but rather these 2nd order neuron fibers emanating from each cord level cross just above that level and then join the main tract bundle ascending in its anterolateral position (see Fig. 13.3).

Dorsal column system

The dorsal column/lemniscal system (see Fig. 13.14) differs dramatically from the lateral spinothalamic system: the dorsal column fibers for vibration, joint position sense, and some aspects of fine touch do not cross in the spinal cord. The 1st order neuronal cell body is, as usual, in the dorsal root ganglion. Its central axonal process enters the cord and (those destined for the "fast-lane") ascends in the ipsilateral dorsal white matter columns of the cord to synapse in the dorsal column nuclei in the caudal medulla. The 2nd order neurons then cross as a group in the medulla and proceed (as the medial lemniscus) towards the thalamus where they synapse with the 3rd order neurons that will project to the sensory cortex. (Note that some conscious proprioceptive fibers travel more laterally than the dorsal columns proper – as one example of actual variance from this schematic presentation.)

Brown–Séquard syndrome

Dissociated sensory loss

Thus, because the fibers in the dorsal column system do not decussate in the cord itself, a cross-sectional lesion of the entire right side of the spinal cord produces: (a) ipsilateral (right-sided) deficits in vibratory, joint position, and touch sensation; (b) a loss of pain–temperature sensation contralaterally, as explained earlier; and (c) an UMN type of motor deficit below the level of the lesion and ipsilateral to it. (The lateral corticospinal tract has already crossed in the medullary decussation; in the cord its fibers descend without further crossing to synapse on anterior horn cells at each segment.) This pattern of findings from a lesion of one-half of the spinal cord, causing ipsilateral deficits in vibration, joint position sense, touch, and also an ipsilateral hemiparesis, but contralateral pain–temperature loss, is called the Brown–Séquard syndrome (Fig. 13.16). It exemplifies dramatically the important diagnostic features of spinal cord tract anatomy. In temperate climates, parts of this syndrome are commonly seen in multiple sclerosis. For further discussion of dissociated sensory loss, see Chapter 14.

FUNCTIONAL ANATOMY OF THE VISUAL PATHWAYS

Visual reception

Visual crossing

The visual receptive system (Fig. 13.17) follows the general principle of crossed representation. Information from the right side of visual space (right visual field) flows to the left hemisphere. However, there are some anatomic twists. Each eye (the left half of each retina) receives light from the right visual field, because light rays from the right side of space must go through the pupil and hence strike the left side of the retina. Thus, incoming stimuli from the visual field of one side register on the body's receptive surface (retinas) on both sides of the body – on the left side of the retinas of both eyes. (Compare this with the reception of sound and smell and with taste and somatosensory stimuli.)

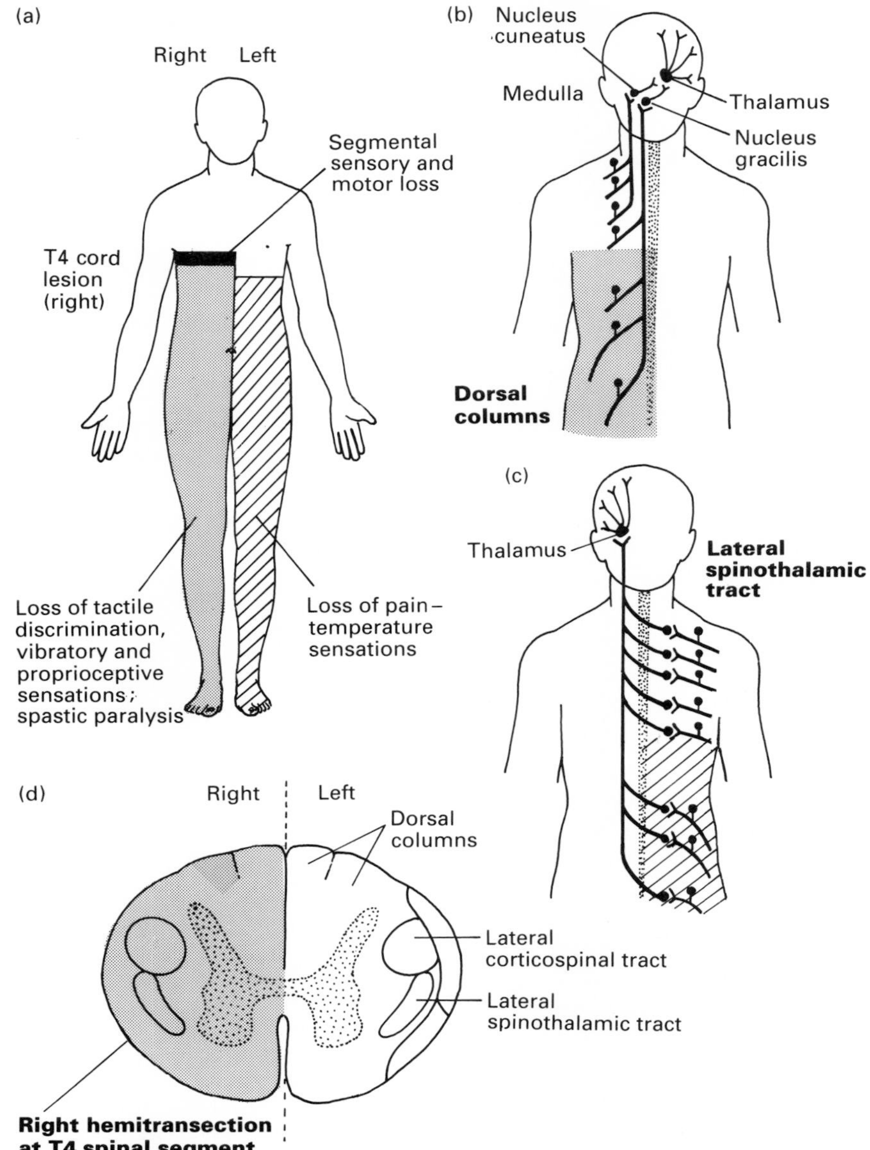

Fig. 13.16 Brown–Séquard syndrome. Principal deficits resulting from a right hemitransectional lesion of the spinal cord, shown here at T4 cord level. (a) Dissociated sensory loss, with deficit (shaded) of "dorsal column" modalities (vibration, some aspects of fine touch, and joint position sense) ipsilaterally below the lesion and spinothalamic (pain–temperature) deficit (shown by hatching) contralateral and almost up to the level of the lesion. Corticospinal motor deficits occur ipsilaterally below the lesion. All segmental functions are affected ipsilaterally at the level of the lesion. (b) In this highly simplified schema, "dorsal column" modalities are conveyed by 1st order neuronal fibers that enter the right side of the cord at each segment and would ascend in the right (ipsilateral) dorsal column without synapse until the medulla, if not blocked by the T4 lesion represented in (d). (c) The 2nd order neuronal pain–temperature fibers cross just above their segmental level of origin to form the right lateral spinothalamic tract. (d) The position of the three main ascending and descending tracts are seen in the cross-section of the cord at T4 (lesion shaded).

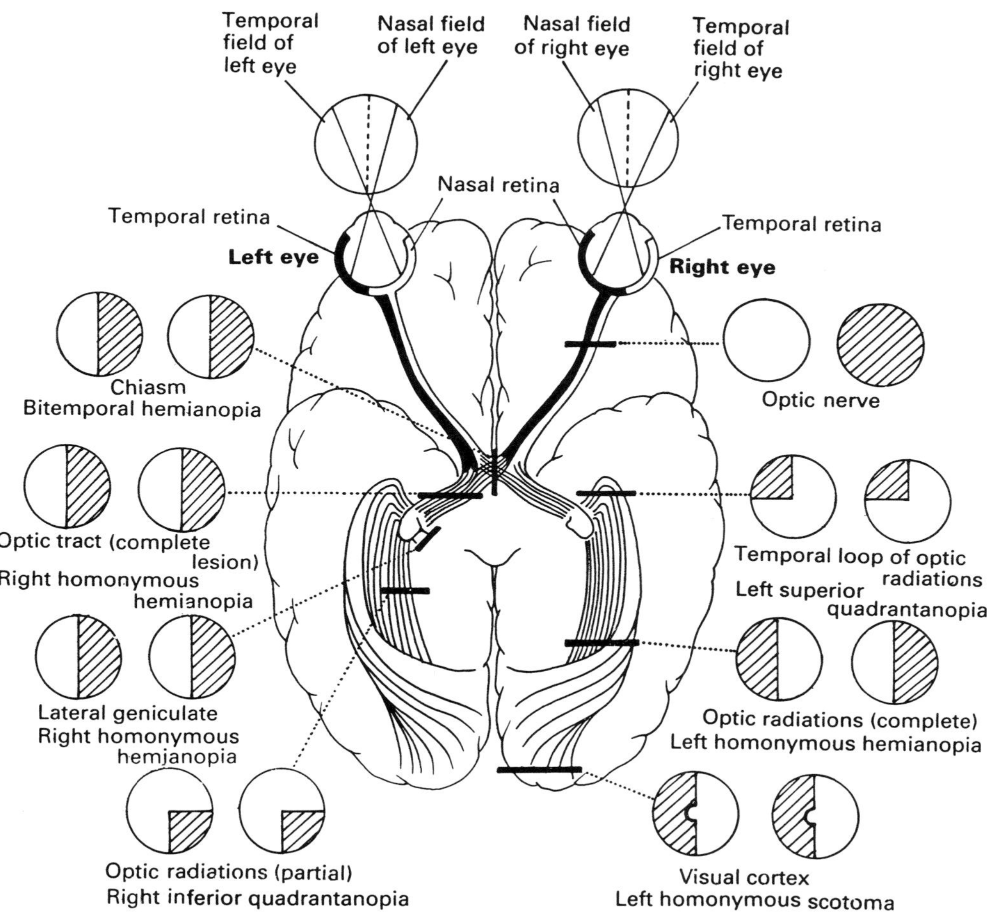

Fig. 13.17 Visual receptive pathways: localizing field defects. Fields are always portrayed from the viewpoint of the patient; the visual field of the left eye is shown on the left side, within which the left hemifield is on the left. In this schematic (for the sake of maintaining right–left relationships) the view of the brain is from the top, as if we are looking through the brain to see the structures at the base of the brain. (The issue of preservation of macular central field representation ("macular sparing") with certain visual cortex lesions causing hemianopia is not addressed here.)

Because of the bilateral reception of visual stimuli, only half of the visual field information needs to cross in the visual pathways to achieve virtually full informational crossing. Thus, half of the fibers of the optic nerve cross in the optic chiasm. These crossing fibers originate in the nasal half of each retina.

Optic nerves

When optic nerve fibers (having originated in retinal ganglion cells) are affected by a lesion, the visual defect appears in the field of that eye only – a monocular defect (see Fig. 13.17). If the lesion is complete, that eye is blind and there is no pupillary light reflex to illumination of that eye. However, the overlap of the visual field of the other eye is nearly complete, so that most visual field information can still be transmitted to the appropriate part of the brain.

Optic chiasm

At the optic chiasm complex deficits may occur because of the close proximity of fibers that are crossing and not crossing from each eye. The classic chiasmal syndrome results from pressure by a pituitary tumor on the medial parts of the chiasm, affecting crossing fibers from each nasal retina. This produces a defect in each temporal visual field—a so-called bitemporal heteronymous hemianopsia (see Fig. 13.17 and Chapter 5, Section on CN 2).

The fibers in the optic nerve, chiasm, and optic tract are continuous, without synapse, even though the names change according to location. The visual receptive fibers finally synapse in the lateral geniculate nucleus, from which the optic radiations arise. These, in turn, synapse in the primary visual cortex of each medial occipital lobe. The pupillary light reflex afferent fibers in each optic tract branch off just before the lateral geniculate nuclei and distribute (via the pretectal area) to both sides of the midbrain, where connection with the efferent limb is made.

Postchiasmal lesions

Unilateral lesions of an optic tract, lateral geniculate nucleus, optic radiations, and primary visual cortex are all similar in two ways: (a) these postchiasmal pathway lesions produce homonymous contralateral field defects (Table 13.3 and Fig. 13.17); (b) the routine direct and consensual pupillary light reflexes are preserved bilaterally.

In the visual receptive system a retinotopic relationship is maintained. At the stage of the optic radiations the fibers spread out, such that fibers representing half of each inferior retina traverse a loop that swings more inferiorly and laterally through the temporal lobe. Those fibers that arise from half of each superior retina take a more superior and direct route, passing through the parietal lobe to terminate in the upper bank (lip) of the calcarine fissure; those that course through the temporal lobe end in the lower bank. Thus, in both the optic radiations and in the primary visual cortex it is relatively likely that a lesion might affect just the superior or just the inferior visual hemifield of each eye, a homonymous quadrantanopia (see Fig. 13.17).

SYSTEMS FOR HEARING, SMELL, AND TASTE

Unlike the visual system, a knowledge of the CNS pathways for the auditory, olfactory, and gustatory systems is not of first-order importance for the nonspecialist. The reason is bilateral representation: auditory information reaching the brainstem is soon distributed bilaterally in the ascending pathways to the medial geniculate body of the thalamus; similarly for taste information reaching the brainstem or olfactory information reaching the temporal lobe. Unilateral lesions affecting the CNS pathways (once bilateral crossing has occurred) produces no deficit

Table 13.3 Clinical correlation of peripheral visual field defects

Type of defect	Principal localizations	Common pathologic lesions (example)
Homonymous hemianopia	Contralateral, postchiasmal: usually optic radiations in temporal/parietal lobes or visual cortex in occipital lobe	Infarction: (a) posterior (inferior) division of middle cerebral artery; (b) posterior cerebral artery; also, hemorrhage, tumor, etc.
Homonymous quadrantanopia	Contralateral, postchiasmal	
superior quadrant	Usually temporal radiations or inferior lip (bank) of calcarine fissure in visual cortex	Infarction, usually embolic; hemorrhage, tumor, etc.
inferior quadrant	Usually parietal radiations or superior lip of calcarine fissue	Same as above
Heteronymous (nonhomonymous); bilateral defects	Optic chiasm (often bitemporal defects)	Pituitary tumor (aneurysms, other tumors also compress chiasm)
	Retinas (bilateral)	Detachment, degenerations, etc.
	Both optic nerves	Optic neuritis, demyelination
Monocular defects	Retina, ipsilateral	Detachment, degenerations, injury, etc.
	Optic nerve, ipsilateral	Demyelination, tumor

detectable by routine clinical testing. Bilateral lesions can cause syndromes of sensory loss, but are rare (for the very important features of peripheral input see Chapter 5, sections on CNs 1, 7, and 8).

THE CEREBELLUM AND ITS CONNECTIONS

Functional zones

The cerebellum is one of the better understood parts of the brain in terms of its wiring diagram, and one of the less well understood parts in terms of exactly what its job is and how it is accomplished. From the standpoint of functional neuroanatomy, two points of view are useful. The first is the functional stratification of the cerebellum into three zones: (a) a spinocerebellar zone that includes the midline vermis and a paramedian region of the cerebellar hemisphere; (b) a lateral hemispheric zone; and (c) the flocculonodular lobe. The midline vermis and paramedian (intermediate) regions are critical in stance, gait, and limb coordination. The lateral zone of each cerebellar hemisphere seems to be more involved with motor planning and learning. The flocculonodular lobe is involved in bidirectional connections with the vestibular nuclei and hence relates closely to balance and orientation of the head and eyes in space.

Inputs and outputs

The second point of view pertains to the main cerebellar inputs and outputs via the three sets of cerebellar peduncles. Each set relates to one of the three rostrocaudal divisions of the brainstem (see Table 13.1). The inferior cerebellar peduncles, forming struts from the medulla to the cerebellum, carry most of the direct and indirect spinal input. Fibers from the vestibular nuclei also gain access here. The middle cerebellar peduncles transmit information from the frontal lobes to the contralateral cerebellar hemisphere: frontopontine fibers synapse on neurons in the base of the pons, which then project across to the other side and through the middle cerebellar peduncles. In contrast, most cerebellar output flows through the superior cerebellar peduncles which carry fibers that decussate in the midbrain and synapse in the red nucleus and thalamus (Fig. 13.18).

Ipsilateral deficits

The cardinal rule of cerebellar localization is based on the crossed output of the cerebellum. Signs of incoordination from a cerebellar lesion are ipsilateral to that lesion for the following reason: a lesion in the right side of the cerebellum affects the output via the right superior cerebellar peduncle, which crosses in the midbrain before it synapses in the left red nucleus and/or thalamus. The thalamus projects to the frontal cortex on that same side (the left). The lateral corticospinal tract from the left motor cortex decussates in the medulla so that the fibers terminate on anterior horn cells on the right side of the spinal cord. This so-called "double cross" of the cerebellar outflow and the corticospinal tract determines that a right-sided cerebellar lesion will be manifest as incoordination on the right side of the body, ipsilateral to the lesion (see Case 8B and Chapter 14).

Posterior fossa compression

As noted earlier in this chapter, an expansive space-occupying lesion in the cerebellum, whether a tumor, hemorrhage, or swollen infarction, may cause increased pressure in the posterior fossa, with compression and distortion of brainstem structures. Respiratory depression and arrest may occur without being heralded by motor, sensory, or other familiar neurologic signs. Cerebellar hemorrhage or other expansive masses represent true neurologic emergencies.

A QUICK TOUR OF THE CEREBRAL LOBES

The functions traditionally associated with the lobes of the brain barely scrape the surface of what actually goes on. Some of these functions relate to the origin or termination of long fiber tracts: the descending motor fibers from the posterior frontal lobe; the somatosensory projections from the thalamus to the anterior parietal lobe; and the optic radiations to the visual cortex of the medial occipital lobe. Other localizations not related to these long tract systems include the speech areas, memory

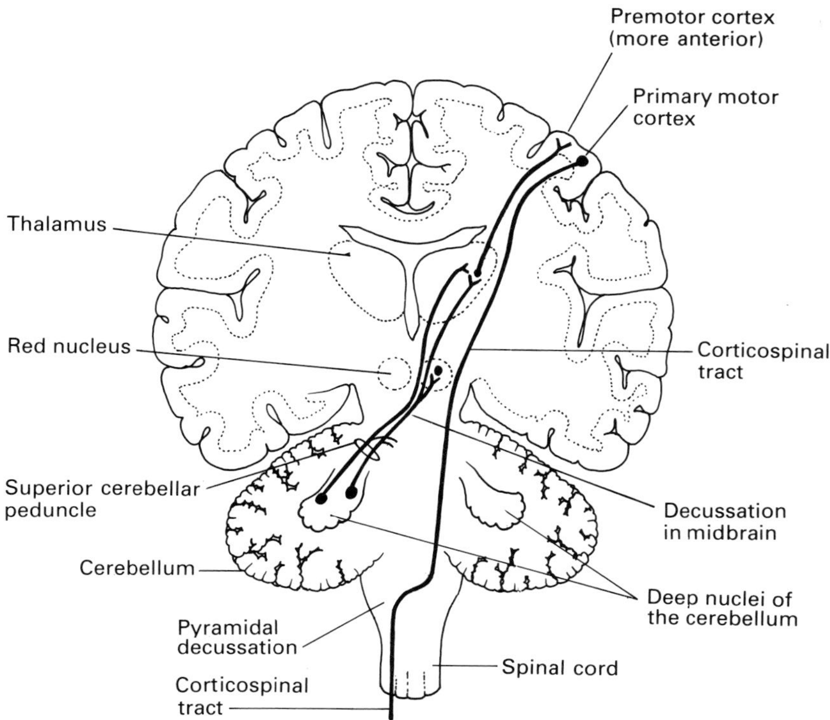

Fig. 13.18 "Double cross" of cerebellar influence on limb coordination: a cerebellar deficit is ipsilateral to the cerebellar lesion. The cerebellar outflow from the deep nuclei (dentate, etc.) travels through the superior cerebellar peduncle, which decussates in the midbrain and then travels close to the red nucleus with some fibers synapsing there and others continuing directly to the thalamus. The thalamus nuclei then project mainly to the premotor cortex. The descending corticospinal tract from the primary motor cortex decussates in the medulla, achieving the second crossing – back to the same side as the lesion. The rubrospinal, fronto-ponto-cerebellar, and olivo-cerebellar tracts (not shown) also cross, but the "double cross" described here is not affected.

structures, centers involved in spatial orientation, etc.

As will be mentioned in the next chapter, "centers" for particular functions seem to represent only essential hubs of neurologic activity, which depend upon connections to other areas as well. In some respects the right and left hemispheres are roughly equivalent, and in other ways their functions are specialized; in Table 13.4, the left hemisphere is assumed to be dominant for motor and language functions. Note that selected functions are categorized here just by lobe (and side), but a wealth of specific information has been accumulated as to more specific localizations. In addition, the inclusion of a broad area such as "personality" on both left and right is not meant to imply necessarily that the roles of the two hemispheres are equivalent (see Further reading section).

Table 13.4 Some of the left and right hemispheres

	Left hemisphere	Right hemisphere
Frontal lobe	(dominant)	(nondominant)
	Personality; attention (certain aspects); ability to change "sets"; initiative, planning, etc.; judgment, evaluation, and modulation of responses, inhibitions	
	Motor; gaze control (frontal eye fields); anterior speech areas (Broca's)	Motor; gaze control (frontal eye fields)
Parietal lobe	Somatosensory; reading (requires angular gyrus of posterior, inferior parietal lobe)	Somatosensory; spatial relationships (especially many visual–spatial faculties, general spatial attention)
	Writing; calculations and right–left distinctions (certain aspects of both); naming body parts	Attention to left side of space and body (mainly nondominant parietal); "insight" into contralateral deficits (c.f. anosognosia or lack of such insight) – mainly nondominant
	Vision (parietal optic radiations) Taste (also ?temporal)	Vision (parietal optic radiations) Taste (also ?temporal)
Temporal lobe	Language (posterior speech areas – Wernicke's)	Nonverbal visual comprehension; prosody; affective, gestural aspect
	Auditory–verbal comprehension; visual reception (temporal optic radiations); limbic/memory functions; smell (?taste)	Auditory perception; visual reception (temporal optic radiations); limbic/memory functions; smell (?taste)
Occipital lobe	Visual perception and associated ability to recognize objects	Visual perception and associations (most visual associative deficits require bilateral occipital–parietal and occipital–temporal lesions)

SUMMARY

A number of items in the core clinical–anatomic knowledge base prove hard for students and residents to remember, especially if they have been away from neurologic problems for a while. The best way to help with this is to build a framework of understanding on which to hang particular pieces of knowledge, so that they make sense. In addition, images, mnemonics, and even silly associations may help. The following memory hooks are baited in several ways.

1 Orientation of the motor and sensory homunculi on the cerebral cortex (see Fig. 13.6): as in human anatomy, the feet are together, which can only occur if they are represented on the adjacent medial hemispheric surfaces; the upper extremities are separated, as they must be on the lateral convexities.
2 Vertebral levels vs. spinal cord segmental levels: the spinal cord must be shorter than the vertebral column for the safe performance of a spinal tap. The fact that a spinal tap is a lumbar puncture reminds you that most of the lumbar region is safe, since the cord usually ends at approximately L1.
3 The organization of the ventricular system: the ventricular system is a sort of waterworks, akin in a rather gross, anatomic way to the urinary system. (As noted elsewhere, CSF has been mischievously called the "urine of the brain.") Picture the two lateral kidneys with outlets (ureters) to one midline bladder with a simple midline outlet tube or aqueduct, the urethra. Two lateral ventricles are the largest source of CSF and they have outlets (foramina of Monro) into a midline 3rd ventricle, which empties into the midline aqueduct of Sylvius. Here the analogy ends, unless we add the iatrogenic extension of a Foley catheter from the urethra into a urine bag that no one has yet been so bold as to call a 4th ventricle.
4 What sensory roots innervate the saddle area of the anatomy, crudely speaking the posteromedial thighs, and perineal area – the contact areas of the rider's "tail"? The cauda equina, or horse's tail, of course. (Actually, the saddle area is innervated mainly by the lower roots of the cauda, including the S2–S5 roots. Their sensory distribution more or less defines the nether erogenous zone – in case you ever need to remind yourself of the extent of this territory of living anatomy.)

PROBLEMS FOR SELF-STUDY

Problems

1 A patient with occipital head trauma, including a fracture through the foramen magnum, develops cerebellar swelling and suffers a respiratory arrest. Tonsillar herniation is found. Unlike transtentorial herniation, cerebellar herniation (and cerebellar pressure on the medulla, in general) is not heralded by distinctive pupillary changes or other eye signs. What is your explanation?
2 A patient presents with a left hemiparesis (face and arm more than leg) and sensory deficits. There is no field cut. A MCA territory stroke is postulated. Which major division of the MCA would be involved?

Comments

1 None of the cranial nerves emanating from the medulla subserves pupillary functions or eye muscles. The descending autonomic pathways in the brainstem are affected by intrinsic lesions, such as infarcts and hemorrhages, but not by extrinsic lesions, except perhaps termi-

nally. In contrast, transtentorial herniation involves CN 3 early, and secondary hemorrhages in the midbrain may affect the CN 3 nuclei, vertical gaze mechanisms, etc.

2 The primary motor and sensory cortical strips are in the superior (anterior) division territory of the MCA, whereas the optic radiations are more posterior. (The lower leg and foot areas of the cortex are in anterior cerebral artery territory.)

FURTHER READING

Neuroanatomy

Carpenter, M.B. *Core Text of Neuroanatomy*. 4th edn. Williams and Wilkins, Baltimore (MD), 1991. A highly respected "small text" of neuroanatomy that more than suffices for most reference needs.

Gilman, S., Newman, S.W. *Manter and Gatz' Essentials of Clinical Neuroanatomy and Neurophysiology*. 8th edn. F.A. Davis, Philadelphia (PA), 1992. Long favored by many medical students, this summary text is packed with information.

Heimer, L. *The Human Brain and Spinal Cord*. Springer-Verlag, New York (NY), 1983. Combines an anatomic overview appropriate for medical students and house officers with clinical correlations, a small atlas, and an illustrated dissection.

Kandel, E.R., Schwartz, J.H., Jessell, T.M. *Principles of Neural Science*. 3rd edn. Elsevier, New York (NY), 1992. Contains a substantial textbook of neuroanatomy in its own right.

Martin, J.H. *Neuroanatomy: Text and Atlas*. Elsevier, New York (NY), 1989. A major anatomic text that is designed to highlight essential concepts and provide frameworks for approaching neuroanatomy.

Brain herniations

Ropper, A.H. Coma and acutely raised intracranial pressure. In: Asbury, A.K., McKhann, G.M., McDonald, W.I., (eds) *Diseases of the Nervous System*. Clinical Neurology. 2nd edn., vol. 2. WB Saunders, Philadelphia (PA), 1992. A summary (Chapter 75) that includes insights from neuroimaging that bear upon the pathogenesis of herniation deficits; heavily referenced.

Vascular anatomy and stroke

Kistler, P., Ropper, A.H., Martin, J.B. Cerebrovascular diseases. In: Wilson, J.D., Braunwald, E., Isselbacher, K.J., *et al.* (eds) *Harrison's Principles of Internal Medicine*. 12th edn. McGraw-Hill, New York (NY), 1991. More details of vascular territories and syndromes (Chapter 351).

Sudarsky, L. *Pathophysiology of the Nervous System*. Little, Brown, and Company, Boston (MA), 1990, pp. 251–76. Cerebral metabolism and ischemia are areas of pathophysiology that are now rapidly advancing beyond traditional views of cellular injury.

Spinal cord and column

Byrne, T.N. Spinal cord compression from epidural metastases. *N Engl J Med* 1992; 327: 614–19. This article relates to the most serious cause of nontraumatic compression.

Byrne, T.N., Waxman, S.G. *Spinal Cord Compression: Diagnosis and Principles of Management*. F.A. Davis, Philadelphia (PA), 1990. An important clinical area in which spinal segmental and long tract anatomy is vital to understand.

Brazis, P.W., Masdeu, J.C., Biller, J. *Localization in Clinical Neurology*. 2nd edn. Little, Brown, and Company, Boston (MA), 1990. Thorough exposition of clinical–pathologic correlations of spinal lesions.

Davidoff, R.A. The dorsal columns. *Neurology* 1989; 39:1377–85. Present-day evidence regarding the anatomy underlying the clinical concept of the dorsal column sensory system.

Cranial nerve control of eye movements

Leigh, R.J., Zee, D.S. *The Neurology of Eye Movements*. 2nd edn. F.A. Davis, Philadelphia (PA), 1991. An authoritative work, but intimidating in its complexity (see also Further reading section of Chapter 17).

Autonomic nervous system

McLeod, J.G., Tuck, R.R. Disorders of the anatomic nervous system. *Ann Neurol* 1987; 21:419–30, 519–29. (See also Further reading section of Chapter 16.)

The cerebellum and its connections

Kandel, E.R., Schwartz, J.H., Jessell, T.M. *Principles of Neural Science*. 3rd edn. Elsevier, New York (NY), 1991. Cerebellar structure and function: current concepts are summarized in Chapter 41.

Major functions of the cerebral lobes

Adams, R.D., Victor, M. Syndromes due to focal cerebral lesions. In: Wilson, J.D., Braunwald, E., Isselbacher, K.J., *et al.*, (eds) *Harrison's Principles of Internal Medicine*. 12th edn. McGraw-Hill, New York (NY), 1991. A more detailed tour of the cerebral lobes and the effects of lesions (Chapter 32).

Alexander, M.P., Naeser, M.A., Palumbo, C. Broca's area aphasias: aphasia after lesions including the frontal operculum. *Neurology* 1990; 40:353–62. The anatomic areas that subserve speech and the lesions that halt it.

Damasio, A.R. Aphasia. *N Engl J Med* 1992; 326:531–9. Authoritative brief review of present concepts of classic Broca's, and the more limited Broca's area aphasia; Wernicke's fluent aphasia; global aphasia, and others. These disorders are set into the context of modern concepts of localization.

Damasio, A.R. Diagnosis of regional cerebral dysfunction. In: Wyngarden, J.B., Smith, L.H., Bennett, J.C., (eds) *Cecil Textbook of Medicine*. 19th edn. WB Saunders, Philadelphia (PA), 1992. Another presentation of focal disorders, knowledge of which has been based mainly on clinicopathologic correlation, but increasingly on correlation with structural and functional neuroimaging (Chapter 448).

Mesulam, M-M. *Principles of Behavioral Neurology*. F.A. Davis, Philadelphia (PA), 1985. Leading text in the field; broad in scope and rich in detail.

chapter 14

Clinical Constructs and Rules for Anatomic Localization

Introduction

Clinicians employ diagnostic constructs based on neuroanatomic facts that are greatly simplified into a reliably useful form. These constructs lie deeply embedded in all writing and teaching about practical diagnostic localization. Thus, while you may not be familiar with the term "construct" in its present context, the idea is not new. This chapter will define the more important ones, show how they are used, and indicate some of their limitations. Further localizing rules will also be described and illustrated by well-known syndromes. (For some of the anatomic underpinnings of these discussions, refer back to Chapter 13, and for a more comprehensive information base consult the sources suggested in the Further reading section of this chapter.)

The emphasis on clinical constructs serves not only to highlight their usefulness, but to help resolve a tension between the clinical past and the clinical future. This is a tension between traditional tools and new, emerging levels of truth. The gulf between the time-tested constructs and progress in neuroscience is rapidly widening. This could lead you either to lose confidence in the old tools and not bother mastering them, or to dismiss "leading edge" advances as clinically irrelevant. Neither response is desirable. Neither the old construct nor the new understanding cheapens or invalidates the other.

As long as the old tools work fairly well, and there is no better system to replace them, you should become skilled in their use, but only with the understanding that they are not and cannot be a full reflection of what is currently known. You will need to solve practical clinical problems, without being paralyzed by the specter of a vast and unmanageable neuroscience data base. At the same time, by virtue of the intellectual challenge of this tension, you will be better prepared to incorporate upgraded constructs as they are developed.

WAYS OF THINKING ABOUT FUNCTIONAL NEUROANATOMY

To gain a more thorough understanding of the relationship of facts, concepts, constructs, rules, and syndromes, consider the following examples of these "ways of thinking" that will be further amplified and illustrated subsequently.

Fact

Facts such as "The corticospinal tract runs from the cerebral cortex into the spinal cord" are never later proved untrue, but may be modified or may diminish in conceptual and diagnostic importance because of new discovery.

Concept

"The nervous system includes a segmental motor organization as well as suprasegmental control systems that influence activity at segmental levels." This concept combines related facts into a coherent notion.

Construct

A construct is a specific scheme based on facts and concepts that simplifies and even distorts reality, but usually works clinically. An application of the concept of suprasegmental and segmental control is the construct of the upper motor neuron (UMN)/lower motor neuron (LMN) chain of motor control. Out of the great complexity of the motor control system virtually every motor dysfunction is first considered in light of the UMN/LMN construct: are there signs or symptoms that fit the pattern that we associate with an UMN lesion (such as weakness of volitional movement, increased tone, hyperreflexia, Babinski sign)? Or, conversely, are there LMN signs, such as weakness, atrophy, and fasciculations in one or more anterior root or peripheral nerve (spinal or cranial) distributions?

Rule

The statement "A spinal cord lesion can cause a sensory level on the trunk that may be lower than, but never higher than the cord segment of the lesion," is a firm clinical rule based upon anatomic knowledge and confirmed by clinical–pathologic correlation.

Syndrome

A syndrome is an aggregate of symptoms or signs (and may include laboratory findings) forming a recognizable pattern, but it does not represention a specific etiology (which is the hallmark of a disease). Temporal lobe herniation results in a characteristic syndrome that may be instigated by various causes.

Two deferred questions

Two seemingly obvious questions have not been addressed, and these deserve a digression before describing suprasegmental/segmental constructs.

Neurologic or not?

First, is the problem neurologic at all? Too often, clinicians subject difficult symptoms, such as pain, to a snap judgment ("This pain is not neurologic"). All pain is neurologic, in a sense, but does it arise from a specific neurologic lesion? The best way to answer this is to analyze the symptom as if it were a primary neurologic problem, and only then make a reasoned judgment. Knowledge of segmental and suprasegmental patterns will assist you in this.

Central nervous system or peripheral nervous system?

Second, is the lesion in the central nervous system (CNS) or in the peripheral nervous system (PNS)? Sometimes the difference between a PNS and a CNS disorder is very obvious, as in the case of an elbow injury with sensory and motor deficits clearly limited to the distribution of the ulnar nerve. But frequently even seasoned neurologists are not able to "eyeball" the character of the complaint: just because a deficit, such as an apparent "foot drop," is focal and limited to the periphery of the body, you cannot presume that it is a PNS lesion.

The CNS/PNS division overlaps the suprasegmental/segmental distinction. All suprasegmental structures are in the CNS, but the segmental apparatus resides in both the CNS (cord or brainstem segment) and the PNS (roots and peripheral nerves). Therefore, if a patient exhibited fasciculations and neurogenic atrophy in parts of C5 and C6 innervated muscles, you would know that the process was segmental (C5 and C6), but you would not be able to ascertain from these data alone whether these cord segments (CNS) or the anterior roots (PNS) were involved. Clinical approaches to diagnosing PNS lesions are discussed in Chapter 16.

SUPRASEGMENTAL/SEGMENTAL ORGANIZATION

The concept of segmental and suprasegmental organization is the foundation of the localizing process (Table 14.1). Segmental organization underlies the output through all spinal and cranial motor roots and input through all spinal and brainstem sensory roots. Suprasegmental pathways modify the control of segmental output and the processing of segmental input. Thus, we think in terms of suprasegmental/segmental chains of function. For example, a facial weakness may be due to a cortical lesion as well as a lesion of CN 7, itself.

A localizing strategy

After eliciting and summarizing the patient's symptoms and signs, formulate an anatomic localization: analyze the data, system by system, for evidence of suprasegmental vs. segmental characteristics. By characterizing the type and distribution of each deficit – motor, sensory, reflex, etc. – we attempt to localize the problem in each of these categories to a segmental level or to a suprasegmental pathway or "center." Then we compare the localizing information for motor, sensory, reflex, or other deficits to see whether a unifying localization can be established. As you

Table 14.1 Selected clinical–anatomic constructs of suprasegmental/segmental organization

Suprasegmental	Segmental
1 Suprasegmental (long tract) pathways cross. However, crossing occurs at different levels in different tracts and may be incomplete. In sensory pathways it is the 2nd order neuron fibers that cross	Segmental fibers do not cross: a neuron on one side sends out its axon to structures on the same side (for exceptions see Table 14.2). Lesions of segmental input or output cause ipsilateral deficits
2 The upper motor neuron (UMN) with its corticospinal or corticobulbar fiber is the suprasegmental link in the UMN/LMN chain of motor control	The lower motor neuron (LMN) with its anterior root/peripheral nerve fiber is the segmental link in the UMN/LMN chain of motor control
3 Sensory tracts are compartmentalized by modality group (pain–temperature vs. fine touch, position, vibration) in the spinal cord and brainstem. This (along with different levels of crossing) forms the basis of dissociated sensory loss	Peripheral sensory transmission is differentiated (sensory receptors, fiber size, myelination) but not compartmentalized by modality. Most posterior root and peripheral nerve lesions affect all modalities, but sometimes to a variable degree
4 In the control of horizontal conjugate gaze, a hemispheric gaze center activates the brainstem (pontine) gaze center of the opposite side (see Table 17.1 and Fig. 17.1)	The pontine gaze center coordinates gaze to its own side by integrating the segmental outputs of CNs 3 and 6, which innervate the horizontally acting medial and lateral rectus muscles, respectively

will see, the beauty of determining a segmental localization is that the lesion must be at that level and on the same side as the deficit. When the deficit appears to be suprasegmental, the lesion could be anywhere along the CNS pathway; lacking a segmental intercept, a suprasegmental localization can only be achieved clinically by putting together the information available from all systems – or by laboratory testing.

The upper motor neuron/lower motor neuron model

Construct: voluntary motor activity is governed by an UMN/LMN chain of motor control.

This construct is the first and foremost tool for analysis of the common motor problems of weakness, altered tone, and atrophy, as described in Chapter 6. The UMN/LMN distinction (Table 14.2) works well in case after case, notwithstanding the fact that a two-neuron pathway (as implied by the UMN/LMN coupling) is not really the predominant pattern. The critical point is the suprasegmental/segmental linkage for any motor deficit; consider both the UMN and LMN components. In actuality many fibers descending in the lateral corticospinal tract do not

Table 14.2 The upper motor neuron/lower motor neuron construct of voluntary motor function

	Upper motor neuron		Lower motor neuron		
	Nerve cell body	Axon/tract	Synapse/ nerve cell	Axon	Synapse
Spinal output (trunk, limbs)	Motor cortex (areas for limbs, trunk, and parts of neck)	Lateral corticospinal tract (crossed in medulla)	Anterior horn cell (α motor neuron)	Anterior root, peripheral nerve (uncrossed)	Neuromuscular junction (NMJ), trunk, limb muscles
Cranial output (head, neck)	Motor cortex (areas for head and parts of neck – see Fig. 13.6)	Corticobulbar tracts (entirely or partly crossed in brainstem)	Motor nuclei of brainstem	Cranial motor nerves (uncrossed, save CN 4 and some fibers of CN 3 – see text)	NMJ, cranial muscles

synapse directly on α motor neurons. Conversely, each anterior horn cell is connected synaptically with many neuronal processes other than the corticospinal fibers. Moreover, the lateral corticospinal tract operates in parallel with other descending tracts which actually mediate some of the characteristic UMN features. The chief clinical findings of UMN vs. LMN disorders include:

Suprasegmental
Upper motor neuron weakness (functional groups), increased tone; disuse atrophy. (Simple and complex reflexive movements may occur.)

Segmental
Lower motor neuron weakness (muscles of one or more segments or nerves); neurogenic atrophy; fasciculations.

Characterizing a motor deficit

Building upon the UMN/LMN model, an approach to motor localization addresses the following questions.

Distribution

1 What is the distribution of weakness or other motor signs? One-sided? Lower body/legs only? Cranial motor functions affected, or just from the neck down? When weakness of all or most of one side of the body (hemiparesis) is recognized, the likelihood of a UMN (corticospinal tract) lesion is virtually certain, but when just one limb, or part of it, becomes weak, we need to take a closer look. Does the deficit involve multiple muscles that are jointly activated to execute useful motor activity (UMN pattern)? Or, conversely, are only muscles affected that are innervated by one or two motor roots, a peripheral nerve trunk, or a nerve branch (LMN pattern)?

Characteristics

2 Are there characteristic motor and reflex signs that we associate with UMN lesions (such as pathologic hyperreflexia, clonus, or the Babinski sign) vs. the characteristic LMN motor signs such as segmental weakness, fasciculations, and neurogenic atrophy (see Tables 6.2 and 9.1)?

Correlations

3 Are there correlative non-neurologic localizing signs? (Such evidence is not definitive, but may help to focus attention or guide imaging.) For example, a diabetic patient presents with mild bilateral lower leg weakness and severe focal tenderness at T11 vertebral spinous process. While the weakness could be on an LMN basis, due to severe diabetic neuropathy, the thoracic spinal tenderness directs attention to the possibility of a cord lesion involving motor tracts – an UMN basis. An abscess compressing the upper lumbar cord should be ruled out. (Deficits of diabetic polyneuropathy might coexist.)

UMN pattern of weakness of voluntary movement

UMN lesions produce weakness in a group of functionally related muscles – never, if the deficits are sufficient to be fully recognized, in just one muscle. The UMN control over movement requires coordinated changes in agonist, antagonist, and synergist muscles. These must necessarily enlist different nerves over two or more segments. Of the muscles acting on the leg at the knee joint, the extensors are lumbar innervated (L3, L4) while those acting in flexion are mainly lower lumbar and sacral (L5, S1, S2). Thus, weakness of all movement of one leg implicates at least five segments and two major peripheral nerves. An LMN mechanism would be relatively unlikely, though not impossible.

Extensive unilateral weakness

The most obvious UMN pattern of distribution, the hemiparesis (Fig. 14.1), requires an "economical" solution. How much more efficient to produce a hemiparesis by a single tract lesion than by nipping in turn every segment on the side of the body where weakness appears! The totally one-sided character of the weakness over so many segments renders the latter mechanism extraordinarily unlikely. (The problem is more difficult when limbs on both sides are involved.)

Crossed cerebral motor control

Construct: suprasegmental control pathways from the cerebral hemispheres to the brainstem and spinal cord are crossed.

Lateral corticospinal tract

As described in Chapter 13, the prototypic long tract pathways upon which we focus in diagnostic localization cross sides at some point in their descent or ascent (see Figs 5.1, 6.1, 13.13, 13.14). Diagnostic analysis must contend not only with the fact of crossing, but the level of crossing. A lesion in the lateral corticospinal (pyramidal) tract above the medullary level of decussation will cause weakness below and contralateral to the lesion. Conversely, a lesion below this "pyramidal" decussation produces ipsilateral weakness below the level of the lesion. In either case the deficit is suprasegmental in type.

Corticobulbar tracts

The exact point of crossing in the brainstem of each of the corticobulbar tracts is less well defined, but is generally thought to be close to the synapse with the intended cranial nerve motor nucleus (see Fig. 5.1). Thus, you can assume that a lesion rostral to the nucleus interrupts the

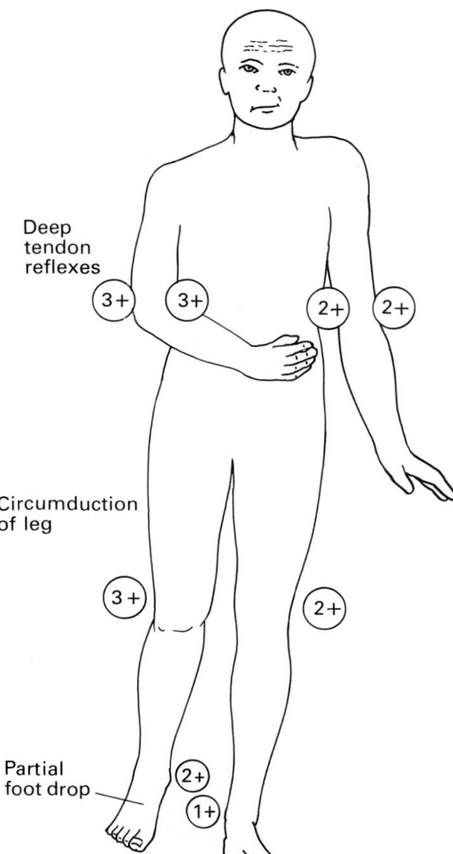

Fig. 14.1 Patient with right hemiparetic posture. The (weak) right arm is flexed (increased flexor tone) and leg extended with plantar flexion of the foot, due to weakness of dorsiflexion and increased tone of plantar flexors. The lower right face is weak. The associated signs of right hyperreflexia (biceps, triceps, knee, and ankle) are indicated, and a right Babinski sign would be expected.

corticobulbar tract before it crosses, thereby affecting the cranial nerve function on the opposite side in a suprasegmental pattern. In contrast, a lesion at the level of the nucleus will affect LMNs; the deficit will be ipsilateral to the lesion and segmental in type.

Other early motor signs

While weakness of voluntary muscular exertion constitutes the prime sign of an UMN lesion, it is not invariably the first sign (see Cases 6A and 14A). An increase in tone or a reflex change, such as a Babinski sign, may precede a recognized loss of strength. These signs follow the same crossing pattern as does weakness.

As with other useful clinical constructs, the generalization of crossed suprasegmental motor control is partly fictional. In localizing a lesion responsible for weakness, we pretend that the lateral corticospinal tract is the sole operative suprasegmental pathway. Other tracts (the so-called extrapyramidal system, to be described later) are more complex. Not all of these other descending motor fibers cross, and of those that do, not all cross in the brainstem. The degree of crossing of particular groups of fibers is related to the role of the musculature which they influence. The greater the degree of fine motor control, the more the suprasegmental pathways are crossed – the lateral corticospinal tract being the prime example. Fine motor control requires fractionation of movement and the ability to control right and left sides independently. Fractionation involves subdividing large, "blunt" movements such as a handgrip into a subtle activation of individual fingers, as in playing a piano, with each hand functioning separately. In contrast, the axial musculature of the trunk and some limb girdle and proximal musculature utilized for posture and gross movement, require less subdivision of control. The suprasegmental pathways governing these functions tend to be more balanced between crossed and uncrossed fibers.

Degree of crossing relates to function

Segmental and suprasegmental sensory pathways

Construct: in the segmental inflow of sensory information in the peripheral nerves, the different sensory modalities are not strictly compartmentalized. In the spinal cord the two main modality groups of pain–temperature and touch–vibration–position are carried in widely separated tracts that cross at different levels. Therefore, in focal PNS lesions all sensory modalities tend to be affected to some degree, whereas focal cord and brainstem lesions typically cause dissociated sensory loss. In the cerebrum (thalamus and cortex) the separate pathways again merge. (Note that, in actuality, the fibers of the incoming segmental roots do not conform to a stereotypic pattern of synapsing or joining monolithic tracts. Most incoming fibers branch widely, some of these branches descending or ascending to other segments. While the segmental/suprasegmental distinction is blurred in this way, the classic construct remains useful.)

Severe focal injury or disease of a peripheral nerve typically involves ipsilateral deficits of all sensory modalities (as well as motor function) – although sometimes to a varying degree (see Chapter 16). Certain compressive processes may differentially affect the spectrum of nerve fiber sizes (with varying amounts of myelination). In addition, some diseases involve particular fiber types more than others. The touch–vibration–position modalities run in larger, more heavily myelinated fibers; pain–temperature (and autonomic) information travels in smaller, thinly myelinated or unmyelinated fibers. For these reasons, even in the PNS a pathologic process often does not cause uniform deficits in all sensory modalities. Throughout the area of sensory loss, however, the degree of impairment of different modalities is maintained. That is, you will not find a predominance of fine touch impairment in one part of an affected region and mainly loss of pain sensation in another.

Peripheral nerve trunks carry all modalities

Effects of fiber size/ myelination

CNS compartmentalization

The CNS compartmentalization of sensory modalities into the dorsal column/lemniscal pathways (see Fig. 13.14) vs. the spinothalamic pathways (see Fig. 13.13) partially underlies the striking phenomenon of dissociated sensory loss in the spinal cord and brainstem. The different patterns and levels of crossing of fibers in the two systems also explain sensory dissociation (see Fig. 13.16). Because of these anatomic differences, pain and temperature sensation may be abolished in a region of the body where vibration–position–touch modalities are preserved. These latter sensations may themselves be diminished on the other side of the body where pain and temperature sensation is normal (see pp. 305–6 and 309–11).

CLINICAL CONSTRUCTS OF BRAIN LOCALIZATION

Constructs of brain localization summarized in Table 14.3 are discussed below.

A rostrocaudal hierarchy

Construct: the CNS manifests a rostrocaudal hierarchy, with "higher" functions being localized within the cerebral hemispheres and more primitive functions at more caudal levels of the neuraxis.

At the extremes of the rostrocaudal hierarchy are the cerebral cortex vs. the medulla and spinal cord. If a disorder involves language, cognition, and perception (so-called "higher function") we think "cerebral" and especially "cortical." If the issue is loss of respiratory drive, we think of the medulla and cervical spinal cord. More "basic" functions are thought of as being lower in the CNS.

Even within a given function there are "higher" and "lower" levels of control. As an example, urinary bladder control depends on a rostrocaudal hierarchy of function combined with a suprasegmental/segmental organization (see Fig. 13.12). Incontinence may occur on a segmental basis from compression of sacral roots, as by a tumor of the cauda equina. Loss of bladder control may also result from disruption of descending suprasegmental pathways. In the spinal cord, compression or inflammation may damage these pathways bilaterally. More rostral yet, in the cortex of the frontal lobes, suprasegmental control has an important behavioral component. Alcohol and structural lesions can loosen inhibitions against socially impermissible voiding, leading to the irrigation of potted palms and other oft-quoted behaviors that do not reflect the heights of human function.

As noted in Table 14.3, the brainstem neuromodulator (adrenergic, dopaminergic) projections to the cerebral hemispheres serve to modify our ideas of rostrocaudal hierarchy. The brainstem is no longer seen as a passive partner – a mere conduit – in the expression of higher function,

Table 14.3 Some clinical constructs of brain localization

	Clinical constructs	Modifications
1	The central nervous system is organized hierarchically in a rostrocaudal axis, with "higher" functions being localized within the cerebral hemispheres and more primitive functions at more caudal levels of the neuraxis	The discovery of neurotransmitter and modulator projection systems from the brainstem to cerebral areas has helped to modify our ideas of hierarchic control and influence
2	Particular neurologic functions are centered in each of the cerebral lobes, but within a lobe diverse functions may coexist	While cerebral localization explains the effects of many focal lesions, the anatomic substrate of normal function is more widely distributed to other areas connected with the "center"
3	One hemisphere, usually the left, has been considered "dominant." This enables lateralization of lesions affecting certain higher functions that are associated with the dominant or nondominant hemisphere	Dominance is neither monolithic nor immutable in development; dominance tends to be function-specific (e.g. motor, language, particular spatial relations, etc.) so that each hemisphere is dominant for certain attributes
4	Body parts are topographically represented in the brain (somatotopic organization), but not to scale	Somatotopic organization is not limited to the well-known homunculi of the primary motor and sensory cortex, but is pervasive through many other cortical and subcortical structures
5	"Higher functions" such as cognition, language, and the most discriminating types of perception are organized at a cortical level	Language and other higher functions can be disrupted by lesions in subcortical connecting pathways (disconnection syndromes) and more rarely by lesions in deep nuclei
6	The extrapyramidal "system" modulates motor control; dysfunction is characterized by alterations of posture, tone, etc., or by involuntary movements – but not by ordinary weakness	The extrapyramidal scheme of basal ganglionic-centered loops and noncorticospinal descending pathways helps to categorize motor disorders (other than the upper motor neuron or cerebellar patterns)
7	The cerebellum is a center for integrating (and learning) coordinated movements	Coordinated movements depend upon multiple neural systems, such as motor (strength and tone), proprioception, vestibular, and visual

but plays an active role in influencing complex cerebral activity. Other examples of a more interwoven, less hierarchic organization include the involvement of the cerebellum in motor learning, and the cognitive/perceptual roles now identified with parts of the basal ganglia (such as the caudate nucleus) which had previously been associated exclusively with motor control. Therefore, while the construct of a rostrocaudal hierarchy remains useful, you would do well to bear in mind a modified

Table 14.4 Specific signs indicating supratentorial vs. infratentorial compartment

Supratentorial compartment (cerebral hemispheres)	Infratentorial compartment (brainstem and cerebellum)
Anterior aphasias – frontal lobe (see Chapter 10); posterior aphasias – dominant temporal/parietal lobes (see Chapter 10)	Cerebellar signs (such as intention tremor); (note: outflow pathway extends to thalamus) Segmental brainstem signs
Eyes deviated away from the side of a hemiparesis (see Chapter 17)	Eyes deviated towards the side of a hemiparesis (see Chapter 17)
Eyes driving (jerking) away from the side of a discharging epileptic focus	Most instances of nystagmus indicate posterior fossa dysfunction (or a labyrinthine disorder); may be drug-induced rather than structural; vertical nystagmus signifies brainstem/cerebellar dysfunction
Cognitive deficits; impairment of abstract thinking, arithmetic abilities, etc.; memory loss	Cranial nerve signs opposite from long tract signs
Hemianopsia or quadrantanopsia (homonymous)	Hearing deficit (usually ear or CN 8, but ?cochlear nucleus)

image – not so much a neatly layered hierarchy, but rather a marbling of particular functional units in which there is considerable interdependence between more rostral and caudal, cortical and subcortical mechanisms. Table 14.4 provides examples of how certain key neurologic findings indicate localization in the cerebral hemispheres (supratentorial compartment) vs. the brainstem or cerebellum (infratentorial compartment).

Localization of function in cerebral lobes

Construct: particular neurologic functions are "localized" in each of the cerebral lobes (but within a lobe diverse functions may coexist).

Functions long associated with particular cerebral lobes have been summarized in Table 13.4. This information remains diagnostically important from the standpoint of localizing to (a) the supratentorial compartment (the cerebral hemispheres): (b) the right vs. left hemisphere; and (c) the lobe or part of a lobe that is implicated.

Diversity within lobes

Various sections of the frontal, temporal, and parietal lobes differ vastly in function (reflecting different connectivities and different cellular architecture). For example, the frontal lobes contain diverse areas relating to personality, speech, and motor function, to name just a few. The parietal lobes include anterior areas involved in somatosensory perception and more posterior areas relating to language or spatial abilities, as well as many other associative functions. Both temporal lobes contain auditory and olfactory processing areas, as well as important memory and other limbic structures; the dominant temporal lobe includes Wernicke's language area.

Localization: discovery and validity

How have ideas of localization developed, and what does localization of function imply? The acquisition of knowledge about localization has traditionally depended upon fiber tract tracing, electrical stimulation of the cortex, and, above all, upon clinicopathologic correlation. Modern techniques of neuroimaging have enabled not only high-resolution depiction of structural lesions in life, but also demonstration of areas that are activated by the performance of certain tasks or by other arousals (positron emission tomography, single photon emission computed tomography, and newer magnetic resonance techniques).

Centers of function

The earlier methods of clinical–pathologic and radiologic correlation were able to show that localized lesions can disrupt a "center" – a key element of a functional system. However, so-called centers are rarely, if ever, self-contained functional modules. Instead, a more distributive concept applies – not a vague field of anatomic substrate, but rather a network of specific connectivities "centered" at the site of essential components. To turn to the example of memory capacity, the ability to learn and recall new information can be partially or entirely lost with bilateral lesions of the hippocampus. These structures are clearly essential centers of memory function, but memories do not reside there – rather, much more diffusely, in the cerebral hemispheres.

Language/speech centers

Practical neurologic diagnosis still proceeds largely on the basis of localization to single pathways or centers. A good example of such a center is Wernicke's posterior language area in the superior plane of the dominant temporal lobe. However, to show how our ideas of the role of centers can change, there may be no better example than the other language center, the anterior or Broca's area located in the inferior frontal lobe: a lesion limited to Broca's area produces (if any language deficit at all) only a transient and partial anterior aphasic syndrome. For a permanent, nonfluent aphasia, it appears that there must be substantial damage to additional areas, adjacent or more distant. Moreover, loss of speech is not always what it seems. Contrary to expectation, an aphasic patient who does not produce ordinary speech, may be able to curse or sing a familiar song, evidently recruiting pathways that are unavailable to less affect-laden speech (see Case 10B).

Initial steps in cerebral localization

Initial steps in cerebral localization are summarized in Table 14.5.

Diagnostic uses of cerebral dominance

Construct: one hemisphere, usually the left, has been considered "dominant." However, each hemisphere is dominant for particular capabilities. This enables diagnostic lateralization of lesions affecting

Table 14.5 Initial steps in cerebral (hemispheric) localization

Localization	Example of localizing deficit
Supratentorial compartment	An homonymous visual field deficit localizes to the cerebrum but not to only one lobe (see Chapters 5 and 13 and Table 13.3)
Particular cerebral lobe (right or left)	Discriminative types of somatosensory deficits (impaired stereognosis, graphesthesia, etc.): parietal lobes (see Chapter 7)
Lateralization: right vs. left hemisphere (see text on cerebral dominance)	Aphasia: dominant hemisphere, usually left (see Chapter 10); anosognosia (lack of "insight" into deficit) nondominant parietal lobe (usually right) (see Chapters 1 and 10)
Particular part of a cerebral lobe	Wernicke's aphasia: superior part of temporal lobe (dominant) (see Chapter 10)

certain higher functions that are associated with the dominant or nondominant hemisphere.

Dominance is specific to function

Cerebral dominance means that the left or right hemisphere may be predominantly or exclusively specialized for certain functions. Not only are many neurologic functions centered in the cerebral hemispheres, and certain functions localized within particular lobes of the hemispheres, but parts of the right or left hemispheres are specialized *vis-à-vis* each other. In case of damage to one hemisphere, the other hemisphere alone would not be able to compensate completely. (By means of "plasticity" or adaptability of structure and function, lateralized capabilities are not immutable, especially in the developing nervous system.) Anatomic asymmetries between the two hemispheres are associated with at least some aspects of dominance. For example, an enlarged superior plane of the temporal lobe is seen in the hemisphere dominant for language.

Handedness

Historically, the left hemisphere was considered to be the dominant or "major" hemisphere for most people. This view arose from a preoccupation with motor dominance (handedness) and its close linkage to language dominance. Virtually all right-handers and about half of the approximately 10% of left-handers in the population are left-hemisphere language-dominant. In fact, the so-called nondominant hemisphere (usually the right) is actually dominant for certain functions, such as specific spatial capabilities and other nonverbal aspects of mental life which have been popularized as "right brain" attributes.

For practical lateralization of neurologic lesions you need to know the following: (a) the patient's natural handedness (see Chapter 6), in order to define the contralateral hemisphere as motor dominant, with linkage to language and other functions; and (b) the higher functions known to be centered in the dominant vs. nondominant hemisphere (see Table 13.4 and Further reading section).

"Mixed dominance"

Left-sided dominance for language is the most striking example of localization to one hemisphere. However, just as some people, especially those with left-handedness in the family, are ambidextrous (mixed motor dominance), they may also exhibit mixed language dominance. They manifest atypical patterns of aphasia with lesions in their presumed language centers.

Cortical localization of higher functions

Construct: "higher functions," such as cognition, language, spatial relations, and the most discriminating aspects of perception, are based in the cerebral cortex.

An approach to disorders of higher function proceeds from two directions: first, will identification of such deficits enable a specific cortical localization? Second, how will a knowledge of higher functions assist interpretation of cortical lesions discovered by neuroimaging?

Are "cortical functions" cortical?

Impaired higher functions (often called "cortical functions") should, in theory, permit localization to the cortex itself, as opposed to other cerebral structures. Specific cognitive, language, and spatial deficits (in contrast to alterations of consciousness) always point to the cerebral hemispheres of the supratentorial compartment. In most instances, such deficits involve the cortex or the subjacent white matter comprising the cortical connecting tracts, but this distinction is clinically difficult. Few neurologists would be willing to stake a bet on predicting whether "cortical" sensory loss is actually due to a cortical lesion as opposed to a lesion of the relevant thalamocortical projecting fibers. Higher functions may be impaired by a disconnection of two related areas.

Laboratory testing for suspected cortical lesions

On the basis of specific deficits, your clinical diagnostic finger can only point toward the cortex and usually cannot trace the lesion to the cortical gray matter exclusively. The occurrence of seizure activity signifies cortical involvement. Since an electroencephalogram (EEG) directly reflects only cortical electrical activity, a focal abnormality implicates cortical gray matter dysfunction. Imaging, of course, offers the most powerful means of cortical localization.

Cortical lesions and pathologic processes

The demonstration by neuroimaging of a cortical abnormality can contribute to your pathologic or pathogenetic formulations. Localization to gray matter vs. white matter, in particular cortical gray matter vs. subcortical and central white matter, directs you to a body of knowledge about "gray matter diseases" and "white matter diseases." If you discover from neuroimaging that the cortical gray matter appears shrivelled ("atrophied") while no lesions are seen in the white matter, then you can look up a differential diagnosis of diseases predominantly affecting the cortex and thus narrow your search. You might pay particular attention to Alzheimer's disease (a gray matter disease) if the patient displays an array of deficits of higher function. A small, focal cortical computerized tomography (CT) or magnetic resonance imaging (MRI) lesion consistent with an infarct strongly suggests an embolic pathogenesis. Small emboli tend to lodge in cortical arterial branches, while *in situ* thrombosis is rare in the distal arterial arborization.

"Retrodiagnosis"

To reason from the neuroimage to the clinical symptoms and signs might seem to be putting the cart before the horse. However, just this is occurring in practice. Clinicians frequently order neuroimages earlier rather than later in the diagnostic process. Then, having found a lesion, the challenge is to establish its relevance. Consider a right-handed patient with a single, imaged lesion in the right frontal white matter. According to present models of functional anatomy, this will not explain the patient's deficits in recent memory and language capability. Instead, these abnormalities of higher functions would more likely be attributable to a coexistent cortical disease process, whether or not cortical abnormalities are evident by imaging. A knowledge of established localizations of higher functions will repeatedly help you to avoid false correlation of an imaged lesion and clinical event.

Progression of steps in cerebral localization

In summary, despite its limitations, the construct of "higher functions in the cortex" can be put together with the constructs of "a rostrocaudal hierarchy," "localization of functions to specific cerebral lobes," and "cerebral dominance" to help formulate an anatomic localization (Table 14.6): are suprasegmental signs present? Are there symptoms or signs that localize to the intracranial contents? Can you adduce evidence of hemispheric (supratentorial) involvement? Taking into account hemispheric dominance, are there findings referable to a particular cerebral lobe or part of a lobe on the right or left? Finally, in this localizing progression, is there evidence to suggest that the gray matter of the cortex, as opposed to white matter tracts, is the site of pathology? Conversely, working back from an imaged lesion to clinical relevance will test your understanding of functional localization.

Somatotopic representation in the brain

Construct: body parts are topographically represented in the brain but not necessarily to scale.

What do we mean by "representation?" On the sensory side, specific neurons in the cortex (or in deep nuclei) are activated as the result of stimuli to receptors on the skin or in other peripheral structures: the information from a given area of skin reaches neurons in a given area of cortex, so that a body part is represented on the cortical "map." Topographic order is maintained, but typically not to scale or to orientation of the body axis. Similarly, motor representation means that the control of activity of each body part is linked to a specific array of cortical motor

Table 14.6 Brain localization

Deficit	Localizations in supratentorial compartment				Infratentorial localization
	Cortex	Central white matter	Internal capsule	Subcortical "nuclei"	Brainstem or cerebellum
Hemiparesis	Frontal	Corticospinal tract	Posterior limb		Descending motor tracts (cerebral peduncle, base of pons; medullary pyramid)
Hemisensory deficit	Parietal	Thalamoparietal projections	Posterior limb	Thalamus	Medial lemniscus; spinothalamic tract
Dysarthria (worse if bilateral lesions)	Frontoparietal (especially left)	Corticobulbar tract(s)	Genu(?) Posterior limb(?)	Basal ganglia	Corticobulbar tracts; CNs 7, 9, 10, 12; cerebellum
Incoordination	Frontal (weakness, slow initiation); parietal (proprioceptive)	Motor/sensory tracts	Posterior limb; anterior limb (fronto-cerebellar)	Basal ganglia (extrapyramidal deficit)	Cerebellum; vestibular system; motor/sensory long tracts
Visual field cut	Occipital (medial)	Parietal/ temporal optic radiations		Lateral geniculate	
Dementia	Many areas in combinations	Many intercortical tracts in combination		(Thalamus, caudate – rare); nucleus basalis (cholinergic)	
Coma	Diffuse, bilateral	Extensive, bilateral		Thalamic reticular formation (bilateral)	Midbrain and upper pontine reticular formation (bilateral)

neurons. These motor and sensory representations are often pictured as "homunculi." These are little humanoid figures (albeit distorted in their proportions) that are overlaid on a surface view of the brain so as to show the localization of body parts (see Fig. 13.6). How can this construct help clinically?

Cortical localization and vascular territories

In cases of ischemic stroke, a focal deficit, such as weakness in the right hand, points to the area of cortex that is affected (assuming, as is likely in this instance, that the lesion is at a cortical level). Knowledge of the location of this cortical area then permits you to assign a vascular territory. For example, the primary motor control for the hand is in middle cerebral artery territory, whereas the foot area is in anterior cerebral artery territory. Why not just order brain imaging by CT scan to establish the site of the lesion for sure? At the present time immediate imaging by CT does not reveal ischemic lesions (MR technology is solving such problems). Moreover, once imaging identifies a lesion, knowledge of somatotopic representation enables you to assess its relevance: can the abnormality on CT or MRI, or a blockage on an angiogram, account for this particular clinical episode?

Cortex vs. tract

The very fact that a brain lesion produces such focal symptomatology suggests that the lesion is more likely to be cortical. The spreading of the cortical map, or homunculus, over a large surface area increases the probability that a small lesion will affect only a discrete region, such as the hand area. In contrast, a small lesion in a compact fiber bundle deep in the cerebrum or brainstem often produces a more extensive deficit, such as a full hemiparesis. However, this is by no means a perfect rule, since tracts also have somatotopic arrangements (as will be discussed below) and may be only partially damaged.

Localization at surgery

Localization of an epileptic seizure focus (the cortical area from which the electrical discharge originates) provides a classic example of both the existence of cortical representation and its clinical value. In a case of focal epilepsy intractable to medications, a neurosurgeon might plan to remove tissue (presumably abnormal at a microscopic level) that generates focal motor seizure activity beginning in the thumb. To identify at operation the thumb area on the cortex, the neurosurgeon could electrically stimulate the motor cortex (observing what body part twitches).

Modifications

This simple model of somatotopic representation requires modification in a variety of ways, including the following.

1 Some areas of the body have a much larger representation on the cerebral cortex than others. Intricacy of fine motor control or the need for fine topographic sensory differentiation requires more extensive representation.

2 The map of the body appears not just once for motor and once for sensory on the primary motor and sensory strips. Rather, body maps reappear many times in multiple cortical and subcortical areas.

3 Somatotopic representation is "plastic," that is to say, the size and configuration of a body part on the cortical map may change in relation to such variables as peripheral activity and injury; this means that functional connectivities change also, for these are the basis of the maps.

Tract somatotopy

Like the somatotopic organization of white-matter columns in the spinal cord, similar topographic arrangements exist in tracts in the brain. For example, at the level of the cerebral peduncles or the internal capsule the lamination of fibers reflects the spatial arrangement of the structures from which these fibers originated: fibers from cortical face, arm, and leg areas maintain a spatial relationship. In ascending pathways, sensory fibers carrying information from different parts of the body are likewise laminated topographically, but the position varies from pathway to pathway. I do not recommend that you memorize tract somatotopy, but simply remain aware of it for future reference.

The extrapyramidal motor system

Construct: the extrapyramidal "system" modulates motor control, but extrapyramidal disorders are not characterized by true weakness.

Table 14.7 Comparison of motor findings in extrapyramidal vs. upper motor neuron and lower motor neuron disorders

	Lower motor neuron (segmental)	Upper motor neuron (suprasegmental)	"Extrapyramidal" (suprasegmental)
Strength	Weakness in roots' or nerves' segmental distribution; complete lesion causes absolute paralysis	Weakness involves functional muscle groups; reflexive movements despite paralysis	No true weakness; patient may feel weak; may have poor initiation or acceleration of movement, etc.
Muscle bulk	Neurogenic atrophy (disuse atrophy)	Disuse atrophy	May show disuse atrophy if immobile; muscle hypertrophy, due to excessive contraction in dystonias or repetitive involuntary movement
Adventitious movements	None (see Chapter 6, section on fasciculations, etc.)	(Flexor spasms, etc., with upper motor neuron lesions)	Adventitious movements are cardinal extrapyramidal signs: chorea, athetosis, tremor, etc.
Tone	Decreased (or normal)	Increased (normal or decreased, especially acutely)	Usually increased (dystonias); cogwheel rigidity in Parkinson's disease

Noncorticospinal motor deficits

The simplistic UMN/LMN construct fails to explain the occurrence of motor disorders that are not characterized primarily by weakness. Thus, another construct, that of a noncorticospinal (nonpyramidal) or extrapyramidal motor system, has been invoked to account for disorders (Table 14.7) manifested by: (a) involuntary (adventitious) movements; (b) dystonic postures and rigidity; and (c) akinesia (deficits in initiating or sustaining action).

Extrapyramidal anatomy: descending tracts

Anatomically, the term "extrapyramidal" refers to descending motor pathways that are not part of the corticospinal tract in the medullary pyramids (Fig. 14.2). These pathways (sometimes also called "parapyramidal") convey the influence of certain brainstem and, indirectly, cerebral structures to the spinal segments. The rubrospinal tract is one example. Some of the tracts also participate in the control of axial postures and gross proximal limb movements, as part of a "ventromedial" system of motor control. (The lateral corticospinal tracts, along with the rubrospinal tracts, comprise the main component of the "dorsolateral system" that governs more distal, fine movement.) At least two of the features of the UMN profile, hypertonia and hyperreflexia, are partly mediated by

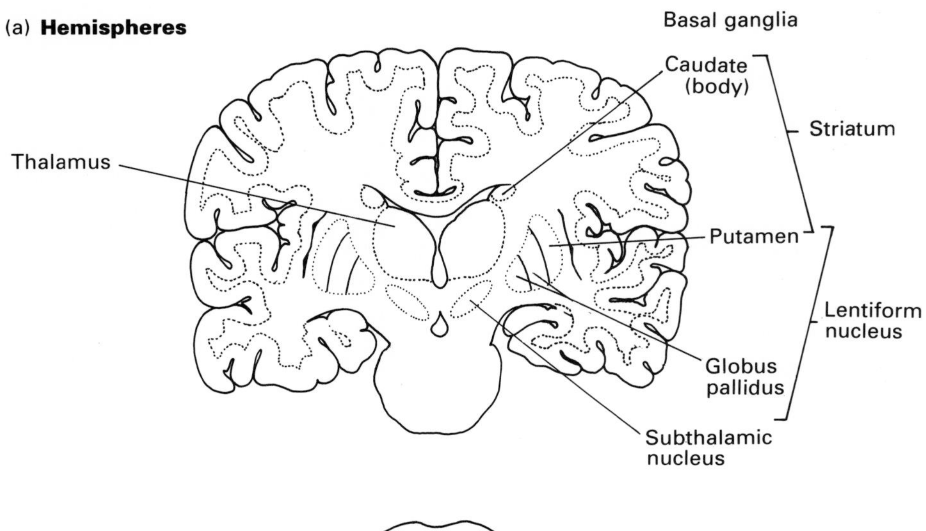

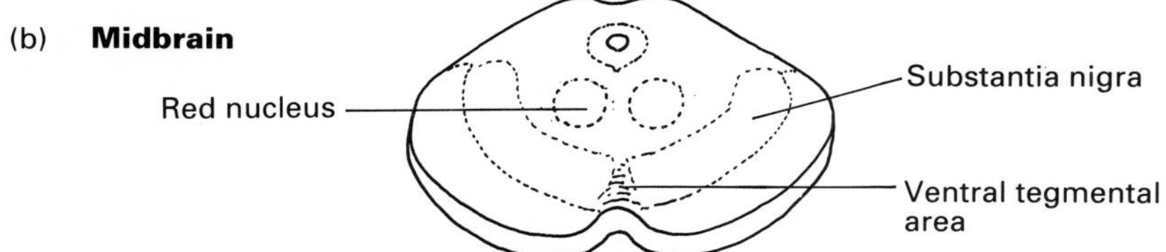

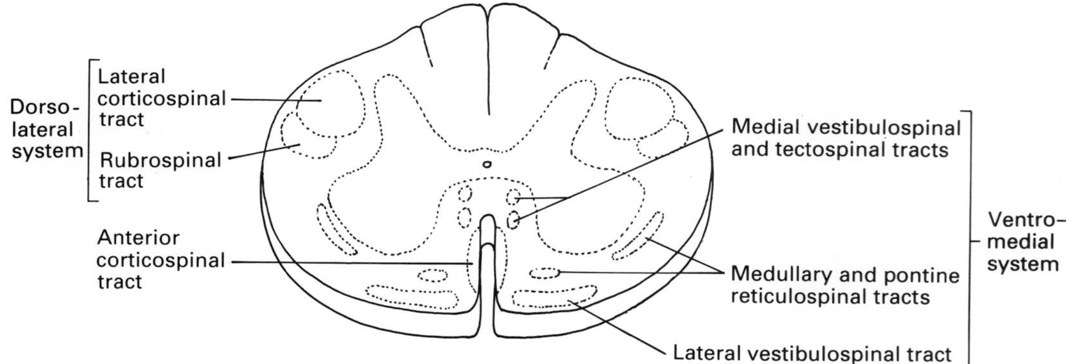

Fig. 14.2 The basal ganglia and the extrapyramidal descending motor pathways. (a) The basal ganglia shown in this section include the body of the caudate nucleus, the putamen, globus pallidus, (external and internal segments), and subthalamic nucleus. (b) Additional components currently categorized with the basal ganglia – the substantia nigra, and the related ventral tegmental area. (c) The so-called extrapyramidal descending pathways of the spinal cord, including rubrospinal, vestibulospinal, reticulospinal, and tectospinal tracts, are shown in their spinal cord locations – the latter three groups being ventromedial.

extrapyramidal neurons rather than the corticospinal tract itself. Somewhat conflicting evidence bearing upon this comes from the effects of "pure" pyramidal lesions. Because extrapyramidal fibers run more diffusely, "pure" extrapyramidal correlations are lacking. In any case, equating the UMN profile with damage to the corticospinal tract is one of the liberties of the UMN construct.

Extrapyramidal disorders: basal ganglionic

Signs and symptoms that are conventionally associated with the extrapyramidal system are mainly those of basal ganglionic disease, e.g. various movement disorders, such as the tremor, rigidity, and akinesia of Parkinson's disease or the chorea of Huntington's disease. For the most part, the basal ganglia, however, do not funnel directly through the extrapyramidal descending motor fibers, but circuitously via the thalamus and motor cortex. Therefore, the motor manifestations of basal ganglionic disease are expressed, at least in part, through the corticospinal tracts, as well as through other, less direct, crossed and uncrossed, extrapyramidal fibers.

Thus, we are left with a loosely defined and rather poorly localized group of anatomic tracts that give the extrapyramidal "system" its name, and another group of structures, the basal ganglia, that are involved in complex motor control "loops." The basal ganglia form the principal anatomic substrate of extrapyramidal syndromes, as epitomized by parkinsonism.

Specific pathways

1 The brainstem extrapyramidal output descends in the reticulospinal, tectospinal, vestibulospinal, and rubrospinal pathways. In the medulla, these are relatively diffuse fibers running dorsal to the pyramids. The transmission of their suprasegmental influence on α motor neurons tends to be multisynaptic and indirect.

Basal ganglionic-centered loops

2 The second set of structures, the basal ganglia, have been implicated in most movement disorders and disorders of posture. As noted, basal ganglionic influences are not simply expressed by way of the extrapyramidal pathways referred to above. The principal output from the basal ganglia projects to "motor-associated" nuclei of the thalamus which, in turn, connect mainly to the premotor and other frontal cortical areas. These, in turn, relay largely to the primary motor cortex which gives rise to a portion of the fibers of the corticospinal tract. Thus, to some extent, the output of the basal ganglia functions in series with the corticospinal tract (dorsolaterally placed in the spinal cord). Other fibers from frontal motor areas, as well as those originating in the brainstem, enter into parallel extrapyramidal pathways that contribute to the ventromedial component of the descending spinal motor system.

Correlation with basal ganglionic diseases

Descriptive knowledge of extrapyramidal disorders has been gained through clinicopathologic correlations: the effects of tumors, infarctions, and degenerative diseases, etc., as well as the use of experimental lesions. While the various loops of motor control include the cerebellum and parts of the thalamus, the extrapyramidal disorders described here are closely identified with pathologic changes and/or neurotransmitter deficits in the basal ganglia, and are quite distinct from most disorders localized to the cerebellum or thalamus. Parkinson's disease and Huntington's disease represent two of the best examples of extrapyramidal disease. Even in these two conditions, about which much has been learned, the actual pathophysiologic basis of tremor, akinesia, chorea, or other manifestations remains a matter of hypothesis and ongoing research.

Integration of "motor" and "sensory" control of movement

Control of movement is not synonymous with motor tracts. At every level of the nervous system, from the muscle spindle to the cerebral cortex, motor and sensory systems interact. Within the motor control loops of the brain, terms like afferent and efferent become increasingly relative and certainly cannot be equated with sensory and motor functions, *per se*.

In summary, the construct of extrapyramidal disorders serves to categorize suprasegmental motor disorders that do not involve a loss of peak resistive strength, but do include rigidity, dystonia, akinesia, or adventitious movements. Clinical diagnosis proceeds by a broad pattern recognition of dysfunction associated with basal ganglionic disorders. Lesions of the descending extrapyramidal tracts themselves lack even this degree of correlation in human disease.

Localizing incoordination to the cerebellum

Construct: the cerebellum is a center for integrating (and learning) coordinated movements, but balance and coordination are dependent on many neural systems.

Despite the fact that we all know more or less what coordination is, the jump to localizing a particular coordination deficit to the cerebellum may prove difficult. Aside from localization by imaging or pathologic examination, no clinical gold standard exists for confirmation of a cerebellar disorder. In addition, we currently have no general physiologic method of distinguishing a cerebellar lesion *per se* from a lesion in the connecting input or output tracts or nuclei. Because of these difficulties, it was emphasized in Chapter 8 that tests like finger–nose, heel–shin, and tandem gait should be considered an assessment of coordination (or balance). These are not specific tests of the cerebellum itself or even of the cerebellar system, since a pure cerebellar test has not been devised. As a practical matter, the construct of cerebellar incoordination depends partly on pattern recognition and partly on exclusion of deficits in other systems.

Clinical pattern recognition

Pattern recognition of cerebellar signs derives from clinicopathologic correlation. The effects of cerebellar lesions are traditionally taken to comprise interruption of the smooth flow and direction of motor activity, including dysmetria, as well as impaired stability of posture and gait (see Chapter 8 for a detailed description of "cerebellar" signs). However, sometimes the pattern is obvious to all observers, while at other times even a roomful of neurologists cannot agree at all.

Exclusion of other deficits

As presented in Chapter 8, incoordination may be tentatively attributed, by exclusion, to the cerebellar system when an impairment of balance or the modulation and accuracy of motor performance cannot be ascribed to other systems: pyramidal, extrapyramidal, proprioceptive, vestibular, visual, or specific peripheral disorders. For example, mild clumsiness of a hand may result from subtle weakness, impaired tactile or proprioceptive sense, or a cluster of extrapyramidal findings that include rigidity and bradykinesia, as well as from cerebellar dysfunction (see Case 8A).

Gait ataxia

An awkward gait and poor truncal balance represent potentially difficult challenges to localization, from the standpoint of either pattern recognition or exclusion. Occasionally, even parietal lobe and anterior frontal lobe lesions enter into the differential diagnosis of gait ataxia. Neuroimaging techniques are now able to provide evidence of structural abnormality, which often solves the diagnostic problem by confirming a cerebellar localization. At the same time, mistaking the clinical relevance of an imaged lesion represents an increasingly common pitfall for the unwary.

Case 14A
Failing gait in a recovering alcoholic

John Pomona, a 57-year-old alcoholic, was referred for progressive ataxia characterized by an unsteady, rather wide-based gait. He arrived with a CT scan showing "moderate cerebellar atrophy, especially in the midline," attributed to his chronic alcoholism. He was no longer actively drinking. An initial examination excluded weakness, decreased joint position sense, vertigo, poor vision, and extrapyramidal signs of parkinsonism, but did reveal asymmetric hyperreflexia in the limbs, without Babinski signs. Nothing on the head CT accounted for these findings. Subsequent reexamination uncovered a spastic increase in extensor and adductor tone in the legs. This caused some tendency of the legs to "scissor" (adduct) during walking, but the effect was partially masked by the widened base that had suggested a cerebellar localization in the first place. An MRI of the cervical spine revealed compression of the cord by a bony spur – a spondylotic cervical myelopathy that was as yet insufficient to produce weakness or sensory loss and did not, for unknown reasons, cause the Babinski signs that would ordinarily have been expected. After neurosurgical consultation, the patient elected to defer intervention in order to assess any further tendency for progression. He remained stable through a 1-year follow-up.

Formulation summary

This case illustrates the following points:

1 an attempt by pattern recognition to attribute a mild and nonprogressive, wide-based gait to mild alcoholic cerebellar degeneration;

2 the identification, during a careful process of exclusion, of clinical signs probably referable to cervical myelopathy – hypertonia, hyperreflexia, and awkward gait;
3 the recognition by cranial neuroimaging of cerebellar changes that appeared consistent with alcoholic cerebellar degeneration (however, this abnormality was inadequate to explain the full neurologic picture);
4 the identification by cervical MRI of the contributory factor of cervical cord compression, presumably responsible for the signs noted in (2), above.

Localization within the cerebellum

Implicit in the use of pattern recognition for cerebellar localization are two features of the clinical neuroanatomy discussed in Chapter 13: first, the functional zones of the cerebellum, especially the predominant role of the midline vermis in stance and gait; second, the crossing of cerebellar output to the midbrain and cerebrum. When combined with the crossing of the corticospinal tract, the net effect is a "double cross." This causes the manifestation of lateralized cerebellar signs to be on the same side as the cerebellar lesion (see Fig. 13.18 and Case 8B). This rule in particular will prove useful not only in "forward" diagnostic localization from signs to lesion, but in "backward" or "retrodiagnostic" correlation of imaged lesion to clinical symptoms and signs.

In summary, how can the construct of cerebellar incoordination be applied in patient care?

Correlative experience

1 The diagnostic use of pattern recognition is based on an inventory of correlations, such as that of intention tremor, with lesions of the cerebellum or its outflow tracts. Seek expert help in characterizing suspected cerebellar signs.

Directed history and examination

2 Since the process of cerebellar localization also depends upon exclusion, pursue the history and examination assiduously to detect symptoms and signs pointing to other neural systems. As in Case 14A, reexamination is a powerful tool.

Imaged lesion

3 Applying the construct of cerebellar localization hinges on the question of whether an imaged lesion is clinically relevant. This highlights the value of bringing neurologic and radiologic expertise together to help in diagnosis.

Control of horizontal gaze

This last construct to be considered brings us back once again to the concept of suprasegmental/segmental organization. The control of horizontal gaze will be discussed only briefly here, as its great clinical importance requires careful explanation (see Chapter 17).

Construct: A suprasegmental (hemispheric) gaze center and a segmental brainstem (pontine) gaze center act to control conjugate horizontal gaze.

According to the clinical construct for horizontal conjugate gaze, the eyes deviate toward the side of a destructive (depressive) hemispheric lesion and away from a destructive brainstem (pontine) lesion. Stimulation of one hemisphere (frontal regions), as in an epileptic seizure discharge, causes the eyes to deviate in rhythmic jerks, away from that hemisphere. These effects should not be memorized as such, but rather understood in terms of a schema that can be easily reconstructed (see Chapter 17 and Fig. 17.1).

This construct is based upon the concept of ipsilateral segmental brainstem function and crossed suprasegmental hemispheric function: the descending long tracts from the hemisphere cross to reach the contralateral "gaze center" in the pons. This pontine coordinating center for conjugate horizontal (lateral) gaze mediates movement of the eyes to the same side. This requires precisely yoked activation of the muscles that move the eyes in the horizontal plane: one medial rectus (CN 3) and the opposite lateral rectus muscle (CN 6). Thus, in this construct, "segmental" control is two-tiered: first, there is activation of the pontine coordinating center that controls conjugate gaze to its own side; second, two separate cranial nerve nuclei are stimulated to innervate the appropriate muscles.

Use of this construct helps to indicate:

1 whether a destructive lesion such as stroke is localized to the cerebrum or brainstem;

2 on which side the lesion is lateralized;

3 from which side a seizure with eye deviation is emanating (but note that this is an imperfect rule).

SOME RULES OF SPINAL AND BRAINSTEM LOCALIZATION

Dissociated sensory loss

Clinical rule: dissociated sensory loss – the separation of pain–temperature and touch–vibration–position deficits – localizes the lesion to the spinal cord or brainstem.

Separate pathways

Dissociated sensory loss results from: (a) discordant crossing – one pathway crosses and another does not, or they cross at different levels; and/or (b) topographical separation of different sensory tracts, so that one may be disrupted but not the other.

Spinal cord tracts

Recall from Chapter 13 (see Fig. 13.14) that in the dorsal column–lemniscal system that conveys vibratory sense, etc., the entire tract of 2nd order neuronal fibers crosses as a group in the medulla just rostral to their nuclei of origin. The lateral spinothalamic tract of the anterolateral system carries pain and temperature information; the 2nd order neuron fibers cross close to (usually a few segments above) each segment of entry where the incoming 1st order axons synapse (see Fig. 13.13). Because of the very different levels of crossing of these two systems, as well as their posterior vs. anterior separation in the cord, dissociation is possible. (The existence of other, less well-defined crossed and uncrossed spinothalamic tract fibers in the anterior columns does not spoil the overall practical value of this model.)

The discovery that a patient has lost the capacity to feel a pain stimulus, such as a pinprick, but can still perceive touch, stands out as one of the more dramatic bedside revelations in neurology. It may seem almost unbelievable to patient and examiner alike. Three classic spinal cord syndromes and a brainstem syndrome illustrate dissociated sensory loss.

Brown–Séquard syndrome

The first is the Brown–Séquard syndrome which was described in Chapter 13 (see Fig. 13.16). With a cross-sectional lesion of one-half of the cord (hemisection), both major sensory systems are affected, but the clinical deficits appear on opposite sides because of the different levels of decussation: dorsal column fibers do not cross in the cord, whereas all fibers in the lateral spinothalamic tract have already crossed.

Anterior spinal artery syndrome

The second condition is the anterior spinal artery syndrome (see Fig. 14.3 and Case 7A) in which the anterior two-thirds of the spinal cord are infarcted over a number of segments. The lateral spinothalamic tract is disrupted, affecting pain and temperature modalities below the lesion, but the dorsal columns remain intact. (The corticospinal tracts are also damaged.) Typically, the lesion extends across both sides of the cord, so that pain–temperature loss is observed bilaterally. Thus, one group of sensory modalities is affected but not the other, because of the topographic separation of the tracts.

Syringomyelic syndrome

In syringomyelia (or hydromyelia), a cavity (syrinx) occupies the center of the cord, disrupting fibers crossing from one side of the cord to the other for all segmental levels at which the cavity exists (Fig. 14.4). The 2nd order neurons of the lateral spinothalamic pathway cross just anterior to the central canal. This renders them vulnerable to interruption by an expansive, fluid-filled cavity. Damage to fibers crossing from right to left thus results in a right-sided dermatomal pain–temperature loss for each segment involved. (However, each band lies one to two dermatomal segments below the level of the crossing fibers, because the fibers ascend as they cross.) Since fibers are crossing left to right as well as right to left, the pain–temperature deficits are bilateral, although not necessarily symmetric. Vibration–position–touch modalities are not affected unless the cavity expands to such a degree that the dorsal columns (along with other tracts) are compressed. The cavity may also destroy central gray matter (including 2nd order neurons of the spinothalamic pathway). Note that since the prototypical vibration–position–touch fibers do not synapse in the dorsal horn before entering the dorsal columns, cell loss in the central parts of the dorsal horn would not affect this pathway. In the anterior horns, α motor neurons may be destroyed, leading to ipsilateral LMN signs referable to those segments.

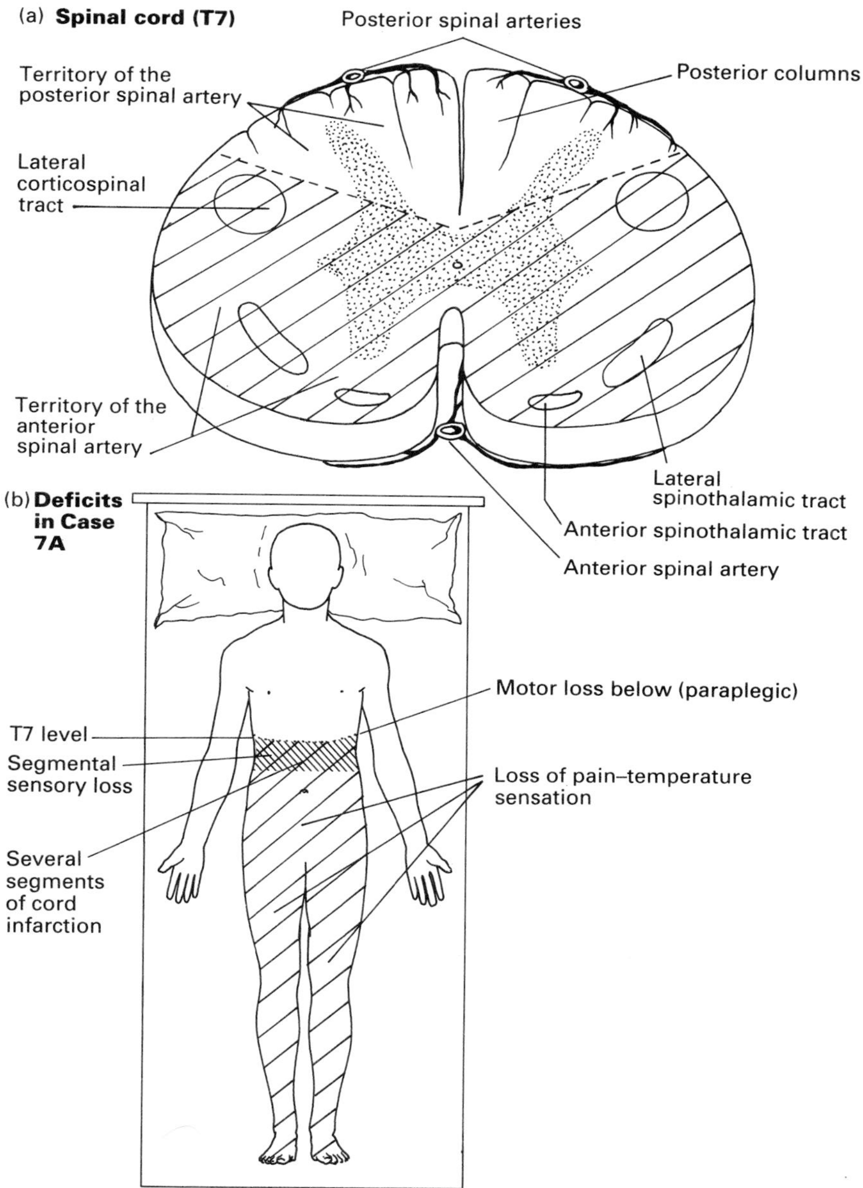

Fig. 14.3 Anterior spinal artery territory and syndrome. (a) The anterior spinal artery (with its collateral supply) irrigates the anterior two-thirds of the cord (diagonal hatching). (b) Deficits in Case 7A, with the uppermost level at T7, due to failure of the anterior spinal artery circulation. All segmental functions are affected in the infarcted cord levels. Deficits in pain–temperature sensation occur below the sensory level, due to interruption of all ascending information in the spinothalamic tracts bilaterally. The posterior columns (and posterolateral columns), serving vibration and some aspects of fine touch and joint position sense are preserved. The lateral corticospinal tract involvement causes paraplegia. Compare with Figs 13.9, 13.16, and 14.4.

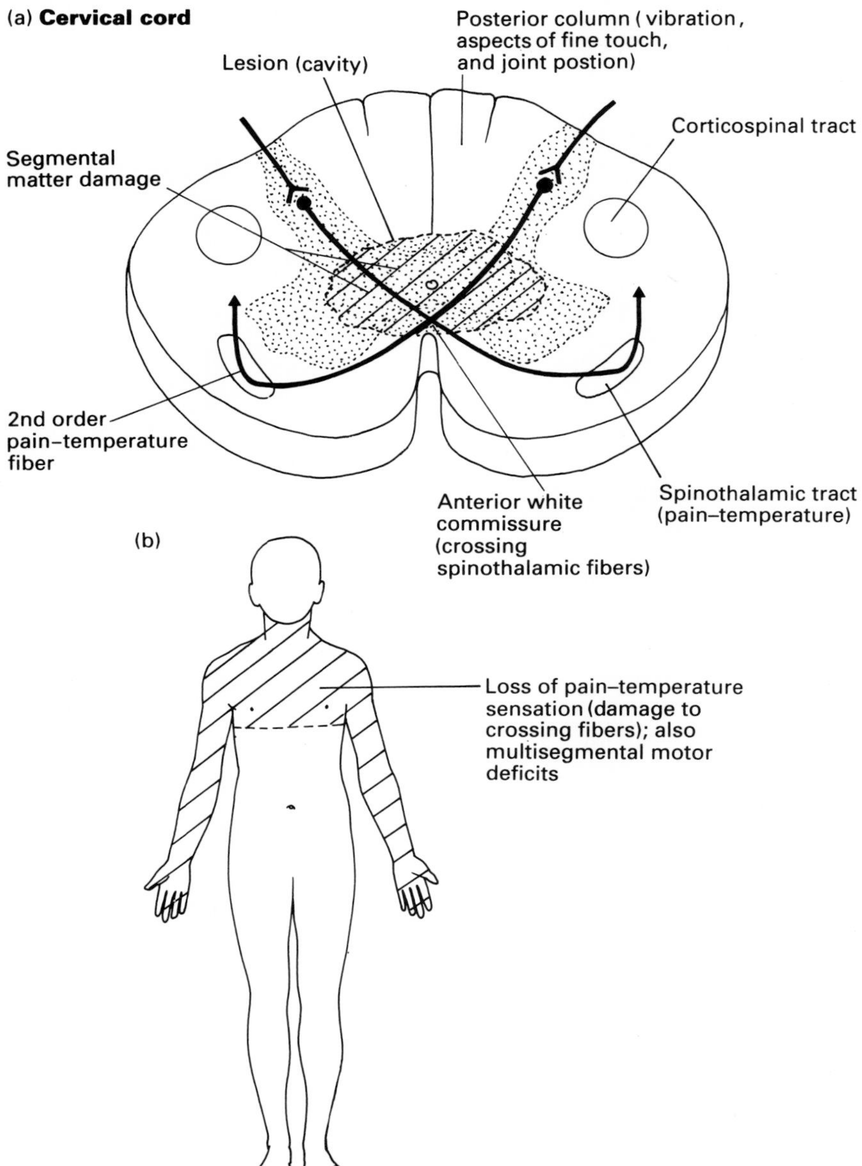

Fig. 14.4 Syringomyelia. (a) In a representative section of the cervical cord, the lesion (a central cavity) involves the anterior white commissure (just ventral to the central canal) through which the 2nd order fibers of the pain–temperature pathway cross. Pain–temperature is lost only at (or slightly below) each segment of damage from the syringomyelic cavity, but is not lost from lower parts of the body since the spinothalamic tracts themselves are unaffected. Lower motor neuron deficits are also variably present in each affected segment, because of damage to the anterior horns of the spinal cord. Compare with the anterior spinal artery syndrome (Fig. 14.3).

Brainstem

Above the caudal medulla in the brainstem, both ascending somatosensory systems have already crossed, but remain separate. The dorsal column–lemniscal pathway is medially placed (in the medial lemniscus) and the spinothalamic tract is located more laterally. Thus, a dissociated sensory loss results from a lesion limited to the lateral medulla, with the pain–temperature deficit appearing on the trunk and limbs contralateral to the lesion. This anatomy accounts for that part of the lateral medullary syndrome in which the dorsolaterally situated infarct affects the spinothalamic tract, but not the medial lemniscus (Fig. 14.5). The following section will amplify the illustrative value of this syndrome by comparing pain–temperature sensation on the face vs. the body.

Lateral medullary syndrome

In summary, each of these syndromes demonstrates an aspect of why dissociated sensory loss localizes the lesion to the cord or lower brainstem. Up to the level of the midbrain the respective tracts are still quite separated. Above the medulla no more sensory decussations occur in tracts representing the limbs and trunk. By the thalamus, the somatosensory modalities largely have merged, although affective aspects of pain have a separate substrate. Thus, in the cerebral hemispheres, sensory dissociation as described here does not occur. (Another distinction is made above the thalamus, namely, the occurrence of discriminative, "cortical" sensory impairments, with primary modalities preserved, or nearly so.) As explained earlier, differential involvement of larger and smaller fibers in the PNS can create a form of sensory dissociation. However, the neuropathic or radiculopathic distribution of the deficit will usually prevent any confusion with a cord or brainstem lesion.

Opposite cranial nerve vs. long tract signs

Clinical rule: an opposite-sided pattern, consisting of a cranial nerve segmental finding on one side, combined with a long tract finding (e.g. hemiparesis) on the contralateral side of the body, localizes the lesion to the brainstem. (This "opposite" or "alternate side" pattern is often referred to as a "crossed pattern," a term that should perhaps be avoided because of confusion with other uses of "crossed.")

Primary midbrain lesion

The combination of a paralysis of CN 3 function on the right and a left hemiparesis indicates that an intrinsic, nonexpansive primary lesion (such as an infarct) must be on the right side of the midbrain. CN 3 nucleus and its exiting nerve are situated in the midbrain, establishing the segmental level: like almost all segmental functions, CN 3 exits ipsilaterally. A lesion affecting the right side of the ventral midbrain, for example, would involve CN 3 exiting, as well as the descending corticospinal tract in the base of the cerebral peduncle on the right (see Fig. 13.10). Since the corticospinal lesion is rostral to the medullary decussation, the segmental 3rd nerve palsy and the hemiparesis are on opposite sides. By literally coordinating the cross-sectional level of the

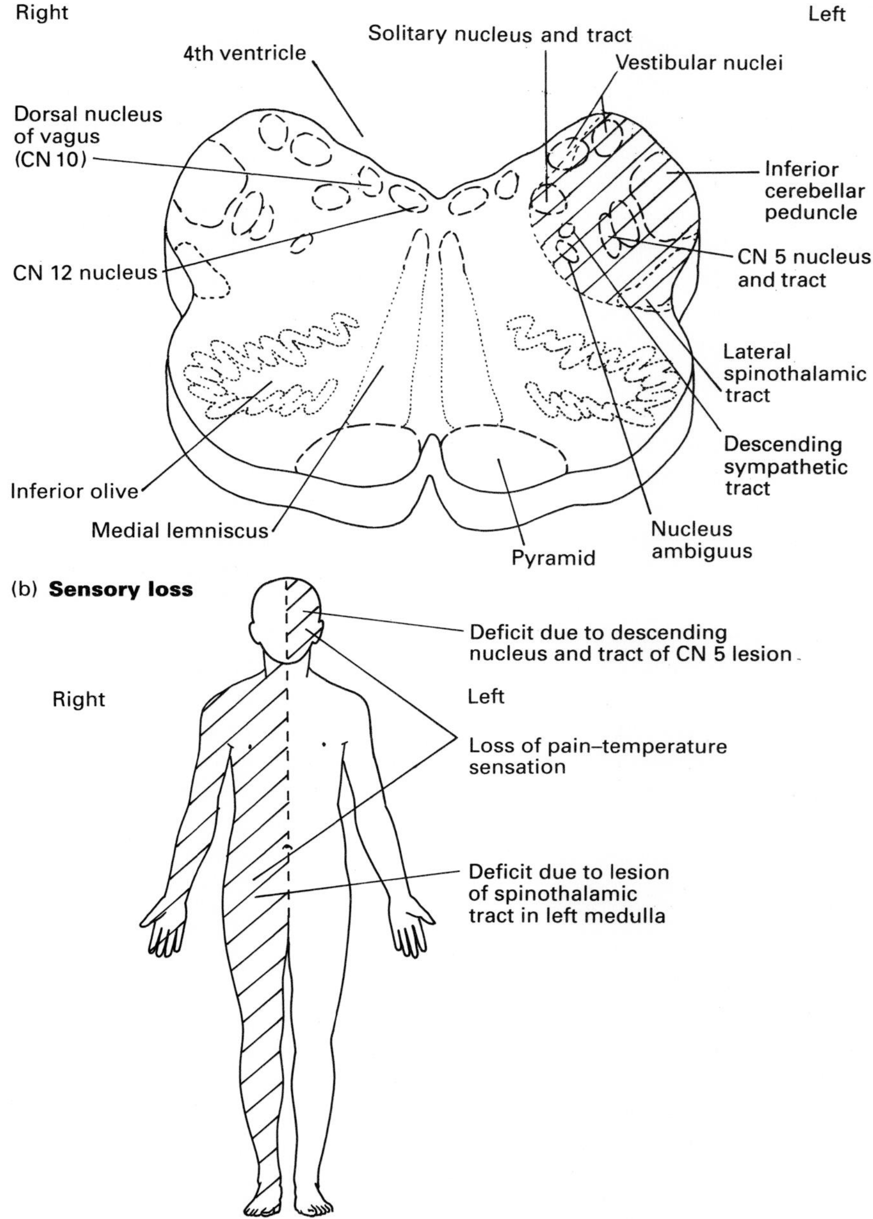

Fig. 14.5 Lateral medullary syndrome: dissociated sensory loss and opposite-sided face and body deficits. (a) Infarction in the dorsolateral medulla (as well as part of the inferior cerebellum, not shown), which is supplied by the posterior-inferior cerebellar artery, a branch of the vertebral. (b) Loss of pain and temperature on the left side of the face, ipsilateral to the lesion due to involvement of the left descending nucleus and tract of CN 5; contralateral pain and temperature deficits in the body, resulting from infarction of the lateral spinothalamic tract, the fibers of which have already crossed at or near every spinal segmental level of entry. The medial lemniscus is not involved. The remainder of the syndrome can be predicted from the other structures within the affected areas (see Further reading section).

segmental finding with the axis of the long tract involved, you can accurately localize the lesion: the CN 3 palsy tells you that the rostrocaudal level is the midbrain, and the left hemiparesis signifies involvement of the right corticospinal tract (in the base of the peduncle).

You should be aware, however, that CN 3 can also be compressed outside the brainstem. If this is due to a transtentorial herniation, then contralateral or ipsilateral signs may result (see Chapter 13). The herniated temporal lobe compresses or stretches and distorts CN 3. The cerebral lesion itself, or the effect of the herniation on the ipsilateral cerebral peduncle, causes a contralateral (crossed) hemiparesis and Babinski sign. However, the shifts involved in herniation can compress CN 3 and the cerebral peduncle on the other side as well, so that any combination of ipsilateral and contralateral signs is possible.

Opposite analgesia

The lateral medullary syndrome, referred to earlier, served as an example of dissociated sensory loss. This classic syndrome also illustrates the rule of opposite or discordant CN vs. long tract deficits, applied to sensation. A lesion of the lateral medulla on the right interrupts the ascending spinothalamic tract, with the expected consequence of a contralateral pain–temperature loss below the head. But this same lesion typically extends to the descending nucleus of CN 5, which receives 1st order fibers serving pain–temperature modalities on the same side of the face. Thus, pain and temperature sensations on the right side of the face are impaired, while these same modalities are affected on the left side of the body (see Fig. 14.5).

Sensory levels on the trunk localize to the spinal cord

Clinical rules: (a) a sensory level on the trunk signifies a spinal cord lesion; (b) the level of the cord lesion may be higher than the sensory level; (c) below the cervical region, the location of a given cord segment is higher than the correspondingly numbered vertebral level.

Sensory level defined

A sensory level is a line above which sensation (in general or for a particular modality) is intact, and below which it is impaired. This clinical line of demarcation may be on a limb, but is most easily visualized on the trunk, where it is generally more circumferential.

Sensory vs. cord level

As stipulated in Chapter 7, the level of the spinal cord lesion can be higher than, but never lower than, the clinical sensory level (due to ascent of sensory information). The main reason that the cord lesion may be higher, sometimes much higher, is that spinal cord tracts are somatotopically organized, such that a partial lesion might affect only some "leg fibers" and not "trunk fibers." For example, a medial lesion in the dorsal columns at C4 cord level might impinge on the most medial fibers transmitting touch and vibratory information from the lower limbs, but leave more lateral fibers from the abdomen and arms intact. Let us say that the initial clinical sensory demarcation is found to be at L1 level,

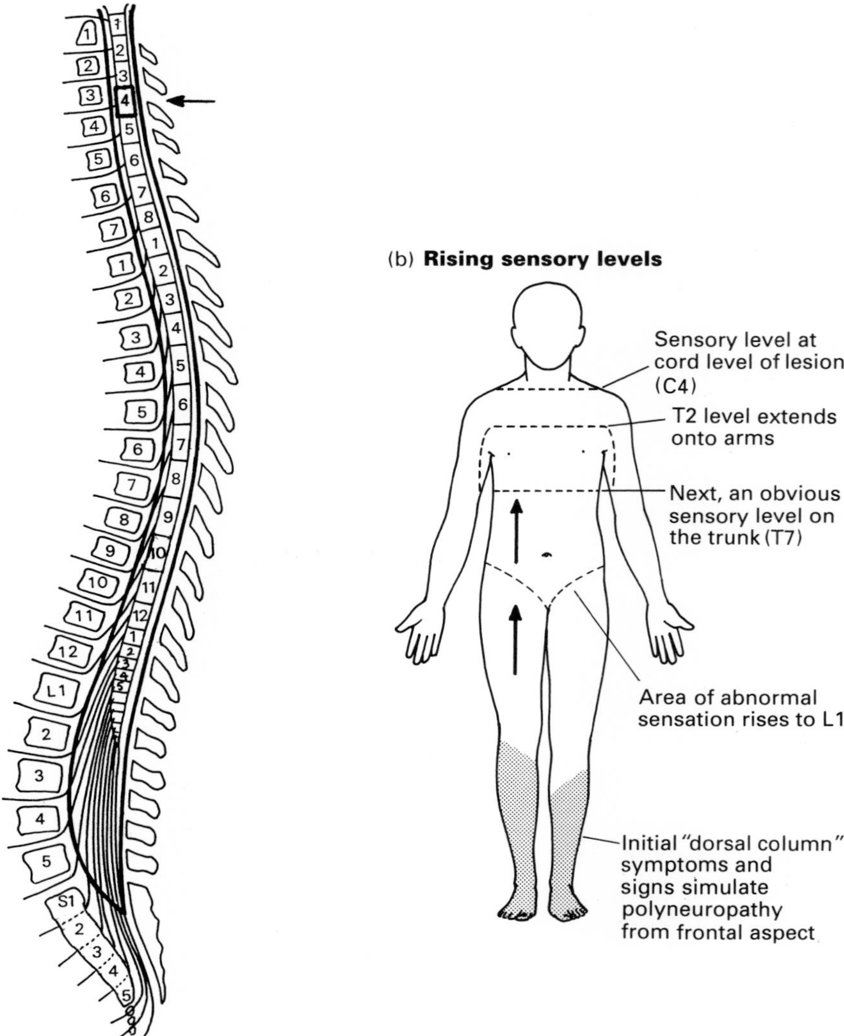

Fig. 14.6 Rising clinical sensory levels – due to an expanding cord lesion. (a) Spinal cord and column showing C4 location of cord lesion. (b) Clinical progression is shown sequentially, from distal to more proximal sensory symptoms and signs. Distal involvement might be mistaken for a polyneuropathy (from the anterior aspect), but note the asymmetry. The medially placed C4 lesion in the posterior columns at first affects only those fibers (fasciculus gracilis) that come from the lowest lumbosacral segments and has yet to involve fibers originating from higher dermatomes. (You can visualize the location of the lesion by placing it on the section used in Fig. 14.4.) As the lesion expands at the C4 level to involve more and more of the posterior column fibers, the clinical level ascends to L1, to T7, then to T2, and finally to the level of the spinal cord lesion (C4). (In reality, the rising sensory levels are not usually so well demarcated, nor so symmetrical, and do not "jump" from one level to another.) Other long tract signs, as well as segmental signs at the level of the lesion, may also be noted in some cases.

using the L1 dermatome as a convenient marker; vibration, some touch sensation, and some position sense are impaired in the lower extremities. Subjective numbness is felt below the groin. All sensation rostral to that level is intact. If we were to make the mistake of thinking that the lesion were necessarily at cord level L1, then we might wrongly direct CT examination to the location of cord level L1. As the C4 cord lesion expands at its level, affecting more and more of the tract fibers, the clinical sensory level will ascend – for example, to the lower sternum (xiphoid), for which we can use T7 dermatome as a marker. Eventually the dermatome of the sensory level will approximate the number of the cord level, in this case, C4 (see Fig. 14.6). Pitfalls in the interpretation of apparent or real sensory levels are summarized in Table 14.8.

Motor and reflex levels

Motor and reflex levels also provide localizing information (Fig. 14.7). In a trauma patient you discover a marked disparity between absent biceps jerks (C5, C6) and brisk triceps jerks (C7, C8), knee jerks, and ankle jerks. This suggests the possibility of a cord lesion at C6 cord level (although there are other possible explanations). A C5 and C6 cord lesion affecting the anterior (and/or posterior) horn cells would obliterate the

Table 14.8 Pitfalls in assessing sensory levels

	Pitfalls	Comment
1	Establishing too low a sensory level by defining it as the transition from no sensation to partial sensation, rather than partially impaired sensation to normal sensation	When moving the touch, pin, or other stimulus rostrally to seek a level, do not stop when the patient says, "I feel it." Compare with a higher level on the trunk, limbs, neck, or face
2	Assuming the sensory level to be at T3 or T4 on the chest, when in fact the level is at T2 to C5 on the arms.	Dermatomes move onto the arms starting with part of T2 and move back onto the shoulders and neck with C4. So testing must move from chest to arms to shoulders, neck, and posterior scalp to find the true level. (Cervical dermatomes on the back can be tested but are very narrow and hard to assess)
3	Presuming that sensory loss in both legs is due to polyneuropathy, whereas if the upper boundary with normal were defined, a sensory level on the trunk would be recognized	Sometimes the error lies in simply not pursuing the deficit to more and more proximal regions. Testing should not stop at the groin (underwear line) or misinterpret the greater sensitivity of skin in the groin area vs. the thighs
4	Confusing a cutaneous sensory level with the cord level of the lesion	As described in the text, the sensory level may be lower, because of partial tract involvement
5	Confusing a cutaneous sensory level or cord level with the correspondingly numbered vertebral level	For cord/column disproportion see Chapter 13 and Fig. 13.9

biceps reflexes, which are segmental. Damage to the corticospinal tract would heighten all reflexes at lower levels, starting with the triceps reflexes (mainly C7). Additional examples, including analysis of the jaw jerk and the superficial abdominal reflexes, are provided in Chapter 9.

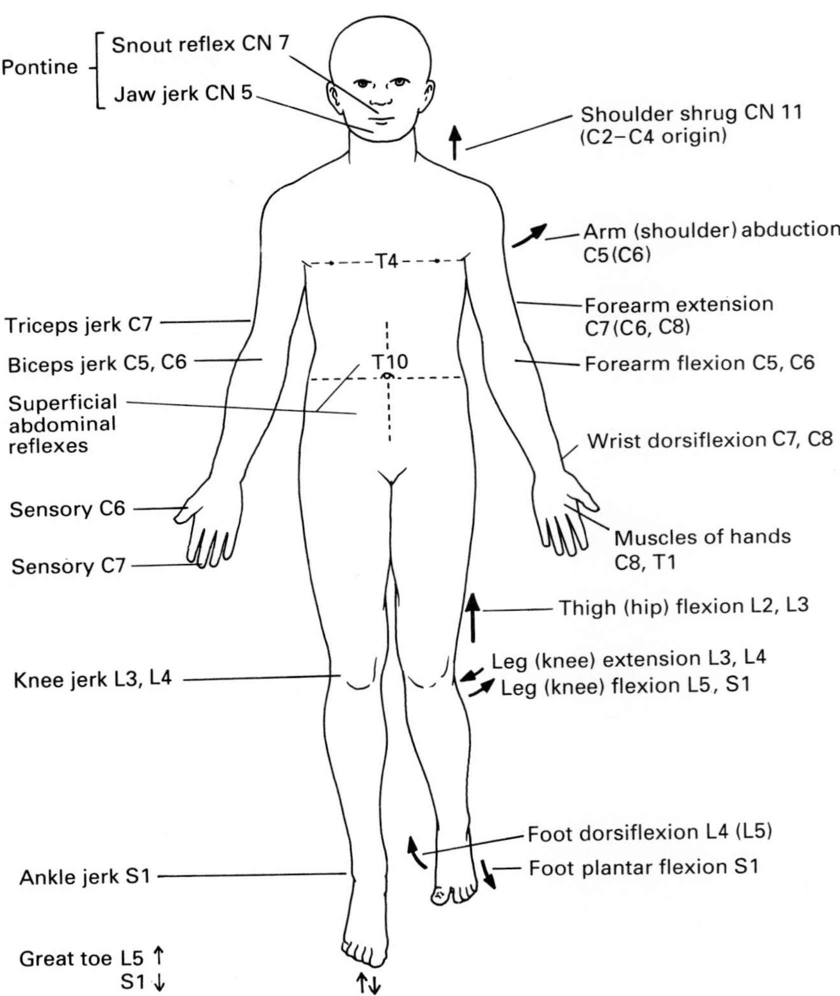

Fig. 14.7 Segmental levels: motor, reflex, and sensory tests or demarcations. Note that key sensory markers, such as C6 for the thumb and C7 for the middle finger (sometimes index finger), only comprise a small part of the dermatome. The roots identified with the reflexes are the main contributors. The most caudal spinal segments (S2–S5 and coccygeal segments) are represented in the "saddle" area – genital, perineal, inner gluteal (not shown).

Localizing value of bilateral symptoms and signs

Clinical rule: bilateral symptoms and signs from a single lesion indicate a spinal cord or brainstem localization (but notable exceptions exist).

Bilateral structures in proximity

Structures on the right and left sides of the brainstem or spinal cord lie close together or in continuity (Fig. 14.8). Nuclei and tracts that are medially placed and adjacent to their opposite counterparts are likely to be jointly affected by a lesion crossing the midline. Examples include the dorsal columns of the spinal cord (especially the fasciculus gracilis on each side) or the medial longitudinal fasciculi of the brainstem (see Fig.

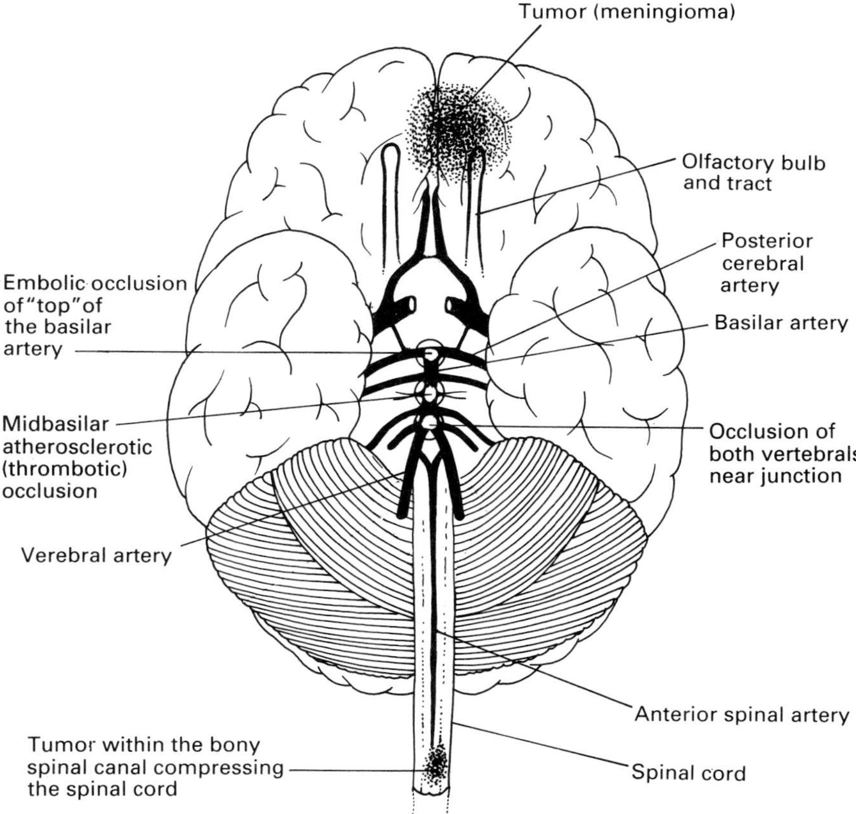

Fig. 14.8 Bilateral symptoms and signs – produced by a single lesion. In this view of the ventral aspect of the brain and upper spinal cord, a tumor (meningioma) is seen anteriorly compressing not only the ipsilateral frontal lobe (and olfactory pathway) but also the contralateral frontal lobe which is adjacent. More typically, parasagittal tumors arise superiorly from the falx. In the spinal column a tumor is placed so as to compress the spinal cord, typically causing bilateral corticospinal and sensory tract dysfunction. In the brainstem, vascular occlusions of the vertebrobasilar system, in the sites shown, are common causes of bilateral brainstem and/or posterior cerebral artery territory symptoms and signs.

5.7g) which connect the nuclei of CN 8 (vestibular) and CNs 6, 4, and 3.

In contrast, most structures of the right and left cerebral hemispheres are separated, but in the following situations medial or midline lesions produce bilateral signs.

In using this rule, the following important modifications and exceptions should be kept in mind.

Midline supratentorial lesions

1 Single lesions of supratentorial midline structures may exert direct or indirect effects, resulting in bilateral signs. A large tumor of the pituitary gland may compress both sides of the optic chiasm. Blockage of the 3rd ventricle (or of the aqueduct or 4th ventricle in the posterior fossa) produces hydrocephalus by preventing CSF egress (see Chapter 13). An acute, obstructive hydrocephalus causes bilateral cerebral dysfunction from the pressure of the paired lateral ventricles upon the two hemispheres; also, downward forces act on the upper brainstem due to the elevated pressure in the supratentorial compartment.

Hydrocephalus

Parasagittal masses

2 Lesions placed at the medial hemispheric surfaces may cause bilateral deficits. The classic example is a meningioma (a histologically benign tumor) arising from the midline dural fold, the falx cerebri. Such a "parasagittal" meningioma can compress the facing cortices of the two hemispheres. Since the leg areas of the somatotopic "homunculus" are represented on the medial surface of the motor and sensory strips, the patient typically presents with bilateral lower extremity symptoms and signs.

Callosal lesions

3 Lesions of hemispheric commissures (bidirectional right–left connecting tracts), such as the corpus callosum, should produce bilateral deficits. Symptomatic cases of this type are uncommon, or uncommonly recognized.

Bilateral vascular distribution

4 Bilateral hemispheric lesions may result from single lesions of the vascular system. The most notable example comes from the posterior circulation in which the basilar artery divides into the two posterior cerebral arteries (that irrigate part of the occipital lobes and other territories, see Chapter 13). Thus, occlusion of the bifurcation of the basilar artery ("top of the basilar") may cause bilateral infarction that includes both the right and left visual cortex, yielding bilateral hemianopsias (cortical blindness).

5 A single mass lesion in the supratentorial compartment can exert effects on the other hemisphere (by subfalcial herniation) and/or on the midbrain and other structures of the tentorial notch. In the syndrome of transtentorial (temporal lobe) herniation (Fig. 13.2), secondary lesions cause the bilaterality.

PROBLEMS FOR SELF-STUDY

The following questions relating to some of the clinical–anatomic constructs are intended to help you to consolidate your understanding of their use.

Questions

1 Long tracts cross. What examples can you cite as exceptions to this generalization?
2 Cerebral dominance. In what instances can the right hemisphere be considered dominant, rather than the left?
3 Somatotopic organization in the nervous system. Why does the homunculus on the cortical primary motor strip look so grotesque?
4 The organization of "higher functions" at a cortical level. In what ways is cortical function dependent on brain activity at lower subcortical and brainstem levels?
5 The extrapyramidal system. How does Parkinson's disease, a model extrapyramidal disorder, differ from a typical "pyramidal" (corticospinal) syndrome, as caused by an infarct in the motor cortex?
6 The cerebellum as a center of coordination. Aside from neuroimaging, how would you go about implicating the cerebellum as the site of a lesion responsible for incoordination of a limb?

Comments

1 Two particular variations on the theme of long tract crossing were encountered in Chapter 5. In the case of facial expression, the upper face (mainly forehead) is under both ipsilateral and contralateral UMN control, i.e. fibers to the part of the CN 7 nucleus that innervates muscles of the upper face. The sternocleidomastoid muscles are presumed to be under the control of UMN fibers that cross twice, or at least some of them do. This enables the right motor cortex to influence the right cervical cord segments that govern the right sternocleidomastoid muscle that turns the head to the left.

   A more general modification of the construct of long tract crossing is exemplified in the motor system by the large number of uncrossed as well as crossed fibers in the descending motor tracts in the spinal cord, especially those of the "ventromedial system" that controls axial and more proximal musculature relating to posture and truncal movements, etc.
2 As described in Chapter 13, dominance should be considered in regard to specific functions; many aspects of attention, spatial relations, nonverbal aspects of speech, etc. are lateralized to the right hemisphere in left speech-dominant individuals. In some left-handers, the right hemisphere is dominant for speech.
3 Cortical somatotopic representation is not mapped to scale, as the amount of cortical area allotted to a given part is related to its function – how much fine, fractionated motor control is needed, for example. Hence the "big mouth." Increasing evidence indicates that there are multiple somatotopic representations in the brain.
4 While most "higher functions" may be centered in cortical areas, cognition is dependent upon a waking level of consciousness and alertness (or so we tend to assume). The brainstem and diencephalic reticular formations are essential for cerebral activation. In addition (to scratch just the surface of this subject), subcortical gray matter nuclei

of the basal ganglia, for example, are intimately connected with the cortex and play roles in cognition and behavior, not just motor function. Diffuse neuromodulatory chemical projections from the brainstem and basal cerebral nuclei also influence functions that we think of as "higher cortical."

5 Although Parkinson's disease contains the word "paralysis" in its other name, "paralysis agitans," the problem of movement is not one of weakness, as we usually think of it in terms of objective loss of power on resistive testing. Impairment of fine, fractionated motor control is the hallmark of corticospinal deficits, (within the larger UMN syndrome), whereas the parkinsonian patient displays combinations of akinesia, tremor, and rigidity. Work on the role of the supplementary motor cortex, as an example, is helping to clarify knowledge of the initiation of movements, a matter relevant to both pyramidal and extrapyramidal disorders.

6 In attempting to localize the source of incoordination, it is essential to exclude all other known mechanisms (such as weakness, spasticity, proprioceptive loss, etc.), before concluding that the dysfunction is probably in the cerebellum or its direct connections. By pattern recognition, certain signs, such as intention tremor, are very suggestive of cerebellar involvement, but should not be taken as absolute. If a lesion in the cerebellum is depicted by neuroimaging, it should be ipsilateral to the ataxic limb because of the "double cross": first, the cerebellar outflow and second, the corticospinal pathway (see Fig. 13.18).

FURTHER READING

Damasio, A.R. Aphasia. *N Engl J Med* 1992; 326:531–9. Traditional views of language localization are revised within the context of distributed neural networks with localized components. Although language has long been classified as a cortical function, the roles of basal ganglionic and thalamic nuclei are being clarified.

Davidoff, R.A. The pyramidal tract. *Neurology* 1990; 40:332–9. Scholarly and accessible review of the anatomy of the pyramidal tract with discussion of modern revisions of corticospinal function.

Davidoff, R.A. The dorsal columns. *Neurology* 1989; 39:1377–85. Present-day evidence regarding the anatomy underlying the clinical concept of the dorsal column sensory system.

Geschwind, N., Galaburda, A.M. *Cerebral Lateralization*. Massachusetts Institute of Technology Press, Cambridge (MA), 1987. Essays on hemispheric specialization.

Landau, W.M. Clinical neuromythology V. Ataxic hindbrain thinking: the clumsy cerebellum syndrome. *Neurology* 1989; 39:315–23. Challenges common concepts of "cerebellar" signs.

Phillips, C.G., Landau, W.M. Upper and lower motor neuron: the little old synecdoche that works. Clinical neuromythology VIII. *Neurology* 1990; 40:884–6. Brief review of Gowers' still-useful insight into the "upper and lower motor" neuronal organization.

chapter 15

An Introduction to Neuroimaging and Laboratory Testing

The process of formulating a neurologic diagnosis has thus far utilized clinical skills that are physically noninvasive. History and examination findings have enabled systematic analysis of the following:

1 localization of the lesion;
2 pathology – type of tissue change;
3 pathogenesis – mechanism of pathologic change;
4 etiology – root cause of the disorder.

Each of these aspects of formulation depends to a different extent on the kinds of data available from the history and clinical examination (see Table 1.1 and Chapter 12). Technologic examinations also contribute to each category of the formulation. Neuroimaging by computerized tomography (CT) scan or magnetic resonance imaging (MRI) definitively establishes the localization of many lesions, but typically provides only inferential evidence regarding specific types of pathologic change and how they came about.

Localization

As an example of the inferential role of imaging with respect to pathology, a low-density lesion with mild mass effect on a CT scan could be a quite recent infarction, tumor, or an inflammatory lesion. Further

Pathology

testing and analysis would establish probabilities, but would not be definitive. Similarly, very small hemorrhages cannot always be differentiated from calcifications on a single CT scan. Thus, in some instances the neuroimage simply defines the physical characteristics of the lesion and the surrounding brain while leaving the pathologic diagnosis ambiguous.

Pathogenesis

"Ancillary" (laboratory and radiologic) tests can also provide information pertinent to the pathogenesis of a lesion, although this aspect of the diagnosis is also inferential. For example, in a case of ischemic stroke a small, discrete, cortical abnormality on a CT scan suggests that the pathogenesis of the infarction is very likely to be embolic. This represents an interpretation, based on the knowledge that focal cortical infarcts almost always result from occlusion of small, distal, arterial branches. Since atherosclerosis and other intrinsic diseases of these branches are rare, the most likely mechanism would be embolic occlusion. A similar process of deduction would follow the detection by CT scan of high-density material (blood) pooled in the subarachnoid spaces, especially around the Circle of Willis and in the Sylvian fissures. This information would suggest that the mechanism of the subarachnoid hemorrhage was probably a ruptured berry aneurysm of or near the Circle of Willis, because of the localization of the accumulated blood.

Etiology

In some instances, knowledge of pathology and pathogenesis provides a link to the etiology, or root cause. For example, cerebrospinal fluid (CSF) containing increased white cells signifies an inflammatory pathologic process. Knowing that infection might be the mechanism of inflammation, a Gram-stained smear is examined, revealing Gram-positive cocci. To identify the exact etiologic agent, the CSF is cultured and grows out pneumococci (*Streptococcus pneumoniae*). These data might also suggest certain etiologic host factors.

If neuroimaging (or other laboratory investigations) reveal or confirm the correct formulation, then should we bother with clinical analysis at all? Why not just order the test?

Guiding test selection

Test ordering requires that you specify: (a) the kind of test (e.g. MRI vs. electrophysiologic nerve conduction studies); (b) the part of the nervous system to be tested (e.g. an MRI of the head vs. spine); and (c) when to do the test (e.g. an immediate CT scan to detect hemorrhage or a delayed scan to visualize an area of infarct necrosis)?

Cross-correlation

Clinical analysis of symptoms and signs enables a preliminary formulation that will guide the choice and sequence of tests to be ordered and help establish their degree of urgency. In addition, just as imaging and other tests can serve to validate the initial formulation, that formulation provides a check on the correlation and significance of abnormal test results – which may not be relevant to the clinical problem.

Two languages

The language of testing should be distinguished from the language of pathology. A good report on a CT scan should state as fact the descriptive characteristics of a high-density (high-attenuation) lesion and then may add the interpretation that this is probably a tumor (for particular specified reasons). Loose use of pathologic terms (e.g. atrophy) to characterize imaged abnormalities (e.g. increased CSF spaces) can lead to misunderstandings. For example, increased ventricular or sulcal size might reflect a developmental problem rather than a degenerative process, as the term atrophy implies.

Skills of neurologic testing

The following sections will be process-oriented and problem-oriented: (a) how to orient yourself with regard to the use of selected neuroimages, laboratory tests, and procedures; and (b) which groups of tests are appropriate to assess particular clinical hypotheses. The two most active skills you will develop will receive special attention: performing lumbar punctures for CSF sampling, and participating in the interpretation of neuroimages. Hints for managing two types of blood tests, anticonvulsant levels and measures of anticoagulation are also offered.

GLOSSARY OF PRINCIPAL CENTRAL NERVOUS SYSTEM IMAGING TESTS

Computerized tomography (CT, CAT): based upon degree of attenuation of X-rays by tissues of varying densities; intravenous iodinated contrast agent enhances areas with increased vascularity, or impaired blood–brain barrier.

Magnetic resonance imaging (MRI): generation of signals depends upon interaction of nuclear particles with a powerful magnetic field (nuclear magnetic resonance). Present uses emphasize structural imaging, but newer rapid magnetic resonance techniques are increasingly able to provide physiologic information, such as changes in blood volume and flow with functional activities.

Positron emission tomography (PET): positron emission from an injected radionuclide is incorporated into metabolically active compounds and permits physiologic mapping.

Single photon emission computed tomography (SPECT): utilizes gamma emitting radionuclides for physiologic mapping; less cumbersome than PET, but generally less sensitive.

Arteriography (arterial dye injection by catheter): conventional invasive arteriography delineates the arterial and venous vascular systems, showing areas of increased and decreased vascularity, displacement of vessels by masses, occlusions, malformations, and aneurysms; also, limited data on dynamics, e.g. circulation time of injected dye, reversals of flow, etc; the digital subtraction angiographic (DSA) technique can augment clarity and decreases invasive risk factors.

Magnetic resonance angiography (MRA): noninvasive magnetic resonance angiographic techniques are rapidly advancing, supplanting invasive diagnostic arteriography for many purposes; the blood columns are depicted by the effect of flow on signal generation.

Myelography: injection of radioopaque dye into the spinal fluid to delineate abnormalities impinging on the subarachnoid space; use has declined, but is still necessary in certain spinal emergencies when MRI is not available; risks include complications of spinal tap, radiation, and rare dye reactions.

Cranial Doppler: images large vessels; excellent selective imaging in infant with open fontanelle.

X-rays (plain): still used to help screen for or define lesions of bone, but supplanted by CT in cranial diagnosis.

Bone scan: radionuclide bone scanning is helpful in screening skull and spine for metastases, infection, and other inflammatory or metabolically active processes that might impinge on the meninges, nerve roots, or central nervous system (CNS).

AN APPROACH TO INTERPRETING CT AND MR IMAGES

Orienting to CT

To identify a scan as a CT, learn to recognize visual characteristics, as well as the label on the envelope or the film itself: CT scans are usually oriented in a quasi-horizontal plane of section (Fig. 15.1). Almost every CT section contains a thick white oval ring representing the full thickness of the skull around the brain's circumference (the appearance of the bony skull is much less striking on MRI scans). If you see the frontal horns, bodies, or occipital horns of the lateral ventricles in a single section or adjacent sections, you will know the plane is horizontal. Similarly, if you see both eyeballs in the same section as parts of the temporal lobes and cerebellum, the plane is horizontal. As you become more familiar with looking at CT scans compared with MRI scans you will recognize the far greater detail of brain structure in the latter.

Light–dark scale

Since the CT scan depends upon X-ray attenuation, which is a function of tissue density, bone appears white – its high density blocks the X-rays from darkening the film. Since all scans include bone and all cranial scans include the CSF-filled ventricles, you can always take advantage of this built-in range: bone light, water dark. Therefore, you will be able to find the white of bony landmarks such as the sella turcica (where the pituitary gland sits) and the petrous pyramids which separate the posterior fossa (brainstem and cerebellum) from the middle cranial fossae (temporal lobes). At the other end of the scale, you will be able to delineate black areas representing not only the ventricles but the subarachnoid spaces. In between these extremes of bone and water will be the shades of gray of the various types of brain substance and of many pathologic tissues. The one type of lesion that stands out most strikingly

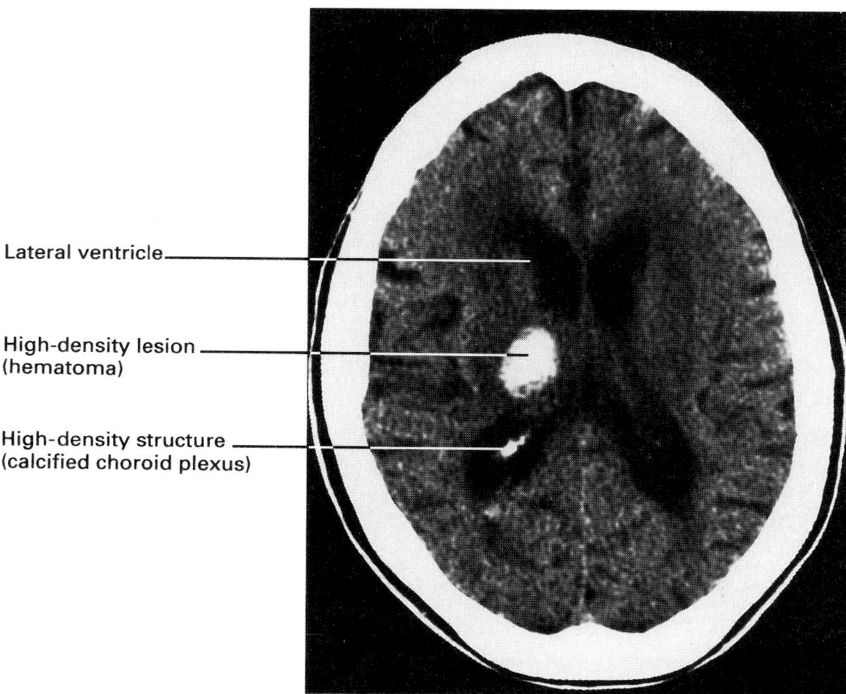

Fig. 15.1 Computerized tomography scan, noncontrast, in the usual near-horizontal (axial) plane. Note the very white (high-density) appearance of the skull (outer and inner tables not differentiated). In contrast, the low-density cerebrospinal fluid in the lateral ventricles appears black. A high-density (white) lesion, consistent with hematoma (hemorrhage), is seen in the right hemisphere in this scan obtained several hours after the clinical onset of stroke symptoms. (Courtesy of Jonathan Kleefield MD.)

is acute intracranial hematoma which shines "like a lightbulb," since the density of the iron-containing hemoglobin complexes in the clotted blood is so high (see Fig. 15.1). (Interestingly, unclotted, intravascular blood is close enough to water density that it does not "light up" without dye enhancement.)

Contrast enhancement

The infusion of iodinated contrast dye enhances the density of intravascular blood, making it appear lighter than surrounding soft tissues. However, CT resolution only enables identification of large arteries, veins, and venous sinuses. (To test your ability to recognize a contrast-enhanced or C+ scan, look at sections near the base of the brain, at which level you should be able to see at least parts of the Circle of Willis.) Compare these sections ("cuts") of a C+ scan with comparable cuts of a C− (plain, nonenhanced) scan. As will be discussed subsequently, more diffuse enhancement also occurs in lesions with increased vascularity, or a faulty blood–brain barrier which permits dye accumulation in the diseased tissues. Take care to differentiate lesions that appear light due to high density (such as calcifications and fresh hematomas), independent of contrast dye infusion. Some areas within tumors may be of relatively high density, but enhance to an even lighter appearance with the addition of dye. The effect of contrast dye is best demonstrated by first performing a C− scan, followed by a C+ scan.

CT vs. MRI

The main limitations of CT scanning of the brain are: (a) inferior resolution and visualization of subtler types of brain pathology; (b) inability to detect brain infarction acutely because of lack of tissue density changes; and (c) relatively poor imaging in the posterior fossa and the pituitary fossa because of artefact from bone, inferior resolution, and only "horizontal" sections readily available.

Orienting to MRI

By comparison with CT, orientation to MRI is more complex, because techniques and planes are more varied, but more informative. You will grow accustomed to seeing coronal sections, but often horizontal and sagittal images will be displayed as well, each supplementing the others with respect to effective delineation of some feature. The next important distinction is between T1- and T2-weighted images. The simplest key is that in T1 images water (CSF) appears dark; in T2 images the CSF spaces and eyeballs appear bright. However, you cannot extrapolate a fluid to bone scale as you can with CT. The signal generation depends on factors that are not intuitively obvious. In general, T1 images may offer some advantages in depicting anatomic detail, whereas many lesions are often better shown on T2. In particular, inflammatory and neoplastic lesions, in which there is increased water content, will be more evident on T2 images. A paramagnetic compound, gadolinium, is currently the substance approved for infusion to highlight lesions with an impaired blood–brain barrier.

Images and communication

It is becoming as important for physicians to participate actively in reading neuroimages as it is now for internists to look at the chest films of their patients. In part, this will keep physicians in close contact with the reality of their patients' status, rather than becoming distanced by the interface of verbal reports that often do not capture the entire sense of the image. Even if computerized reproductions of key images should become routine parts of the patient's record, the physician will still need a habit of informed review. Perhaps the more compelling reason for physicians to become "reader friendly" with neuroimages is to improve communication with the radiologist, neurologist, or neurosurgeon who is providing the definitive interpretation. The clinical information typically provided on requisitions simply does not do justice to the challenge of making the greatest clinical use of the extraordinary data available on these images. As noted previously, the wealth of information on neuroimages has greatly magnified the problem of "retrodiagnosis" – the correlation back from imaged abnormalities to the relevant clinical events or findings. Success in this process often depends upon close consultation between clinician and imaging specialist.

Table 15.1 Principal vascular tests

Component of circulatory system	Noninvasive (or minimally invasive)	Invasive
Intracerebral circulation: medium to small vessels – occlusions and malformations	Magnetic resonance techniques for smaller vessels in development; contrast CT, MRI, or MRA for vascular malformations	Arteriography (pressure injection of dye through catheter via femoral artery); best visualization by "selective" catheterization of specific neck vessel
Intracranial trunk vessels: large arteries, Circle of Willis – stenoses, occlusions, aneurysms	MRA (depicts blood in major vessels); transcranial Doppler (adaptation of Doppler technique, see below)	Arteriography (catheter injection into aortic arch or selectively into neck vessels – common or internal carotids, subclavians, vertebrals)
Neck (and chest) vessels (carotid, vertebral, subclavian arteries, etc. – stenoses, occlusions, kinks, dissections, plaques)	"Noninvasive carotid battery"; ultrasound/ Doppler (images lumen and provides flow data); MRA (as above)	Arteriography (aortic or major branch injection); DSA (can clarify images obtained with lower dye concentrations)
Cardiac assessment for source of cerebral emboli	Echo (ultrasound) (for cardiac chamber, walls, valves, clots); EKG; 24 hour EKG (Holter monitor)	Cardiac catheterization (rarely required) for right to left shunts

CT, computerized tomography; DSA, digital subtraction angiography; EKG, electrocardiogram; MRA, magnetic resonance angiography; MRI, magnetic resonance imaging.

VASCULAR IMAGING AND FLOW ANALYSIS

As summarized in Table 15.1, a variety of noninvasive and invasive techniques are available to assess the vascular system for stenoses, occlusions, malformations, aneurysms, and other changes. The advent of MRI technology has offered hope that all of the common vascular questions that arise in clinical practice may be answered by using MRA (Fig. 15.2) or other MRI techniques at a single sitting. At the present time, however, contrast CT and invasive catheter angiography retain diagnostic usefulness. Not yet mentioned are the so-called "carotid noninvasive tests" which collectively provide data on patency and flow in the carotid arteries in the neck. The battery employed in different laboratories varies, but usually includes ultrasound/Doppler techniques for imaging the carotid lumen and analyzing flow characteristics. These techniques are quite sensitive in the detection of plaques and disruption of flow in the carotid arteries, but are not specific as to the pathology. Complete

Carotid noninvasive tests

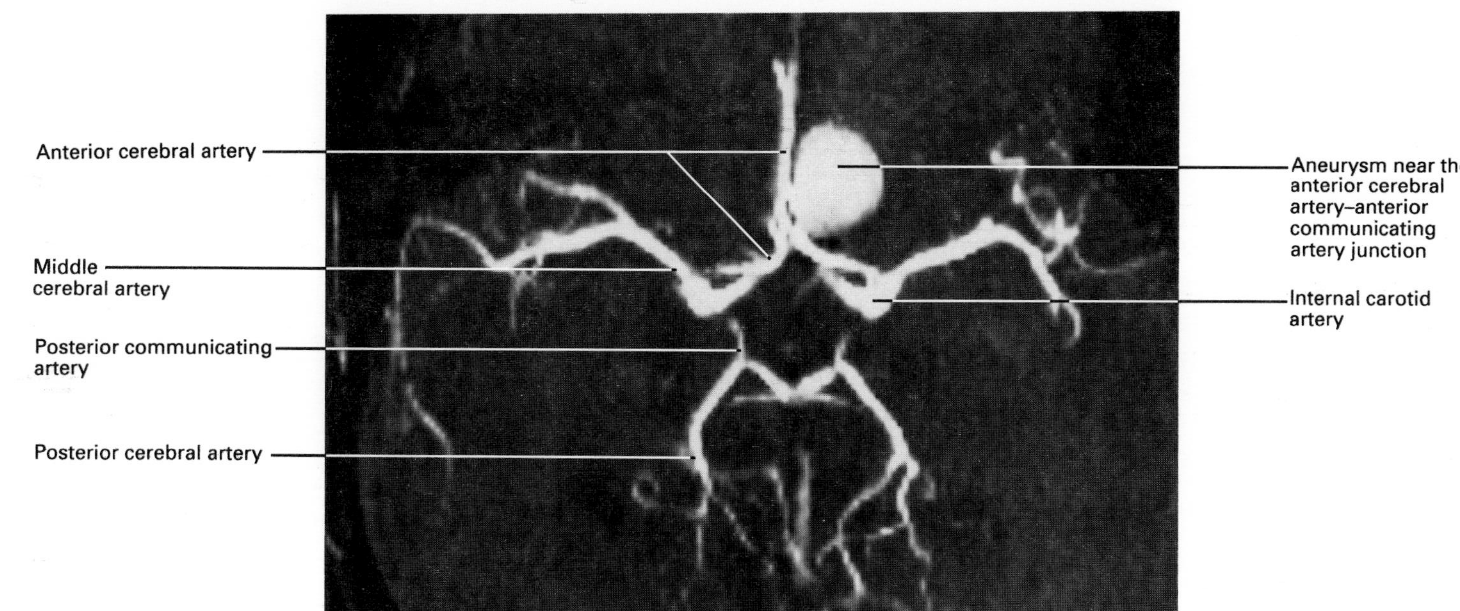

Fig. 15.2 Magnetic resonance angiogram (MRA) of the Circle of Willis. The MRA noninvasively reveals a very large unruptured aneurysm near the anterior communicating artery. As in Fig. 4.1, the intravascular blood appears white because of the technique of imaging (not because of dye, as in a conventional angiogram). (Courtesy of Jonathan Kleefield MD.)

occlusion cannot always be reliably distinguished from very high-grade stenosis (a matter of great import for treatment). Transcranial Doppler techniques have been developed to provide some information noninvasively on large intracranial arteries, but MRA is proving superior.

EVALUATION OF SUSPECTED BRAIN LESIONS

CT and MRI scans dominate the field of brain and spinal cord neurodiagnostic tests (Table 15.2). It is unclear how long CT scanning will persist in use, given the remarkable resolution and burgeoning capabilities that MRI has shown, even in the infancy of the technology. As of this writing, however, CT still represents the more accessible, hospital-based method, at least outside of major medical centers. For emergency brain problems presenting to hospital emergency departments, CT remains a valuable avenue of laboratory investigation. Moreover, CT excels at depicting many of the lesions you will need to identify promptly: intracerebral and intracerebellar hemorrhage, acute epidural and subdural hematoma, hydrocephalus, mass effect and shifts from intracranial space-occupying lesions, and major subarachnoid hemorrhage. Thus, in case of suspected stroke, an emergency CT is often ordered to rule out hemorrhage, but then must be repeated in 2–10 days to visualize infarction. Looking for hemorrhage or mass effects requires only a noncontrast scan that can be completed in minutes. The rapidity of scanning minimizes the effects of head motion of the uncooperative patient, although sedation is sometimes required, nonetheless. In the critically ill patient, clinical monitoring and management of airway, intravenous and intraarterial lines, etc., benefit from relatively easy access to the patient. Finally, patients with cardiac pacemakers or with metal fragments, etc., in the brain, eyes, or elsewhere can be safely scanned, although metal objects may create artefacts.

CT scanning

CT scanning with contrast dye enhancement improves the delineation of areas of hypervascularity and an impaired blood–brain barrier (Fig. 15.3). This serves to highlight most tumors, inflammatory lesions, and hypervascular areas, such as the margins of infarcts. Arteriovenous malformations are well shown. Although parts of the Circle of Willis can be seen on contrast-enhanced (C+) CT scans, only giant aneurysms tend to be visualized, so that MRA or conventional invasive angiography are needed to depict most berry aneurysms. Use of contrast dye carries allergic risk and may provoke renal failure in patients with renal disease and dehydration.

Enhancing lesions

Pathologic changes that are often readily identified on MRI, but less well on CT scans (even with contrast) include plaques of multiple sclerosis, other inflammatory lesions, and various tissue changes seen in brain involvement by AIDS. Although CT scans usually identify at least early signs of major infarction within 24–48 hours, a better topographic

MRI

Table 15.2 General uses of most common neurodiagnostic tests

Part of the nervous system	Localization (where is it?)	Pathologic inference (what is it?)
Central nervous system: brain	MRI (definitive, high resolution); CT (definitive, lower sensitivity); (EEG: cortical localization, see text)	MRI informative, improving; CT not as good as MRI, except for hemorrhage
Intracranial vessels	Localization of vascular occlusion; arteriography, MRA, transcranial Doppler (see Table 15.1; MRA improving for depicting aneurysms)	CT (C+), MRI for AVM; MRA, arteriography for aneurysm, artheritis
Spinal cord (and spinal canal)	MRI (best for most purposes); CT (should know approximate segmental level of lesion to guide CT examination); myelography (defines subarachnoid space)	MRI (as above); CT (C−, C+) less sensitive for cord pathology; quite good for thoracic and lumbar discs CSF for inflammation and specific infection (see Table 15.3)
Peripheral nerve trunks and branches, muscles	NCV (focal abnormality of specific nerves): polyneuropathic pattern (diffuse disease); EMG (specific muscle localization vs. diffuse involvement); MRI (developing as a valuable tool for detecting gross, structural lesions)	NCV (axonal vs. primary demyelinating pathologies); EMG (primary myopathy vs. neurogenic atrophy); MRI (developing use for gross lesions, e.g. tumors).
Peripheral nervous system: roots	NCV ("H" and "F" late responses); EMG of paraspinal and limb muscles innervated by a particular root; MRI and CT can image root compression	EMG (denervation pattern indicates axonal pathology); NCV (late responses sensitive to demyelination); CSF (inflammation, neoplasm, etc. of intraspinal roots)

AVM, arteriovenous malformation; C+, contrast-enhanced CT; CSF, cerebrospinal fluid; CT, computerized tomography; EEG, electroencephalography; EMG, electromyography; MRA, magnetic resonance angiography; MRI, magnetic resonance imaging; NCV, nerve conduction velocity.

picture is presented by MRI (Fig. 15.4). Areas of infarction are also seen sooner by MRI. With new and rapid MRI techniques it will undoubtedly be possible to witness infarcts developing acutely.

The present-day advantages of MRI of the brain can be summarized

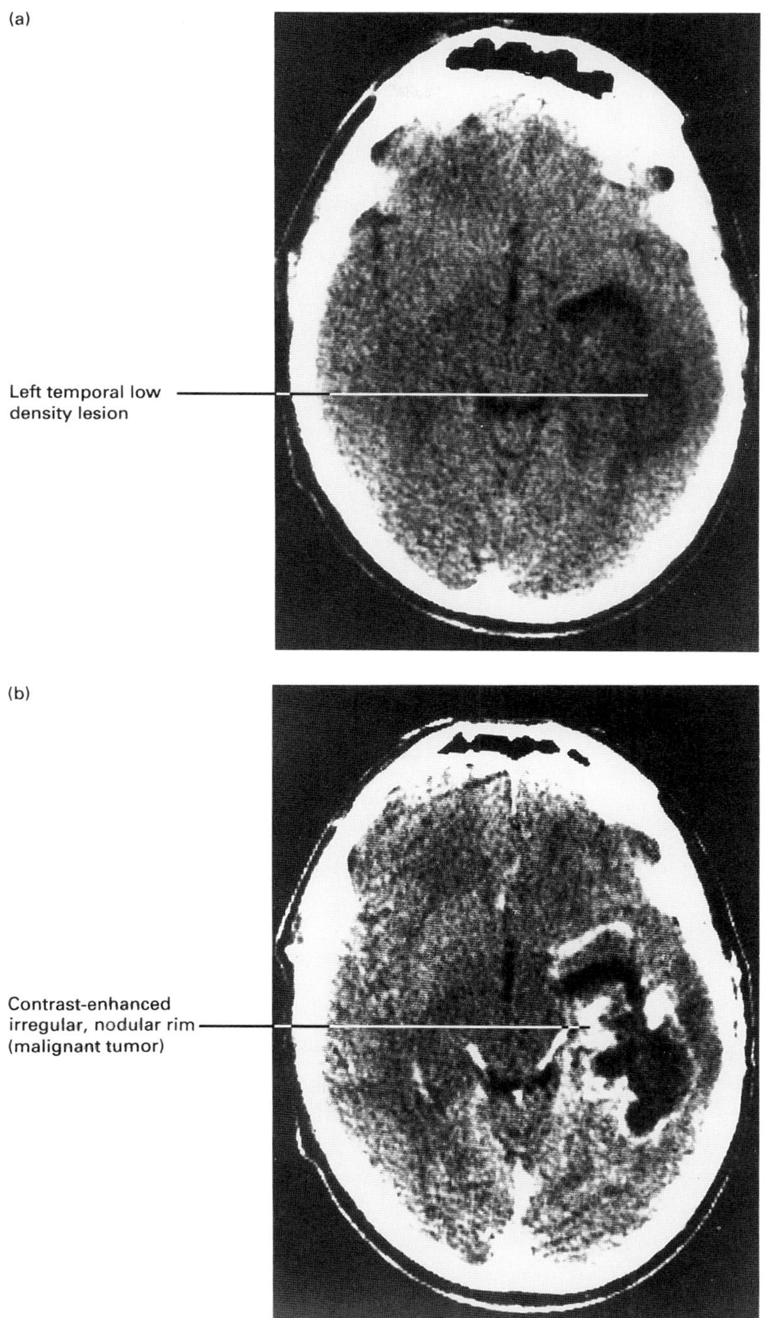

Fig. 15.3 Computerized tomography scans, noncontrast and contrast-enhanced. (a) A highly malignant primary brain tumor (glioblastoma) shows low-density (dark) areas due to central necrosis and edema. (b) The rim shows irregular, nodular enhancement (increased density or whiteness) on the contrast scan, resulting from increased tumor vascularity and alteration of the blood–brain barrier. (Courtesy of Jonathan Kleefield MD.)

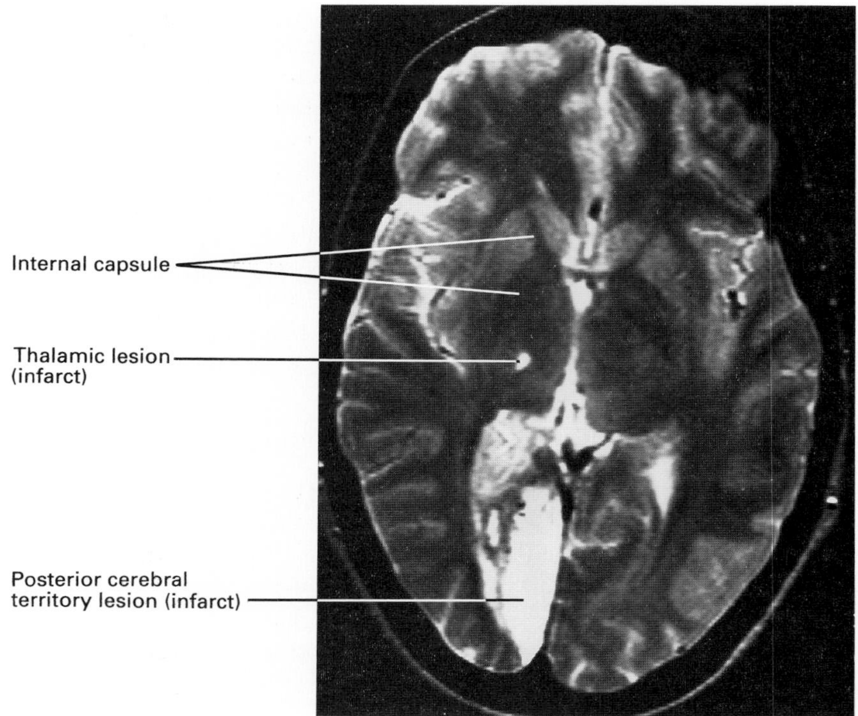

Fig. 15.4 Magnetic resonance image in axial (near-horizontal) plane. Note the detail of brain structure, compared with computerized tomography. In this T2-weighted image, an abnormal, high-intensity signal (white) is seen in the right medial occipital lobe (posterior cerebral artery territory) consistent with an infarct (see Case 5A). There is also a small lesion in the right thalamus, consistent with a lacunar infarct. (Courtesy of Jonathan Kleefield MD.)

as follows: (a) extraordinary resolution of structural detail, which is especially valuable clinically in delineating small lesions, posterior fossa lesions, tumors of pituitary, and lesions of cranial nerves; (b) earlier recognition and more complete characterization of infarction; (c) better detection of some types of pathology, such as multiple sclerosis (MS) plaques; (d) further improvement in depiction of lesions with an altered blood–brain barrier upon intravenous injection of the paramagnetic compound, gadolinium; (e) the opportunity to do serial studies without X-irradiation risk; (f) with the development of rapid and augmented magnetic resonance techniques, the capacity to assess physiologic as well as static abnormalities; currently, small percentage changes in blood oxygenation, volume, and flow can be detected in a given region and correlated with functional activation; (g) a growing capability of MRA to visualize intravascular obstruction intracranially, as well as extracranially, and to detect berry aneurysms noninvasively.

MRI limitations

Current disadvantages of MRI include longer scanning times on many machines, greater expense, and limited availability in many regions. As noted earlier, MRI is not presently available to patients with cardiac pacemakers and with metal in the body that might be moved by the magnetic field. Patients with claustrophobia, usually in the context of a panic disorder, tolerate poorly the confined space of present MRI scanners. These problems will largely disappear due to improved scanner design. Finally, the subtle or long-term effects of powerful magnetic fields on the human body remain uncertain, although there are no present indications of adverse effects of MRI scanning. Caution is advised in pregnancy, although no detrimental consequences have yet been confirmed.

SOME CLINICAL–PHYSIOLOGIC TESTS OF THE CNS

Electroencephalography

Electroencephalographic scalp electrodes record cortical electrical activity, providing a topographic display of normal and abnormal potential changes over time. Various computer-assisted techniques can enhance this electrical profile.

Magnetic stimulation of the nervous system

Magnetic stimulation of the cortex (or spinal cord and roots) is a developing technique used to assess neural pathways. Cortical stimulation can activate limb movement without depending on patient cooperation. Central motor conduction is accessible for study, comparable to central sensory evaluation by measurement of evoked responses. Magnetic stimulation should not be confused with magnetoencephalography, a developing method of magnetic field recording for physiologic cortical mapping.

Evoked potentials/evoked responses

External visual, auditory, or somatosensory stimuli evoke potentials in way-station nuclei or specific receptive cortical areas; these potentials are recorded from surface electrodes and computer processed. The three standard types of evoked potentials are: visual evoked responses (VER), brainstem auditory evoked responses (BAER), and somatosensory evoked responses (SER). These techniques provide a profile of conduction times along these sensory pathways; delayed or absent responses indicate lesions that are nonspecific pathologically. The procedures involved are noninvasive and not uncomfortable. (See Further reading section at the end of the chapter.)

CSF flow studies (radionuclide cisternography)

In the evaluation of communicating hydrocephalus the flow pattern of isotope injected into the CSF can be studied to assess the patency and dynamics of CSF pathways. The use of this test has declined, and its value in diagnosing treatable normal pressure hydrocephalus (NPH) is controversial.

Vestibular tests

Laboratory assessment of the vestibular system (especially for vertigo) may include electronystagmography (ENG), often combined with caloric testing as well as other techniques. ENG is a way of recording ocular movements, such as nystagmus, by means of surface electrodes. In caloric testing the inner ears are stimulated by irrigation of the external ear canals and tympanic membrane with water at different standardized temperatures. This causes vertigo (and nystagmus) that is uncomfortable but not dangerous. The object is to assess the responsiveness of the labyrinths and the function of their CN 8 connections with the brainstem vestibular–ocular systems.

Audiometry

Audiometry assesses hearing capability (rather than physiologic mechanisms) and is totally risk-free and without discomfort. It includes simple pure-tone hearing acuity at a range of frequencies, as well as other tests of auditory function, according to the indication for testing.

Formal visual fields

Testing of formal visual fields is also simply a technologic elaboration of "bedside" testing. It provides improved accuracy and sensitivity of visual field assessment, when performed by trained personnel. The light stimulus can be varied in intensity, wavelength, size, position, and motion to evaluate central and peripheral fields.

ELECTROENCEPHALOGRAPHY (EEG)

Summary of indications

Scalp recording of the electric potentials from the cerebral cortex can provide valuable and unique information, not available from structural imaging. In routine practice, two uses dominate: detection of (a) paroxysmal discharges that underlie clinical epileptic seizures; and (b) diffuse background slowing which is the hallmark of many toxic–metabolic and some degenerative disorders and inflammatory processes. In addition, other accepted uses include localizing discrete cerebral lesions by means of focal slowing or other changes (an indication largely outmoded by imaging); recognition of a small number of particular diseases and syndromes characterized by telltale EEG patterns; and finally, special situations, such as brain death determination and monitoring of cortical activity during operations on the carotid artery (endarterectomy).

EEG terminology

The field of EEG testing is filled with unnecessary mystique. Nonneurologic clinicians are frustrated by the language of EEG interpretation and reporting. The Greek letter designations for different wave frequencies (δ, θ, α, β – from slow to fast) epitomize this communication gap. What you need to know, and what a good report summarizes in plain language, is the following:

1 whether the record is technically inadequate for any reason, such as patient's medications;
2 the occurrence of paroxysmal activity;
3 significant general background slowing;
4 the presence of focal abnormalities, either slowing or paroxysmal activity;
5 distinctive patterns that characterize particular diseases or syndromes.

Frequency of potential changes, as measured in Hz, is a key parameter and generally much more important than amplitude (Fig. 15.5).

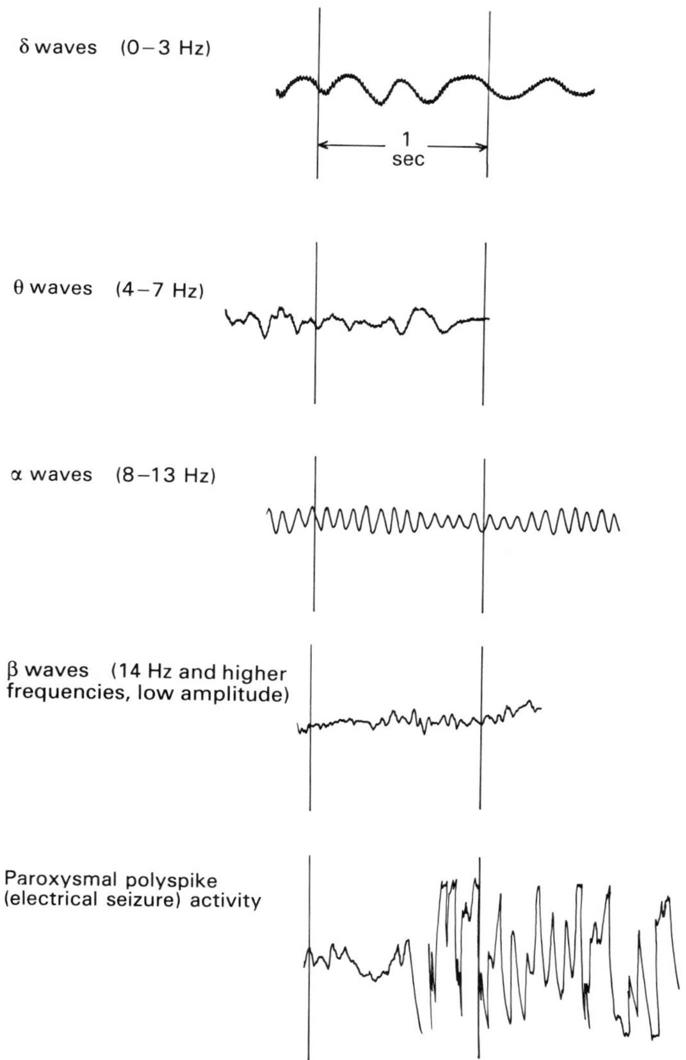

Fig. 15.5 EEG frequencies. Note the frequency ranges, from slow (low frequency) to fast (high frequency): δ 0–3 Hz (cycles per second); θ 4–7 Hz; α 8–13 Hz; β 14 Hz and higher, low-voltage activity. β activity predominates frontally in the alert state; α dominates posteriorly with eyes closed and the mind at ease. Small amounts of scattered θ slow activity may be seen normally in the waking state. Greater prominence of θ and δ slow-wave activity are abnormal awake, but normal in sleep.

Spikes, a prime manifestation of electrical seizure activity, are a type of high-frequency discharge; slow waves are obviously low-frequency. If abnormal frequencies, especially spikes, emerge episodically out of a more stable background – like a lightning storm on a calm day – then paroxysmal activity is present. Paroxysmal discharges carry great weight in the diagnosis of a seizure disorder, but cannot stand alone. Clinical correlation is essential. (The diagnosis of an epileptic seizure disorder cannot be made by imaging techniques, although the underlying lesion that gives rise to an epileptogenic focus can be detected and characterized.)

Sleep study

The usual indication for a "sleep study" is suspicion of a seizure disorder. (A sleep study also includes a waking record.) Sleep is restricted on the night before the EEG test, the degree of deprivation varying according to the protocol of different laboratories. Although commonly ordered for the purpose of enhancing the yield of paroxysmal activity, research has not produced convincing evidence of the efficacy of ordinary sleep studies. Two factors are involved: (a) the state of sleep deprivation as an activating condition; and (b) the state of sleep during the EEG.

To be consistently effective, a far greater degree of sleep deprivation is necessary than the 3–12 hour reduction of a night's sleep that most EEG laboratories request. Thus, although sleep deprivation of profound degree may "activate" clinical seizures and paroxysmal discharges on the EEG, the requisite conditions are not ordinarily achieved. The state of sleep itself is induced more easily if the patient is tired from reduced sleep the night before. Since some patients have seizures only in sleep or in drowsy states, it makes sense to reproduce these conditions favoring increased paroxysms during EEG recording. However, the degree of improved yield and benefit in relationship to cost remains unclear.

Increased slowing normally occurs in sleep. Thus, when the main objective is to detect slowing of general background activity, the patient should be fully awake and should not have been sleep deprived.

Hyperventilation and strobe

Hyperventilation is an activation procedure that may elicit abnormal patterns of slowing or paroxysmal responses, especially in the case of petit mal (3/second spike-wave) epilepsy. Stroboscopic (photic) stimulation – flashing lights at various frequencies – may induce a paroxysmal response or even actual clinical seizure activity in patients vulnerable to activation at particular frequencies. Blue- or green-tinted lenses will diminish or eliminate most photoparoxysmal activity.

Seizure diagnosis

Diagnosis of a seizure disorder depends on a history and preferably observation of convulsive episodes (motor seizures with loss of consciousness) or other episodic motor, sensory or behavioral events. Nonetheless, the identification of a paroxysmal EEG abnormality provides important diagnostic support and may help to categorize the disorder in a way that is valuable for choice of therapeutic agent. For difficult cases of suspected complex partial seizures, nasopharyngeal (NP) electrodes (passed through the nostrils) are used to detect and clarify discharges emanating from the medial temporal lobes and adjacent areas.

Episodic "blackouts"

An EEG is commonly ordered to help differentiate episodes of loss of consciousness or body posture. Some such "sinkers" may be of epileptic origin. As noted, even the discovery of paroxysmal activity should always be evaluated in clinical context. We treat the patient, not the EEG. Because of reduced diagnostic sensitivity, due to limited time sampling of a standard sleep EEG, prolonged 24 hour or overnight continuous EEG monitoring (like Holter electrocardiogram monitoring) is sometimes indicated. This can be done on an ambulatory basis or, if professional observation and concurrent videotaping are desired for behavioral correlation, the patient can spend prolonged time in an EEG/ sleep laboratory.

Medications

Anticonvulsant medications should not be stopped because of a planned EEG. Abrupt discontinuation can provoke seizures or even status epilepticus (continuous or frequent seizures without regaining consciousness). On the other hand, a clinical decision to taper off an anticonvulsant drug may entail an EEG test to determine the occurrence of paroxysmal activity without medication. While the EEG is a useful adjunct, the presence or absence of any paroxysmal activity does not strongly predict whether seizures will resume without medication. Anticonvulsant drugs, whether they act on the focus itself or work to prevent spread of seizure discharges, do not routinely normalize an EEG. Therefore, EEGs performed while the patient is on medication still retain substantial value for diagnosis of paroxysmal discharges and for localization of a seizure focus. Other drugs, especially psychoactive medications, such as anxiolytics and antipsychotics, typically increase the amount of fast-frequency activity in the background record. If these drugs are clinically necessary, they should not be stopped before an EEG and their effects will not, as a rule, prevent essential EEG information from being obtained.

Generalized slowing

When a patient shows mental and behavioral changes, and neuroimaging is noncontributory, EEG serves to detect diffuse cortical dysfunction, especially that produced by toxic–metabolic derangements that may have been missed on initial blood or urine tests. Thus, finding diffuse EEG slowing in this context would send the clinician "back to the drawing board" to look again for metabolic disorders, as well as widespread cortical disease processes not evident on MRI or CT scanning. With the availability of CT and MRI, the relative value of EEG for detection of tumors and other focal abnormalities has receded dramatically.

Summary

Finally, some generalizations and guidelines about the use of EEG are as follows.

1 The main reasons for ordering an EEG are clinical suspicion of a convulsive disorder; history of episodic nonconvulsive alterations in consciousness or behavior; suspicion of a toxic–metabolic or other diffuse cerebral disorder.

2 A sleep study is commonly recommended if a seizure disorder is suspected (although the cost/benefit ratio is uncertain).

3 Do not stop anticonvulsant medications because the patient is to have an EEG.

4 Correlation between paroxysmal activity on EEGs and clinical seizure disorders is quite imperfect. An EEG may be normal in a patient with seizures. Conversely, paroxysmal discharges on the EEG do not in themselves constitute a clinical seizure disorder. Possibly asymptomatic spiking will be shown to merit treatment, but sufficient evidence is lacking to date.

EVALUATION OF SUSPECTED SPINAL CORD AND ROOT COMPRESSION

The main reasons for spinal column imaging are suspected compression of the spinal cord, of the cauda equina, or of intraspinal roots as they exit through intervertebral foramina (see Figs 13.9 and 13.15). The degree of urgency of diagnosis and intervention follows that same order: compression of the cord represents an absolute neurologic emergency because of the permanence of damage to the cord as CNS tissue. The roots of the cauda equina are PNS tissue with the potential for regeneration; however, their close anatomic proximity means that damage to multiple roots in the cauda equina tends to produce severe and widespread deficits. Pathology at an intervertebral foramen typically affects just one root; diagnosis is less urgent, but it is often difficult to ascertain whether a disc protrusion is actually affecting a root and responsible for the patient's pain and other symptoms and signs. Because of the prevalence of disc pathology, its relevance to symptoms must be established by careful clinical correlation (see Chapters 16 and 19).

Preeminence of MRI

MRI is rapidly becoming established as the preferred method of imaging for spinal cord and root compression. Plain films show bony changes, and thus reveal fractures and dislocations, disc-space narrowing, osteophytes, and lytic and blastic neoplastic lesions. Radionuclide bone scans also can show neoplastic, inflammatory, and other changes of bone, but neither technique visualizes the spinal cord or roots themselves. Thus, demonstration of skeletal lesions by plain films or bone scan often requires further elucidation by MRI or CT examination. MRI is currently an expensive technique for initial screening and surveys, but will eventually supplant plain films entirely for neurologic purposes. CT scanning is presently more widely available, but to minimize radiation and the length of the study, the clinician should be able to identify the region of the spinal column to be studied.

Identification of segmental level for CT

In the common situation of bilateral lower extremity weakness (paraparesis) or sensory loss with a level, a lesion causing cord compression might be located anywhere from lumbar cord levels on upwards. Without segmental neurologic signs, local pain or tenderness, or bony lesions established by plain film or bone scan, the radiologist would not know where to focus the CT examination (see Chapters 13 and 14, sections on segmental signs and sensory levels). Another limitation of spinal CT imaging, aside from inferior resolution of detail *vis-à-vis* MRI, is that the shoulders often obscure features of the lower cervical spine, especially in the C7–T1 region. MRI does not suffer from this technical disadvantage. Even more important, MRI can be used to screen the entire spinal column in sagittal sections for compressive lesions. Having thus identified the level of a suspected or definite lesion, cross-sectional images can then clarify the picture and provide details. Nevertheless, current MRI images do not necessarily correlate perfectly with anatomic pathology, and in certain instances CT examination or CT combined with myelography proves more accurate, especially with regard to disc pathology. Myelography (see Table 15.1) is rapidly becoming outmoded for most purposes, but remains effective for ruling out spinal cord compression as an emergency when MRI is not available or CT is inadequate for the particular case.

ELECTROMYOGRAPHY AND NERVE CONDUCTION TESTS

Electromyography

Electromyography (EMG) records muscle activity by means of extracellular needle electrodes inserted into muscle. Spontaneous muscle firing at rest and during voluntary contraction is measured, noting features such as amplitude and duration of the compound muscle action potentials. EMG study distinguishes between the two main forms of muscle disorder, primary muscle disease (myopathy), and muscle disorders secondary to abnormalities of neural innervation (neurogenic muscle disorders). Actually, the use of the terms primary and secondary may create some confusion, in that some non-neurogenic (so-called primary) myopathies are caused by systemic diseases, such as hyperthyroidism, and as such are not truly primary to muscle itself: they are simply not secondary to neural lesions.

Sensitivity and specificity

In the hands of a competent electromyographer, EMG testing is quite sensitive: in a muscle disorder, EMG testing will usually be specific as to myopathic vs. neuropathic origin, but only a small number of diseases or syndromes write a unique signature on the EMG record. EMG testing enables more precise localization of peripheral nerve lesions than can be achieved by nerve conduction testing alone. Analysis of the pattern of denervated muscles indicates not only whether the deficits are attributable to a particular nerve trunk (Chapter 16), but also where the lesion is located – since muscular branches leave the nerve successfully along its course. In contrast, the results of EMG alone usually do not specify the type of myopathic process or the cause of neurogenic changes. (Muscle biopsy sometimes solves the former, and nerve conduction studies may help with the latter.)

Localization

In the diagnosis of radiculopathies from spinal disc protrusion or other causes, EMG testing also provides localizing information. Denervation in the paraspinal muscles of the back indicates the proximal location of the segmental pathology, since the motor fibers to the paraspinal muscles branch off early from the spinal nerves.

Nerve conduction velocities

Nerve conduction velocities (NCV) are calculated from the time required for a stimulus to traverse a measured distance. In some situations, such as the distal ends of nerves, the time interval between stimulus and muscle twitch is measured, this latency being compared with established norms.

This simple summary underestimates, however, the capabilities of modern nerve conduction techniques. In addition to motor nerve conductions, sensory nerve conductions are helpful, especially distally. Another tactic is to stimulate nerve fibers involved in monosynaptic deep tendon reflexes, thereby including the proximal components – the posterior and anterior roots – which are otherwise hard to study physiologically. Sophisticated studies can localize certain myopathic-like disorders to the neuromuscular junction, and differentiate one from another (for example, myasthenia gravis from the Lambert–Eaton inverse myasthenic syndrome). These studies utilize rapid, repetitive nerve stimulation with EMG recording of the muscle responses, which varies with repetitive stimulation because of pre- or postsynaptic abnormalities at the neuromuscular junction.

Uses of NCV

The two major values of nerve conduction studies consist of: (a) localizing focal nerve lesions, as occur in particular nerves (or roots) as a result of trauma, entrapment, or occasionally focal inflammatory, ischemic, or neoplastic disease; (b) detecting diffuse polyneuropathies (or radiculopathies) and indicating whether these are axonal or demyelinating. Since the myelin sheath of nerves enables fast conduction, a diffuse demyelinating disease process that interrupts this sheath at various places along each axon (segmental demyelination) causes major slowing in nerve conduction velocities. In contrast, diseases that affect axons (and myelin only secondarily) will show normal or nearly normal NCVs as long as some large, myelinated axons remain intact. When the severity of the disease is such that all axons are profoundly affected, the result is no conduction, rather than major slowing.

This brief account does not do justice to the useful data that may be derived from electrophysiologic studies of the PNS, but further readings on EMG/NCV are suggested at the end of this chapter. Chapter 16 offers a general clinical approach to the PNS.

As a practical matter, three steps need to be taken after an EMG/NCV study has been decided upon.

1 Communicate the clinical problem and objectives of the study clearly to the electromyographer (a physician, usually a neurologist or physical medicine specialist, who is often assisted by a technician).

2 Prepare the patient for some discomfort during the study, mainly from the insertion of EMG needle electrodes. Most patients do not find any one insertion or electrical stimulation of a nerve to be very uncomfortable, but in aggregate the study may prove to be so. Thus, the level of discomfort depends upon the location and the number of muscles (and nerves) to be tested, as well as the attitude and personality of the patient and the electromyographer. (Also reassure the patient as to the safety of the study. Most laboratories are now using disposable needles.)

3 The sites of EMG examination and muscle biopsy should be kept strictly separate: a biopsy taken where an EMG needle had previously been inserted may well show iatrogenic damage.

CSF EXAMINATION AND LUMBAR PUNCTURE (LP)

The prime indication for CSF examination is suspicion of infection, and LP (spinal tap) is the easiest and safest access to CSF.

In Chapter 13, Fig. 13.8 outlines the CSF pathways. The quality and type of cells and protein exudate in the CSF reflect the pathology of tissues bordering these pathways. An excess of white blood cells, called a pleocytosis, is ordinarily the cardinal laboratory finding in meningitis or encephalitis (inflammation of the brain itself). (This traditional marker may be absent in immunosuppressed states, such as HIV infection.) Typically, an increase in CSF protein accompanies infection. Bacterial meningitis often induces a fall in CSF glucose, which may also be seen in fungal infection and other disorders. In addition to the determination of cellular constituents, protein, and sugar, a CSF smear is prepared and stained for microscopic examination to identify bacteria, mycobacteria and fungi, and CSF is cultured appropriately (Table 15.3). Specific antibody and antigen tests can also be performed to identify particular infectious agents promptly.

Other CSF abnormalities

CSF examination holds a unique place in the diagnosis of meningitis and encephalitis, but it continues to have other indications, despite being eclipsed by neuroimaging as a more general diagnostic tool. (Diagnosis of tumor and intracerebral hemorrhage, for example, are now in the province of CT and MRI; in fact, suspicion of space-occupying masses is considered a relative contraindication to LP.) CSF sampling may also be indicated for the following: (a) specific proteins, such as oligoclonal immunoglobulins (e.g. in MS); (b) neoplastic cells from intraventricular or meningeal tumors, either primary to the nervous system or metastatic; (LP is done after imaging indicates sufficient safety); (c) pressure measurements (after imaging to rule out mass effects that might lead to herniation, see Chapter 13); such pressure determinations are pertinent in the evaluation of hydrocephalus and suspicion of a form of intracranial hypertension known as pseudotumor cerebri, but should ordinarily be undertaken only after neurologic consultation; and (d) ruling out small amounts of subarachnoid blood from a suspected aneurysmal leak, despite negative neuroimaging.

Table 15.3 Outline of cerebrospinal fluid testing

Test	Method	Comment
During LP		
CSF pressure	Measurement with manometer; observation of rate of flow out of needle	Measurement with patient horizontal; if sitting, shift to horizontal, or subtract height of CSF column from needle to base of skull
Unspun CSF		
Clarity of CSF	Observation of unspun CSF	Compare tube no. 1 and tube no. 4 (or last tube) for pinkness (blood) or other turbidity
Cell count	Unspun CSF in counting chamber: RBC and WBC count; differential count of WBCs possible, but more definitive on stained sediment	RBCs indicate intrinsic hemorrhage or traumatic tap; in the latter, the RBC count usually declines dramatically from tube no. 1 to no. 4. More than a few WBCs indicates significant inflammation – usually infection
Culture ("bacteriology")	Plating/inoculation of unspun CSF on/into appropriate media	CSF for culture requires sterile and prompt handling; coordinate with laboratory
Spun CSF (centrifuged)		
Clarity of supernatant	Observation of spun CSF (supernatant) vs. clear water standard; suspended cells removed by spinning, leaving dissolved pigments.	Discoloration is usually due to *xanthochromia* – hemoglobin breakdown pigments from bleeding prior to LP; very high protein, bilirubin in jaundiced patient, and iodine contamination also cause discoloration
Bacterial/fungal morphologic identification	Gram stain of CSF sediment for microscopic examination (also, acid-fast and fungal stains)	Visual identification of Gram-positive and -negative bacteria, mycobacteria (by acid-fast stain), fungi
WBC differential count	Wright–Giemsa stain for WBC morphology on sedimented cells	Proportion of polymorphonuclear leukocytes (PMNs, polys) vs. lymphocytes critical in diagnosis

Table 15.3 *Continued*

Test	Method	Comment
Chemistries ("routine") on supernatant	Protein, glucose	Normal protein (20–40 mg/dl): increased with tumors and inflammation; normal glucose above 40 mg/dl and greater than 60% of blood glucose (unless latter is very high)
Special tests on supernatant	Protein electrophoresis, serologic tests for syphilis, antibody and antigen tests for specific microorganisms, etc.	See Further reading section at end of the chapter for guidance on indications for special tests
Cytology	Techniques to concentrate and examine cells in CSF	Diagnosis of neoplasms shedding cells into CSF; special studies of inflammatory cells

CSF, cerebrospinal fluid; LP, lumbar puncture; PMN, polymorphonuclear leukocytes; RBC, red blood cell; WBC, white blood cell.

LP risks

As noted, the main contraindication to LP is a space-occupying intracranial lesion. Other risks arise from blood coagulation defects that might cause bleeding within the spinal canal; introduction of bacteria into the CSF from cutaneous or subcutaneous infection, or from bacteremia. Also, headache, nausea, dizziness, and rarely double vision may follow an LP.

In cases of intracranial mass, the contraindication to LP is not absolute, but in most instances there is no compelling indication, either. Where either CT or MRI is available, a good, conservative working rule is that a cranial scan should precede an LP. (Note that in any acute situation, lack of papilledema on funduscopic examination does not rule out raised intracranial pressure; see Chapter 4.) As with any rule, there are exceptions, and the important one here is in the case of suspected meningitis, especially bacterial meningitis. Bacterial meningitis constitutes a true emergency, requiring rapid diagnosis and antibiotic treatment. The clinician faces a choice between two principal options: (a) performing the LP without a prior scan, because coexistent mass lesions are quite rare; and, even in the presence of increased intracranial pressure, neurologic deterioration consequent to the removal of CSF is unusual; (b) in case of strong suspicion of a coexistent mass, such as an abscess in the temporal lobe or cerebellum, broad-spectrum antibiotic coverage might be started intravenously (after blood cultures) to be followed by immediate cranial imaging and then LP, if considered sufficiently safe. This option violates the practice of obtaining a sample of CSF before starting therapy, but immediate therapy is guided by the Gram-stained smear and other rapid-identification tests, as well as clinical experience.

If greatly increased CSF pressure (such as 300 mm of CSF or higher) is unexpectedly encountered, it is wise to stop withdrawing fluid and then request help. Some experts favor simply removing the needle after a minimum of CSF is collected, while others suggest injecting sterile normal saline back into the subarachnoid space. In either case, treatment with intravenous mannitol, an agent that lowers intracranial pressure, can be initiated before removing the needle or immediately thereafter. The preferred management depends on the level of pressure and each patient's clinical situation.

LP technique

It is beyond the scope of this chapter to detail the complete routine of LP in the adolescent and adult. (LP in the infant and young child requires special guidance.) You will best learn the ordinary step-by-step procedures from an experienced clinician. However, even many skilled house officers are not fully aware of some of the "tricks of the trade." Since LP is the one neurologic procedural test that you may commonly perform yourself, you should make every effort to become truly competent. The following hints will promote success and help minimize the repeated attempts and failures that are painful for the patient and frustrating to the operator (Fig. 15.6).

Explanation

1 Since patients feel very vulnerable to a procedure to be performed "behind their back," especially given the gruesome popular mythology of spinal taps, offer careful explanation and reassurance. Some patients express anxiety about "how big a spinal needle is," usually meaning the length of the needle; you may wish to emphasize its thinness verbally and not brandish it in view. (Informed consent is required.)

Position yourself

2 Make yourself comfortable, so that you can concentrate on performing a successful tap while helping the patient to relax. (An assistant who is "on the patient's side" – relating face to face – is a great asset.)

Avoid spinal sag

3 Position the patient in the fetal position near the edge of the examination table or bed and, if necessary, support the trunk with a pillow, so as to avoid a sag that curves the patient's spine. (Note that bowing the lumbar and thoracic spine in flexion is very helpful for "opening up" the posterior interspaces, but there is no advantage to flexing the neck. In fact, holding the head in flexion may compromise ventilation.)

Do not hide landmarks

4 It is advisable to expose a wide area of lower back and hips so that the body landmarks of the spine and the iliac crests remain in view. To accomplish this, do not use a drape with a small window. The key sterile drape is the one tucked under the patient's trunk, and over which you will be working. Because of the larger expanse of exposed skin, "prep" (cleanse) the skin widely with antiseptic solution before draping.

Anesthetize well

5 When infiltrating local anesthetic, allow time for it to take effect, before injecting deeper. You should use a very fine needle (usually a no. 25 or no. 26 if available) for the skin wheal and subcutaneous injection,

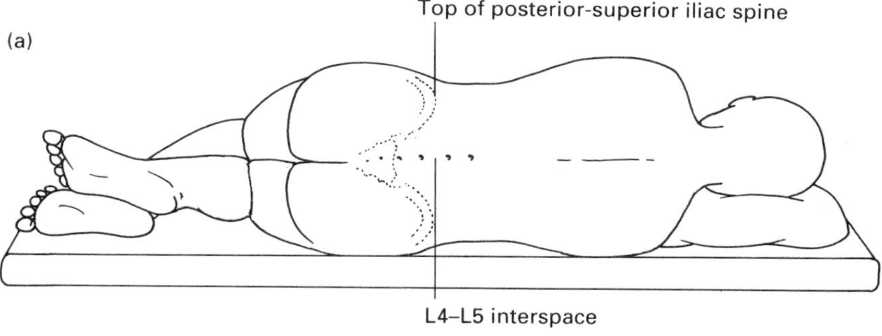

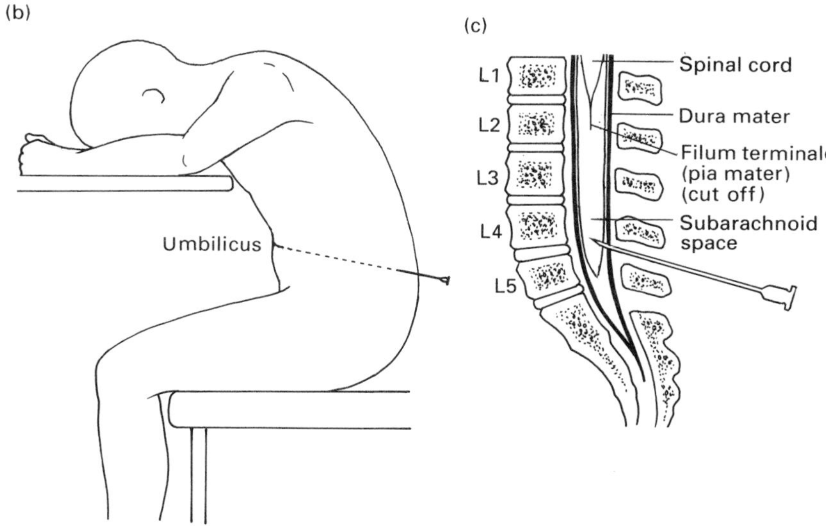

Fig. 15.6 Lumbar puncture. (a) In the lateral decubitus position the L4–L5 interspace is identified near the line from the top of one posterior-superior iliac spine to the other. The body is fully flexed (not emphasized in this view) and the hips and shoulders remain squared. (b) In the seated position the head and arms are supported and the back rounded. (c) Schematic of the lumbar interspaces in midsagittal plane. The spinal needle is slanted so that the needle tip points toward the umbilicus, which allows passage between the spinous processes. (The cauda equina is not shown.)

then change to a thin, but longer needle for deeper infiltration. It should be noted that the injection of local anesthetic entails some discomfort which may be as great or greater than the pain of an unanesthetized LP, performed by a very skilled operator. You should use local anesthetic in most cases until you reach that point, and then individualize.

LP needle gauge

6 In many patients, and for most purposes, you can use a thin no. 22 or no. 21 gauge spinal needle. If this is not available in the LP kit provided, one can usually be obtained separately. In some older people with tougher intervertebral tissues, it may be wiser to use a heavier no. 20–18 needle. Also, a thicker (lower gauge) needle may be indicated: (a) if your main aim is to make an accurate pressure measurement; (b) if you anticipate more viscous fluid (as from high protein); or (c) if you expect very low CSF pressure due to dehydration or other causes.

Cephalad slant

7 The usual guideline is to aim the LP needle for the umbilicus, so as to achieve the slant towards the head that will facilitate slipping between the spinous processes. If your infiltrating needle appears to be on a good line, not encountering any bony resistance, then try to follow that line with the LP needle. If you must shift course, retract the needle to the subcutaneous space where it will become more mobile, and redirect it. (Should your initial starting point on the skin be mistaken, you will need to start over, using the same or a new skin wheal.)

Avoiding deviation

8 While the cephalad slant of the needle allows penetration between the spinous processes, the greater problem is to avoid misdirection towards the right or left side of the patient's body (the up–down plane as the patient lies on one side). The keys here are firm support under the patient's trunk; checking to see that the spinous processes are in a straight line and not sagging; maintaining vertical alignment of the right and left shoulders and of the iliac crests at true right angles to the bed or table; when inserting the needle, be sure that it is at a true right angle to the vertical plane of the back. (It is very easy to slant the needle inadvertently towards the patient's right or left side – this is the foremost reason for hitting bone rather than the subarachnoid space within the spinal column.)

Coping with a dry tap

9 If you believe that your LP needle is well-positioned, but you are still encountering a "dry tap" proceed as set out below.

Depth — Check not only the direction, but the depth of the needle. Inexperienced operators are often reluctant to insert the needle as deeply as may be necessary, especially in a bulky person. Advance or withdraw just a few millimeters at a time, checking for flow each time.

Rotate needle — Rotate the needle in case its opening is up against a spinal root of the cauda equina, i.e. the needle may be well placed, but the CSF inflow is temporarily blocked.

Aspirate — Aspirate very gently with a syringe attached to the spinal needle, in case of very low pressure or viscous fluid.

Interspace Recheck the interspace of entry. It is common to place the needle inadvertently in the L5–S1 interspace, thinking that it is L4–L5. The top of the iliac crests are supposed to be the guide to L4–L5, but it is not always clear which interspace is actually on this line; make this determination with the back in the fully flexed position. In some patients the thecal sac, or end pouch of the spinal meninges, is relatively short, and may be missed by too caudal a puncture, such as at L5–S1. Inexperienced operators are often especially fearful of using too high an interspace, that is, too far up the spine, with risk of hitting the spinal cord. L3–L4 is a perfectly acceptable interspace as well as L4–L5. Even if one were to enter L2–L3, it should ordinarily be safe in the adult, as the cord rarely ends lower than L1–L2.

Tilt If the bed or table can be mildly tilted, head up, without buckling it, you can enlist gravity to distend the lumbar subarachnoid space more fully with CSF. (Measure the CSF pressure in the horizontal position.)

Sitting position Resort rather early to changing the patient to the sitting position, with legs over the side and shoulders slumped forward over a pillow on a tray table or other support, as in Fig. 15.6(b). (You may need to "reprep" and drape.) In the upright position, it is easier to be sure the spine is not twisted and that your needle is not deviating to the right or left of midline. (One disadvantage of this position is that occasional patients are susceptible to fainting; also, the CSF pressure measurement must be adjusted.)

More expert help Certainly by this time, and probably earlier, you should obtain help from a more experienced operator (even if you are being properly supervised up to this point). Aside from any professional who is known to be especially skilled, consider calling a neurologist (or neurosurgeon) or an anesthetist – the latter usually being readily available and highly skilled because of experience with spinal and epidural anesthesia.

Fluoroscopy With the cooperation of a radiologist, perform the tap under fluoroscopic guidance in the X-ray department. Some bony anomalies or other anatomic peculiarities can only be detected radiologically.

Traumatic tap

The spinal needle occasionally punctures a small vein, causing bleeding into the CSF in the subarachnoid space. Except in patients with blood coagulation deficiencies (who should not have LPs without special consideration), the bleeding from a traumatic tap is rarely harmful to the patient's spinal contents. However, the red blood cells (RBCs) in the CSF sample create confusion as to whether intrinsic, disease-related hemorrhage has occurred or an iatrogenic traumatic tap. As indicated in Table 15.3, the RBCs from a traumatic tap usually "clear," that is, they diminish in number as successive aliquots of CSF are collected in four or more tubes. Clearing occurs because: (a) the bleeding usually does not continue; and (b) later aliquots contain more clear CSF that moves down from a spinal level above the site of the traumatic bleeding. Blood that has been present in the CSF for many hours to days (usually blood from pathologic nervous system hemorrhage) undergoes RBC lysis and pigmentary change. This causes xanthochromic (usually straw-colored) tinting of the CSF.

Retap

When the object of the LP is to identify increased white blood cells (WBC) as a sign of infection, traumatic blood in the CSF complicates interpretation of the WBC count: normal WBC constituents of the traumatic blood appear in the CSF cell count. While the expected number of WBCs (in proportion to the number of RBCs counted) can be calculated, it is sometimes advisable to retap promptly at a higher (but safe) interspace.

BLOOD TESTS

Primary neurologic conditions usually cannot be diagnosed by blood test. Nonetheless, many blood tests are relevant to neurologic diagnosis and management because of the impact of systemic disease on the nervous system and musculature. It is beyond the scope of this book to discuss this wider world of blood tests, appropriate use of which will depend upon your growing knowledge of diseases. However, two categories stand out as particularly important and problematic in the care of patients: anticonvulsant "blood" levels and measures of anticoagulation. Aside from more routine blood counts and chemistries, these are the two types of blood test of neurologic importance that you will probably order most and need to manage best.

Use of anticonvulsant levels

"Therapeutic" range

The modern management of anticonvulsant (antiseizure) therapy relies on determination of serum levels of the medications in use. So-called therapeutic ranges have been established, meaning statistical ranges of concentrations within which many patients will receive therapeutic benefit. Above this range an increasing number of patients will experience "dose-related," toxic side effects (although these may also occur within the therapeutic range). Below this range an increasing number of patients in a population with epilepsy will experience seizures.

The problem is that the individual patient cannot count on protection within the therapeutic range, nor will the patient necessarily lack protection below the range. Use of the therapeutic range is helpful as a general guide, especially when beginning therapy. Over time it may become possible to approximate an individual patient's own therapeutic range and toxic threshold for a given drug. (Note that "free" or unbound serum levels confer advantages in certain situations; the guidelines to be described still generally apply.)

These concepts can be translated into some concrete guidelines.

Use specific concentration

1 Always refer to a specific level, a number (serum concentration) in discussing the patient's therapeutic and laboratory status, rather than referring to a test being "in the therapeutic range." For example, if a patient has a seizure while on a medication with a therapeutic range of 10–20 μg/ml, and the patient's level is 12, do not record this simply as a therapeutic level. (It was not, in fact, therapeutic for the patient!) This patient might require a level of 15, 18, or even 22.

Keep tests in clinical context

2 Beware of the "numerical imperative" – a sense of compulsion to raise or lower the dose of a patient whose level is below or above the therapeutic range (and therefore assumed to be inappropriate). Respond to every anticonvulsant level by taking into account the clinical context. You should not automatically assume that a level of 22 is toxic, because it is reported as such or is just above the top of the therapeutic range. Some patients will tolerate such a level perfectly well and may require it for control. Likewise, patients whose seizures have long been optimally controlled with mildly "subtherapeutic" levels do not necessarily stand to benefit from an increased dose and serum concentration.

Dose–level relationship

3 Do not presume that a direct relationship exists between serum level and dosage. Depending on the kinetics of the drug's metabolism, a small increment in drug dosage may cause a major change in blood level. For example, in the case of phenytoin (one of the most commonly used anticonvulsants), a 33% increase in dosage (from three pills per day to four) typically leads to a much larger percentage increase in serum level, often resulting in toxicity.

Anticoagulant monitoring

Monitoring of a patient on anticoagulant therapy (designed to prevent thromboembolism) is a multifaceted issue, but in the context of laboratory testing a few points should be emphasized. The prothrombin time (PT) is a measure of anticoagulant effect used when the patient is on oral anticoagulation (warfarin sodium, known also by the trade-name, Coumadin). Because of variability in control standards, laboratories are adopting the International Normalized Ratio (INR) as a more reliable PT measure for maintenance monitoring (see Further reading section). The partial thromboplastin time (PTT) is used when the patient is on parenteral (intravenous or subcutaneous) heparin.

Flow sheet

1 Maintain a running flow sheet that juxtaposes the anticoagulant dose and the PT (or INR) or PTT result. Using a single PT value in isolation is a particularly dangerous basis for picking the next dose, because of a delayed effect of each dose on the blood clotting system. Always consider the progression or trend of dosages and PTs.

Individualize test frequency

2 The frequency of PT determinations must be individualized. Too often in ambulatory maintenance therapy (once a desired PT has been achieved), an arbitrary frequency of testing every 2 weeks, or even every 4 weeks, is established. In fact, individual requirements may change due to interactions from other medications, concurrent illnesses, etc. Because of the danger of straying too far above or below the target PT (often 1.5 times control), the issue of frequency is critical; scheduling of PTs must continually be subject to reassessment and adjustment. Also, bleeding complications in the context of lowered coagulation do not follow the usual expectations in terms of symptom profile. Be vigilant!

PROBLEMS FOR SELF-STUDY

Problems

1 A CT scan is reported to show a small hemorrhage (hematoma) in the right frontal lobe. What evidence would you want in order to satisfy yourself that the observed lesion really is a primary hemorrhage?
2 A CT scan shows a low-density lesion at the tip of the left temporal lobe in a patient with known cardiovascular disease. Would you accept the initial interpretation of this as an infarct?
3 An MRI reveals quite enlarged ventricles. No tumor or other mass lesion blocking the ventricular system is seen. What more would you like to know about this?
4 An EEG was reported normal in a patient believed to be having epileptic seizures. What else might you do to elucidate the issue?
5 A patient is sent for an EMG to confirm damage to the sciatic nerve, postulated to have occurred the previous day, as a result of an intramuscular injection. What do you think the test will show?
6 A lumbar puncture is planned to test for neurosyphilis of the CNS. Because of difficulty in obtaining CSF in the usual lateral decubitus position, an attempt is made in the sitting position. CSF is obtained, but spurts out under increased pressure and is pink in color. What would you do?

Comments

1 (a) The density (attenuation) reading provided by the CT machine suggests whether this lesion is more in the region expected for clotted blood or for calcification.

(b) Is this a contrast-enhanced scan? Might this be a vascular structure or enhanced lesion? If so, compare with a noncontrast scan.
(c) Is there anything unusual in the location, morphology, or surrounding area that would suggest secondary hemorrhagic infarction rather than primary hematoma, bleeding into a tumor, or calcification? Request expert help in making these distinctions.
(d) Compare with a subsequent follow-up scan. A hematoma will become less dense (less white) as it is resorbed over days to weeks.

2 The interpretation would depend upon some knowledge of the timing of the scan in relation to the relevant clinical event, which might be hard to establish. An infarct occurring that same day would not yet be visible. If the lesion were chronic, it might well be the residual appearance of a traumatic contusion and hemorrhage, for which this is a site of predilection. Not all chronic low-density lesions are infarcts!

3 Enlarged ventricles can be broadly termed hydrocephalus, but this does not necessarily imply obstruction within the ventricular system – and in this instance no internal blockage is seen. Ventricles may passively enlarge due to surrounding tissue loss (hydrocephalus *ex vacuo*). If subarachnoid CSF spaces are also enlarged, and the clinical diagnosis and age are consistent with brain atrophy, then you may not need to do more than a follow-up scan at a later time, if indicated. An alternative explanation for the hydrocephalus would be an impediment in the subarachnoid spaces to CSF flow and resorption, causing ("normal pressure") hydrocephalus, a communicating form of obstructive hydrocephalus (see Chapter 13). Close clinical–neuroradiologic consultation can usually establish the correct diagnosis and course of action in problems like this.

4 A normal EEG does not rule out a seizure disorder. Determine whether the EEG included a sleep study, which sometimes shows paroxysmal activity not seen on the waking record (see text). If the problem in demonstrating abnormalities is one of temporal sampling error, the study might be repeated or a prolonged EEG performed. If the problem is spatial – the focus is too far from the recording electrodes – nasopharyngeal electrodes could be employed in a repeat tracing. Also, an empirical trial of therapy should be considered, if the clinical indications are sufficient.

5 The proximal sciatic nerve is not accessible to the usual motor nerve conduction tests. If the lesion is partial, with a great many fibers entirely preserved, all nerve conduction tests, both immediate and delayed, might well be normal. Damage to some axons, with distal (Wallerian) degeneration, would produce denervation changes on EMG testing, but usually not before 10–14 days or longer. An EMG, guided in part by motor deficits on examination, should be done at a later time, if then indicated.

6 First, replace the stylet while you think about the next step. Request help. Reconfirm that a CT or MRI done prior to the LP had excluded a mass lesion. The increased CSF pressure might be due to the added hydrostatic column in the sitting position and the pink color to a traumatic tap. If no mass lesion was seen, and assuming the patient has not experienced any sudden clinical change, then no emergency steps are necessary before remeasuring the CSF pressure after carefully returning the patient to the lateral decubitus position. If the pressure is normal, remove the CSF sample and needle. Analyze the CSF for clearing in successive tubes and for xanthochromia, etc. The serologic tests for syphilis can be done on a traumatic sample, but you might consider retap at the next higher level to enable a truer WBC count. If the CSF pressure is actually elevated, request neurosurgical consultation, consider steps to lower intracranial pressure, and plan emergency reimaging (see text).

FURTHER READING

Aminoff, M.J. Evoked potential studies in neurologic diagnosis and management. *Ann Neurol* 1990; 28:706–10. Applications of sensory evoked potentials and of motor potentials evoked by magnetic stimulation are categorized according to how they contribute to diagnosis and management.

Dodson, W.E. Level off (Editorial). *Neurology* 1989; 39:1009–10. Confronts the common misunderstanding of antiepileptic drug levels and recommends appropriate utilization.

Donnan, G.A. Investigation of patients with stroke and transient ischemic attacks. *Lancet* 1992; 339:473–7. Brief, critical evaluations of neurodiagnostic tests for stroke and transient ischemic attacks.

Engel, J. Jr. *Seizures and Epilepsy*. F.A. Davis, Philadelphia (PA), 1989. A comprehensive work that includes accessible information on the EEG.

Fishman, R.A. *Cerebrospinal Fluid in Disease of the Nervous System*. 2nd edn. WB Saunders, Philadelphia (PA), 1992. A deep well of information on the nervous system's own fluid.

Gilman, S. Advances in neurology. *N Engl J Med* 1992; 326:1608–16, 1671–6. Review of selected advances in neurology with an emphasis on structural and functional neuroimaging.

Hirsh, J. Oral anticoagulant drugs. *N Engl J Med* 1991; 324:1865–75. Use and monitoring of oral anticoagulant therapy, including the INR, which is still unfamiliar to many physicians dealing with PTs.

Matthews, P.M., Arnold, D.L. *Diagnostic Tests in Neurology*. Churchill Livingstone, New York (NY), 1991. A source for studying the broad array of so-called ancillary (laboratory and imaging) neurologic tests.

Mayo Clinic. Clinical neurophysiology. In: *Clinical Examinations in Neurology*. 6th edn. Mosby, St. Louis (MO), 1991. Good sections on EEG and EMG.

Mazziotta, J.C., Gilman, S. (eds) *Clinical Brain Imaging: Principles and Applications*. F.A. Davis, Philadelphia (PA), 1992. Comprehensive status report, by technique and by category of disorder, in this fast-moving field.

Pritchard, J.W., Brass, L.M. New anatomical and functional imaging methods. *Ann Neurol* 1992; 32:395–400. Reviews advantages and disadvantages of PET, SPECT, and various magnetic resonance techniques.

Tyler, K.L., Martin, J.B. *Infectious Diseases of the Central Nervous System*. F.A. Davis, Philadelphia (PA), 1993. From customary types of meningitis, encephalitis, and abscess with characteristic CSF formulas to AIDS-related infections that betray the traditional rules of CSF response (also see Further reading section of Chapter 4).

part 4

Further Diagnostic Skills

chapter 16

An Approach to Peripheral Neurology

Introduction

Our thoughts and emotions may be uppermost in our minds, but many of the mundane symptoms of daily life originate in the peripheral nervous system (PNS) – the numb leg from sitting on a hard surface too long, or the arm that you slept on that did not "wake up" when the rest of you did. More importantly, clinical problems of the PNS impact the work of most medical and surgical practitioners, not just neurologists. If central nervous system (CNS) anatomy is learned "stroke by stroke," as the saying goes, then the most relevant PNS anatomy is learned "pinched nerve by pinched nerve."

Of the many facts that apply to localization in the PNS, only a few are used commonly, so the following general approach may be helpful.

1 You should be aware of pertinent definitions (Table 16.1) and the overall organization of the PNS, so that relevant facts can be placed in an understandable framework (Tables 16.2 and 16.3).

2 This chapter emphasizes frequently used information. The facts you need repeatedly will eventually be remembered; others can be looked up as required.

3 Avail yourself of a good and convenient reference source (see Further reading section of this chapter).

PNS problems in clinical practice

Many of the neurologic conditions that come to the attention of non-neurologic specialists and generalists result from PNS lesions – the traumatic nerve damage seen by various surgeons and emergency physicians, the "pinched" nerve roots whose owners flock to orthopedists' offices, and the diabetic neuropathies cared for by internists and family physicians. Likewise, obstetricians commonly deal with the "pinched" nerves of pregnancy and delivery, not only in the back and pelvis, but in the carpal tunnel of the wrist, where the median nerve is vulnerable to compression by swollen tissues. Focal peripheral nerve lesions often can

Table 16.1 Schematic glossary of peripheral nervous system and neuromuscular system

Dorsal (posterior) root		
Central process: axon (root fiber) from sensory neuron in dorsal root ganglion (DRG) that enters cord (central nervous system) to synapse or join a tract (see Fig. 13.15)		
DRG: aggregation of 1st order sensory neuron cell bodies (outside cord)		
Peripheral process: axon from 1st order sensory neuron in DRG; first called a "root fiber," then called a "spinal nerve" or "peripheral nerve fiber" after joining with motor fibers to form a mixed peripheral nerve (see Fig. 13.15)	*Mixed peripheral nerve*: formed by ventral and dorsal roots (including autonomic fibers). Usually called just "peripheral nerves." A few large branches are formed by only sensory fibers; all nerves segregate by function at some branch point	*Sensory receptors*: specialized or "free endings" of sensory nerves which transduce stimuli into electrical signals
Ventral root (anterior/motor root)		*Muscle*: specialized contractile tissues
Consists of axons of CNS anterior horn cells which help form mixed peripheral nerves and innervate muscles		

Table 16.1 *Continued*

Root disorders	Peripheral nerve disorders	Muscle disorders
Radiculopathy: any pathologic abnormality of a nerve root	*Neuropathy*: any pathologic process manifest in a peripheral nerve	*Myopathy*: any (non-neurogenic) disease of muscle.
		Dystrophy: any of the genetic, degenerative myopathies
Radiculitis: an inflammatory radiculopathy	*Polyneuropathy*: a diffuse, symmetric involvement of peripheral nerves, but may affect motor, sensory and autonomic fibers differentially. (see Fig. 16.11).	*Myositis*: inflammatory myopathy *Polymyositis*: systemic inflammatory myopathy (autoimmune)
"Pinched nerve": a common term usually implying compressive (or other mechanical) radiculopathy, as from disc disease	*Mononeuropathy*: one nerve involved (see Figs 16.4a, 16.5, 16.6).	*Dermatomyositis*: polymyositis with skin involvement
"Sciatica": a common term for radiculopathic symptoms referable to one of the lumbosacral roots that form the sciatic nerve	*Mononeuropathy multiplex*: multiple (two or more) mononeuropathies	

Table 16.2 Functional organization of the peripheral nervous system

	Root	Peripheral nerve trunk	Muscle
Motor	Anterior root distributed to more than one nerve and muscle	Contains fibers from more than one root: innervates more than one muscle	Most muscles innervated by only one nerve containing fibers from two or more roots
Sensory	Posterior root fibers serve all sensory modalities	Sensory fibers (more than one root) are mixed with motor and autonomic fibers	No sensory deficit; muscle innervated by pain fibers and afferents from muscle spindles, etc.
Reflexes	Each deep tendon reflex (DTR) usually subserved by two roots (see Fig. 14.7) Biceps jerk: C5, C6. Triceps jerk: C7, C8 Knee jerk: L3, L4 Ankle jerk: S1 (S2)	DTR subserved by one peripheral nerve trunk: BJ: musculocutaneous nerve TJ: radial nerve KJ: femoral nerve AJ: Sciatic nerve	DTRs not decreased out of proportion to strength (in contrast to polyneuropathies, polyradiculopathies)

Table 16.3 Anatomic relationships of nerve roots and peripheral nerves

Nerve roots	Peripheral nerves
The dorsal and ventral roots are in the peripheral nervous system, but not yet joined into mixed peripheral nerves (see Fig. 13.15)	Mixed peripheral nerves (sometimes called "spinal nerves" before entering plexuses) are formed by ventral and dorsal roots joining outside of the spinal column (see Fig. 13.15)
Adjacent dorsal roots overlap in their distribution of innervation, such that severance of one root does not produce a band of complete sensory loss (see Fig. 16.2)	Peripheral nerve sensory branches partially overlap adjacent nerve territories, but each has a central "autonomous zone" in which all sensation is lost if the nerve is severed (see Fig. 16.2)
A single dorsal root contributes fibers to two or more mixed peripheral nerves in the limbs; the spinal nerves (e.g. intercostal) that do not enter a plexus typically contain fibers from only one root (see Fig. 16.2)	A major peripheral nerve in the limbs contains fibers from two or more adjacent roots (motor and sensory); a process of sorting and resorting occurs in the plexuses (e.g. brachial)
A dermatome chart artificially shows only the central band of the entire cutaneous innervation of each dorsal root (Fig. 16.1); since each root territory overlaps the adjacent ones, the overlapping territories are split (on the map) – part included in one dermatome and part in each adjacent one	A peripheral nerve distribution map splits overlapped innervations in order to approximate exclusive territories (e.g. Fig. 16.5)
Fibers of a motor root (e.g. right L5 ventral root) innervate more than one muscle via the same or different peripheral nerves	The motor fibers in a mixed peripheral nerve trunk are usually derived from more than one spinal segment (via more than one ventral root) and innervate multiple muscles; each muscle typically is innervated by only one peripheral nerve
If a root is severed, the result is a motor and/or sensory loss; some disease processes affect both ventral and dorsal roots; for example, a herniated disc can affect both roots just before exiting the spine or multiple roots (in the lumbosacral region) descending in the cauda equina	If a mixed peripheral nerve is damaged, both motor and sensory function are usually affected (some diseases affect larger vs. smaller fibers differently and motor vs. sensory function differently)

be specifically treated, but also benefit from the regenerative capacity of the PNS. In addition, localization of a lesion to the PNS relieves the added worry that the cause might have been in the CNS.

Prevention

Issues of prevention loom very large in respect to PNS disorders, because so many problems result from trauma and toxins. To put it differently, work and habits are the key to a host of PNS lesions:

occupational exposures and repetitive motion injury; recreational nerve compression and trauma; alcoholism and poor nutrition, etc.

NEUROLOGIC ASSESSMENT OF THE PNS: A FOCUSED APPROACH

In Chapter 6 and 7 the motor and sensory examinations were discussed and a general approach was presented: you were encouraged to test functions, such as forearm flexion or distal pin sensitivity, rather than testing particular nerves or muscles. A general method does not presuppose any localizing experience or any recall of specific innervations. Analysis follows subsequently: is there any pattern in the findings? What needs to be looked up to guide more detailed testing?

There comes a point, however, when the diagnostic process should capitalize on the efficiency of a more focused approach.

The process of eliciting symptoms arising from the PNS benfits from the fact that the patient's history ordinarily is not subject to the distortion peculiar to some brain disorders (see Chapter 1). Nonetheless, a patient's perception of PNS symptoms often does not conform to "textbook" expectations.

Barriers to PNS diagnosis

Two somewhat paradoxical attitudes often hinder peripheral neurologic problem-solving: the first is intimidation by the knowledge base. Like every student or graduate clinician, you probably hold a mental image of vast charts of dermatomes, maps of peripheral nerve territories, tables of muscle innervations, hellish plexuses, and maybe even a few ultimate minutiae (like the gemelli muscles), dangling in limbo. But do not be daunted: if you can elicit the patient's symptoms well, you can easily look up individual muscle examination techniques and anatomic facts. The specific innervations that pop up recurrently you will come to remember as a matter of course. All of this is made easier, however, if you have gained a general organizational framework and devised a working strategy.

Excessive and forgettable facts

The second expectation is that focal root and nerve lesions will cause deficits that conform neatly to the maps and charts: trace a line around a sensory deficit and the diagnosis is as good as delivered; pull on a few muscles and the strong ones will pop out in obvious contrast to the weak, flabby ones.

Textbook deficits

Why is the delineation of abnormalities often less clear and more frustrating?

1 Most root and nerve lesions diminish but do not obliterate function, because most lesions are partial in degree. Where sensory deficits are mild, boundary demarcations may prove hard to establish. Similarly, particular muscles may exhibit borderline weakness, so you will not have complete confidence in your localizing data.

Lesions partial in degree

Lesions partial in extent

2 Many lesions are incomplete in extent, sparing some fibers, so that the affected area will not include the entire nerve distribution. Even a well-defined deficit will not look just like the published map. The important point to establish is whether the deficit is within a distribution, not whether it fills out the entire territory.

Individual anatomic variations

3 Even allowing for the limitations of textbook maps, individual patient variations occur. For example, in the common cutaneous syndrome of "meralgia paresthetica," the numbness or discomfort in the distribution of the lateral cutaneous nerve of the thigh varies in topographic configuration. In short, do not insist on the exact textbook picture, but do beware if a deficit greatly exceeds the customary boundary, especially in one direction.

Characteristic symptoms of peripheral nerve and root disease

The cardinal symptoms of PNS disease include pain or discomfort, "numbness," and weakness. In addition, autonomic changes (such as a sense of coldness or altered sweating) sometimes add to this trio. Primary nerve pain radiates along the course of a root or a nerve, which is not entirely the same as the sensory distribution of the nerve. However, when a pain "settles in" to an area, the location is usually within the sensory distribution.

Pain and discomfort

Characteristically, in nerve root disease, the pain does not reach into the most distal part of the sensory distribution. For example, most L5 or S1 root pains usually do not extend into the toes, where numbness is often experienced. Nerve or root pains beget vivid descriptions: burning, icy, electric, knife-like, gnawing, like-a-toothache, etc. Coughing, sneezing, or straining aggravate radicular pain. Typically, tenderness does not accompany pain or only in minimal degree. Painful muscle spasms and cramps are often triggered by root and nerve disease, although they may also result from metabolic derangements and primary disorders of muscle. Note that pain in certain sites (such as the shoulder) that might suggest a primary root problem may represent referred pain from thoracic or abdominal viscera.

"Numbness"

Paresthesias (tingling, "pins and needles") or altered cutaneous sensitivity are characteristic sensory symptoms, but are not specific to the PNS. "Numbness" is a broad and imprecise, but useful term that can include paresthesias and/or testable deficits of touch or pain. The intended meaning must be clarified in every instance.

Weakness

There is nothing in a patient's report of the quality of weakness that will reliably differentiate a PNS vs. CNS lesion. Patients tend to emphasize the functional impairment, "I'm tripping over my left foot" or "I can't open jars anymore." The kind of anatomic specificity that is needed to localize a PNS lesion comes from a good examination. (See subsequent sections on muscle testing and motor diagnosis.)

Underlying conditions, antecedent events, and risk factors

Trauma

Most peripheral nerve problems arise from overt injury, inapparent injury from repetitive motion, pressure on nerves or nerve entrapment, toxic exposures and certain specific diseases. A good history should include inquiry about blunt or penetrating injury, including lacerations, fractures, or major bruises. Scarring from an old injury may result in the appearance of neuropathic symptoms and signs months or years later. Nerve damage from repetitive motion is a form of nerve trauma that usually falls into the category of entrapment neuropathies. A prime example is the carpal tunnel syndrome in which the median nerve at the wrist is subjected to intermittent mild compression, which eventually may become chronic, as tissues thicken in the bony and fibrous tunnel through which the nerve passes in the wrist. The superficial location of certain nerves predisposes to acute or chronic compression.

Postures

Accustomed postures, such as leaning on one elbow or crossing the legs, cause repetitive, low-grade, chronic compressive injury at sites of vulnerability. Most acute postural compressions occur in the context of obtundation or coma that may have been drug-induced. Common sites of pressure palsy include the radial nerve as it wraps around the humerus; the sciatic nerve in the buttock; and the common peroneal nerve (after division of the main sciatic trunk) as it winds laterally around the fibular head just inferior to the knee. Here it can be injured by compression, bruising, or by damage from a fibular fracture.

Review of systems

Entrapments: nerves may be restricted or compressed by overgrowth of soft tissues due to particular disease processes. For example, abnormal thickening of tissue in rheumatoid arthritis, hypothyroidism, or acromegaly can cause neuropathies such as the carpal tunnel syndrome, mentioned above.

Neuropathies due to specific diseases: most cases of polyneuropathy and mononeuropathy multiplex (as well as some simple mononeuropathies) result from a specific disease. Diabetes is a good example. Virtually all diabetic patients will eventually develop some degree of polyneuropathy that may become symptomatic or may just show up on an examination as decreased ankle jerks or blunted sensation in the feet. Occasionally, diabetic patients note the sudden onset of a single nerve palsy (a mononeuropathy). Alcoholic–nutritional polyneuropathies are frequently seen in some population groups; human immunodeficiency virus (HIV) neuropathies are increasing, and neuropathies associated with neoplasia and its treatment are relatively common.

Family history

Genetic diseases: genetically determined polyneuropathies may represent the only neurologic abnormality, but frequently are just one manifestation of a multisystem disorder of the PNS and CNS. Both dominant and recessive forms occur, but often the family pedigree gives no clue to the latter.

Are other people affected?

Toxic neuropathies: most systemic toxins that affect nerves do so symmetrically in the pattern of a polyneuropathy. Topical exposure typically causes focal damage. At work the employee may or may not know "what's in the barrel" – the potential toxins to which groups of employees may be exposed. At home, cleaners and other solvents, glues, etc., are often handled naively – without adequate attention to skin or eye exposure, or to ventilation. Even a vitamin excess can result in a neuropathy, as in the case of pyridoxine (B_6). Toxins in the general environment – the air or water – are most often unknown to the individual and hence not reported in the history (see Case 2A).

SENSORY EVALUATION IN SUSPECTED PNS PROBLEMS

"Inside"/"outside"

In using the patient's symptoms as an initial guide to your examination, try to elicit the distinction that I refer to as "inside feeling" (or inner feeling) vs. "outside feeling" (or outer feeling). This is not a sense of how superficial or deep a symptom feels. Rather, the distinction is similar to that between pain and tenderness. An "inside" feeling is a symptom consisting of paresthesias or other sensations that are felt independently of any cutaneous stimulus. An "outside" or "skin" feeling is a sign, an alteration of sensation recognized by stroking or otherwise testing the skin. The patient may have already noticed by self-examination that an area of the skin seems "distant," or "leathery," or "like sandpaper" to the touch. Abnormal "inside" and "outside" symptoms and signs often coexist.

Feelings of "difference"

If the patient, by self-observation, has discovered and can map out for you a cutaneous deficit, then you hold the advantage of a good starting point for your own examination. You can confirm and further define the boundaries. As emphasized in Chapter 7, an observant patient's "feeling of difference" to touch or pin stimulus can suffice to map a deficit, even when you cannot obtain consistent results on "sharp/dull" or "feel it/don't feel it" testing.

Validity of symptoms

Sensory symptoms that are only felt "inside," without cutaneous sensory alteration, retain their subjective validity, but mapping often proves more difficult. In some instances a patient can describe a perfect outline of the area of paresthesias, such as just "the left upper lip to the corner of the mouth," but at other times the best the patient can do is to describe tingling "in the right hand" without being able to specify which fingers, etc. Since lesions frequently first present with only pain or paresthesias, you cannot afford to ignore these "inside feelings" – or downgrade their significance. A patient who complains of low back pain which radiates down the back of the right thigh into the calf, and who experiences paresthesias in the lateral toes, almost surely has a radiculopathy (probably S1 root). This hypothesis would not be invalidated by failure to identify any definite motor, sensory, or reflex signs.

Demarcate the complete topography

After mapping out the "index" or presenting area of sensory abnormality, ascertain its broader topographic relationships. Does its distribution suggest a dermatomal pattern (Fig. 16.1)? Bear in mind not only the overlap of adjacent dermatomes, but the distribution of a given posterior root to more than one peripheral nerve (Fig. 16.2, Tables 16.2 and 16.3). One of the most important relationships to understand is that of dermatomes and peripheral nerve territories in the same region (Figs 16.2–16.4). Also, two peripheral nerve territories can look very similar if all surfaces are not examined (Fig. 16.5).

If the sensory changes are in one hand, do they extend to other areas on the same limb? Are the face, trunk, or leg on the same side of the body affected, suggesting a CNS lesion? The systematic approach to comparative testing suggested in Chapter 7 (see Fig. 7.1 and Table 7.1) will help answer these questions.

For example, consider an index deficit of severe sensory loss on the medial aspect of the left leg. You have mapped it out, finding that it falls within the distribution of the saphenous nerve. By extending the search for sensory deficits, you find an area of loss on the anterior thigh that falls within the sensory territory of the femoral nerve in the thigh (Fig. 16.6). This establishes a combined, severe sensory loss referable to a proximal lesion of the femoral nerve.

Other functions affected?

The next step is to compare the sensory deficit with abnormalities, if any, in other domains: are there local or regional motor, reflex, or autonomic alterations? If you now find very weak quadriceps function and an absent knee jerk, a review of the anatomy will confirm the diagnosis of a femoral nerve lesion. An L4 root lesion would show some similarities, but the deficits would not be profound or well demarcated, because of the complementary role of adjacent nerve roots (see Tables 16.2 and 16.3). A partial femoral nerve lesion might be harder to differentiate, but can be done clinically and by electromyography (EMG).

A BRIEF GUIDE TO SELECTIVE MUSCLE TESTING

Isolated muscle testing

The key to testing a particular muscle is to isolate its function as much as possible. To recall an example used in Chapter 6, if you wish to test the biceps in the arm, you should stabilize the upper arm with one hand while pulling on the forearm. Position the forearm (in supination) so as to maximize the contribution to flexion by the biceps *vis-à-vis* the contribution of the brachioradialis muscle. To differentiate further the roles of different muscles with closely allied function, palpate each muscle as the patient exerts resistance. For example, while testing forearm flexion, palpate the biceps and brachioradialis (you will not be able to distinguish the brachialis).

In using the following lists, remember that each root contributes to the innervation of more than one muscle; testing the muscles listed helps

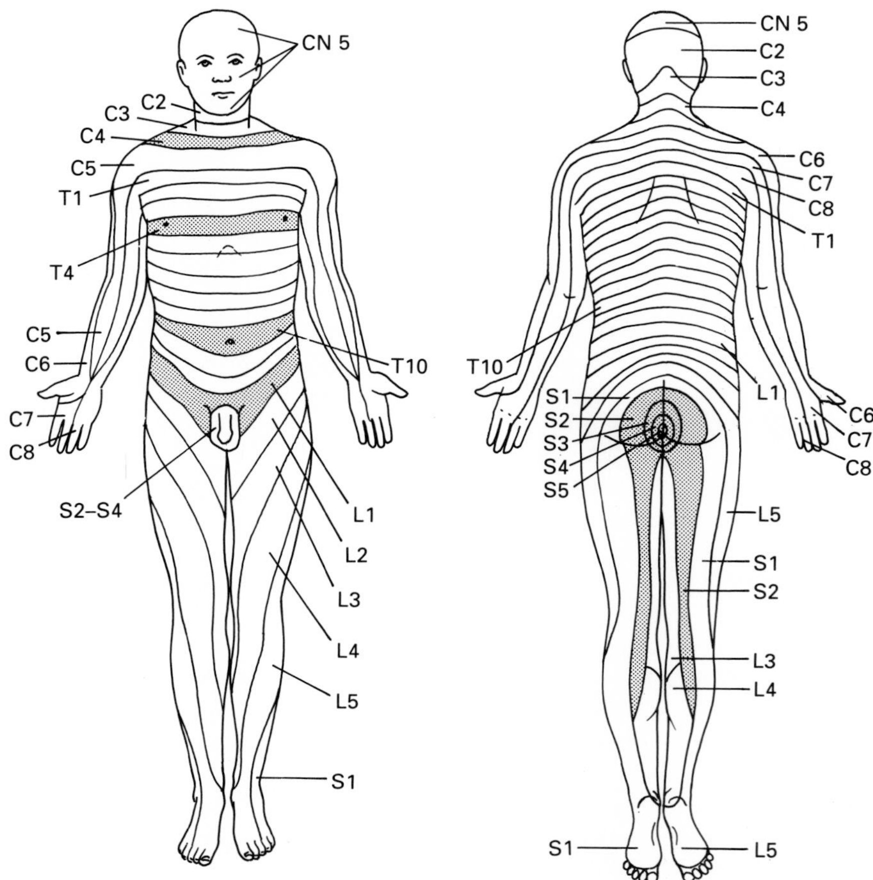

Fig. 16.1 Dermatomes, anterior and posterior views. Different dermatome charts vary considerably, mainly depending on the type of data used in construction. See text regarding the relation of dermatomal stripes to actual posterior root sensory territories. Note that there is no C1 dermatome. C4 is in the "shoulder pad" area. T1 and T2 demarcate the upper extremity from lower dermatomes appearing only on the chest and back. T4 is at the nipple line and T10 at the umbilicus. L1 is at the groin, separating pelvis from thigh. S2–S5 posteriorly represent the "saddle area."

Fig. 16.2 (*opposite*) Posterior roots, spinal nerves, and peripheral nerves. (a) Three adjacent thoracic posterior nerve roots enter spinal (intercostal) nerves which distribute in overlapping fashion to the abdomen (not represented anatomically). Loss of any one root alters sensation but does not cause total anesthesia in overlapped areas. (b) Three adjacent posterior roots L4, L5, and S1 are shown in this schematic diagram to contribute to the common peroneal nerve. (The anterior roots and lumbosacral plexus are not depicted.) Because of distribution of root fibers in the plexus, the fibers of L4, for example, are found in both the common peroneal nerve and the saphenous nerve (from the femoral). Adjacent roots overlap, so that severance of one entire root usually does not produce a band of complete sensory loss. In contrast, severance of a peripheral nerve, such as the common peroneal, produces total sensory loss in a central "autonomous zone." This occurs because the L5 dermatome and perhaps small

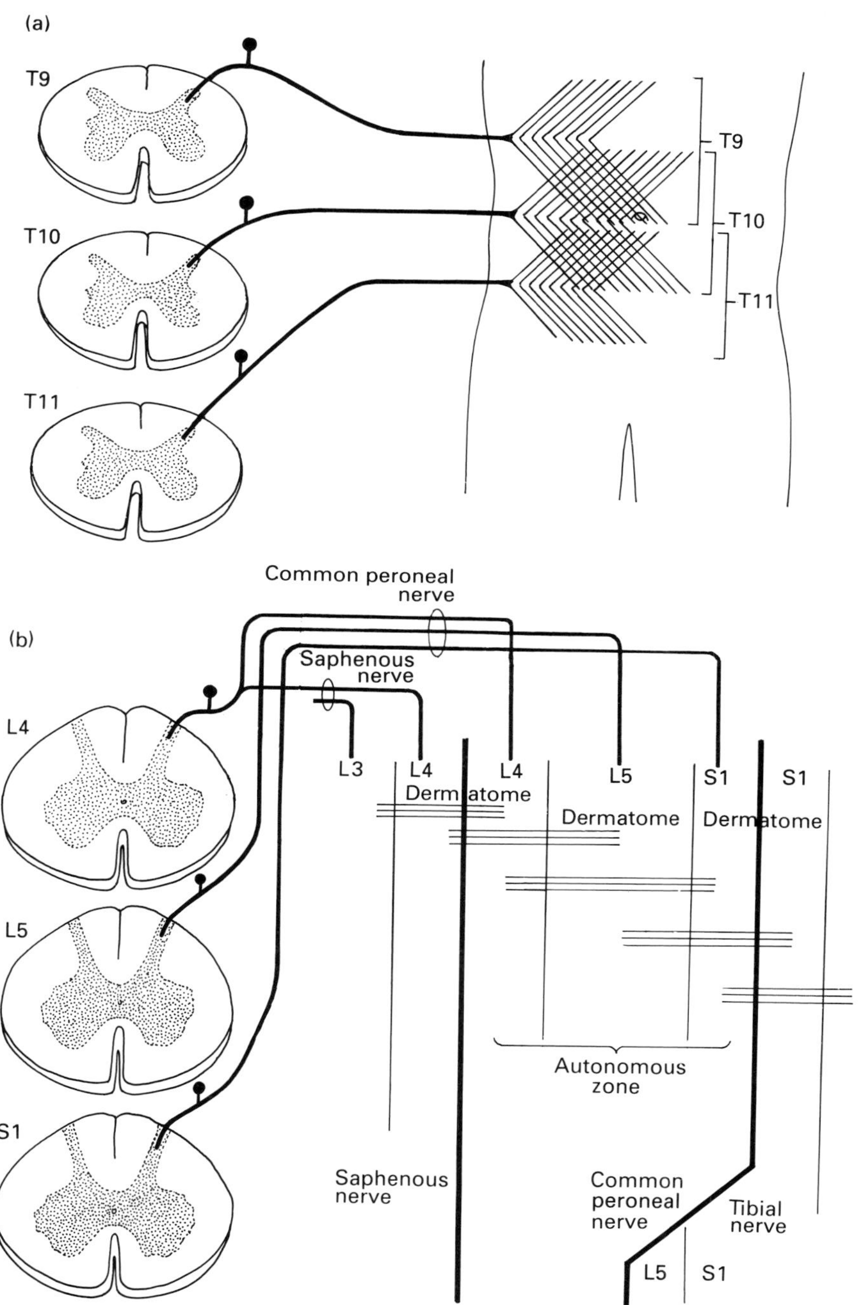

adjacent parts of L4 and S1 contained within the peroneal territory are not overlapped by L4 from the saphenous and S1 from the tibial. Note that contributions of different roots are not uniform throughout a peripheral nerve territory, as suggested by the appearance of L5 in only part of the tibial territory. (For the actual peripheral nerve territories, see Fig. 16.5.)

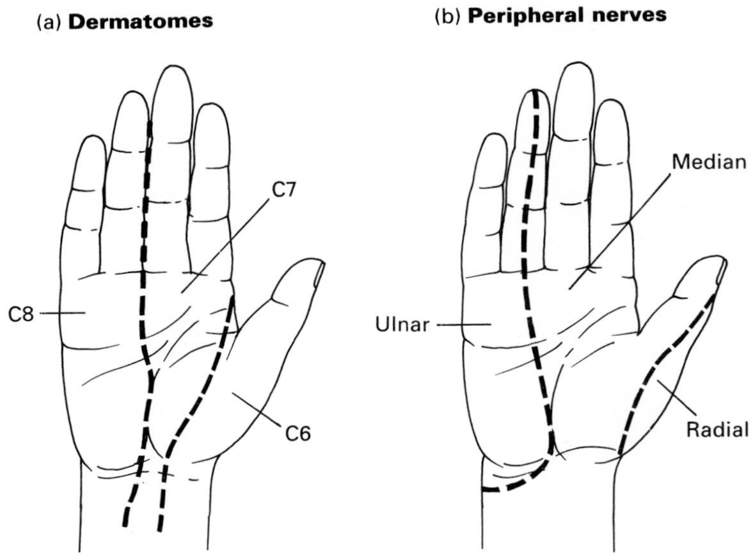

Fig. 16.3 Peripheral nerve sensory territories and dermatomes: The hand. On the palmar aspect note the differences between the part of the C6 dermatome shown in (a) and the small radial nerve territory on the thumb (shown in (b)). The C8 vs. ulnar territories are further depicted in Fig. 16.4.

Root-oriented testing

with initial screening for a given root. For roots C5–T1, and L4–S1 the following motor tests are suggested (but note that in most instances a single root does not innervate the muscle exclusively):

C5 root (C4–C5 interspace)	Deltoid muscle (C5, C6); abduction of the arm (at 60–90° from trunk)
C6 root (C5–C6 interspace)	Biceps (and brachialis) muscles (C5, C6); forearm flexion in supinated or semisupinated position
C7 root (C6–7 interspace)	Triceps (C7, C8); forearm extension
C8 root (C7–T1 interspace)	Ulnar flexor of the wrist (C7, C8, T1)
T1 root (T1–T2 interspace)	Abductor of the 5th finger (C8, T1)
L4 root (exits L4–L5 interspace) (see text that follows)	Anterior tibial muscle (L4, L5); dorsiflexion of the foot
L5 root (L5–S1 interspace)	Extensor of the great toe (L5, S1)
S1 root (fused bony sacral segments)	Gastrocnemius (S1) – soleus (S2); plantar flexion of the foot

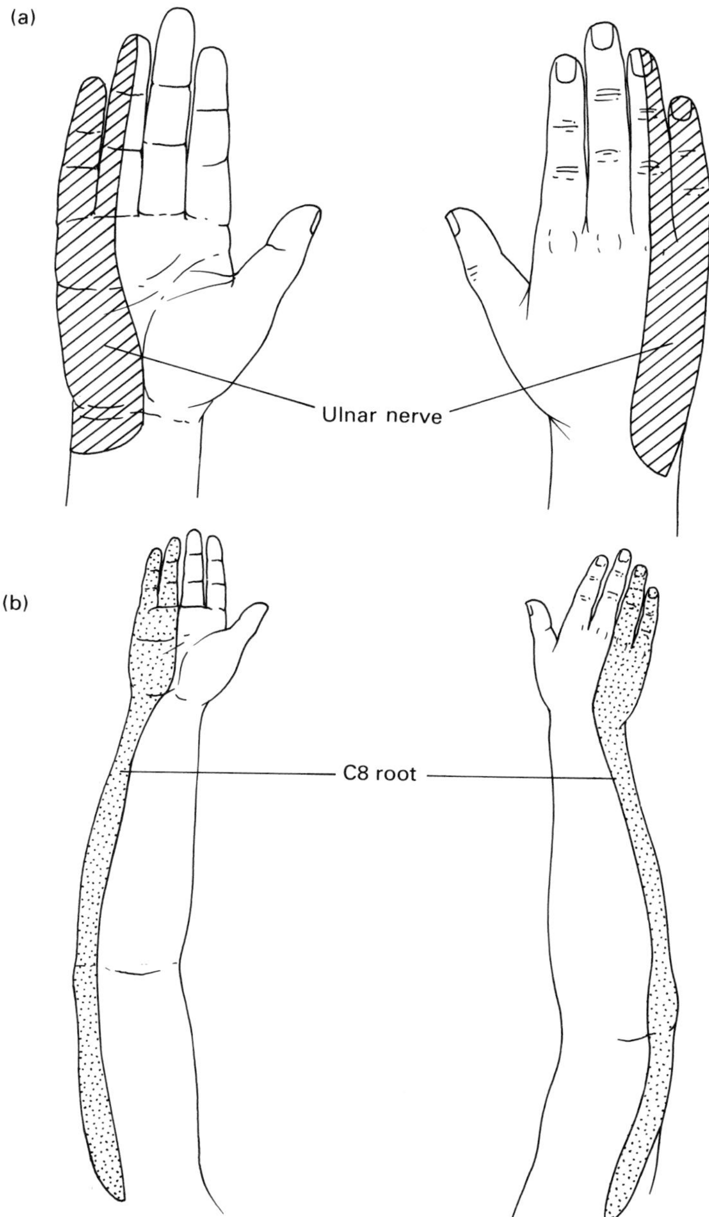

Fig. 16.4 Ulnar nerve sensory distribution vs. C8 dermatome. (a) The ulnar nerve territory includes the 5th finger and the adjacent half of the 4th finger. The ulnar nerve territory is limited to the hand. (b) The C8 dermatome includes all of the 4th and 5th fingers and extends up the forearm and arm. Note that fibers of C8 are distributed to both the ulnar and adjacent median nerves, with the C8 fibers in the ulnar nerve innervating the ulnar half of the 4th finger and the C8 fibers included in the median nerve innervating the other half, adjacent to the middle finger.

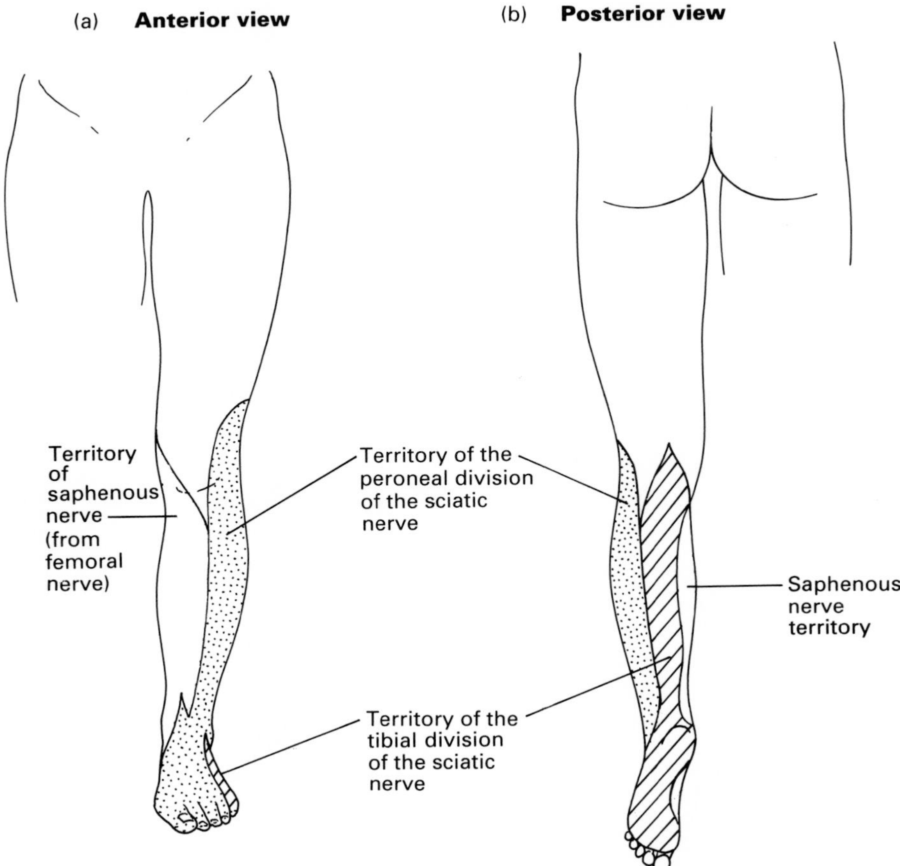

Fig. 16.5 Sensory territories of the peroneal and tibial divisions of the sciatic nerve. (a) In the anterior view the territory of the sciatic nerve as a whole (peroneal and tibial divisions together) appears almost identical to the territory of the peroneal division alone (the common peroneal and its branches). They are distinguished by noting the thin strip along the lateral aspect of the foot which is innervated by the sural nerve from the tibial division. (b) The posterior aspect reveals the large additional territory of tibial nerve branches on the sole of the foot and posterior leg.

As noted in Chapter 13, in lumbosacral disc disease the nerve root affected is typically not impinged by the disc at the root's interspace of "exit," but by a protruding (herniated) disc at the next higher level. The L4 root is usually affected by an L3–L4 disc, the L5 root by an L4–L5 disc, and the S1 root by an L5–S1 disc. The L5 root, for example, is impinged as it passes the L4–L5 interspace, after which it moves laterally to exit at L5–S1 (where it could also be impinged). However, the S1 root must be affected by an L5–S1 (or higher) disc, as there is no disc within the fused sacrum.

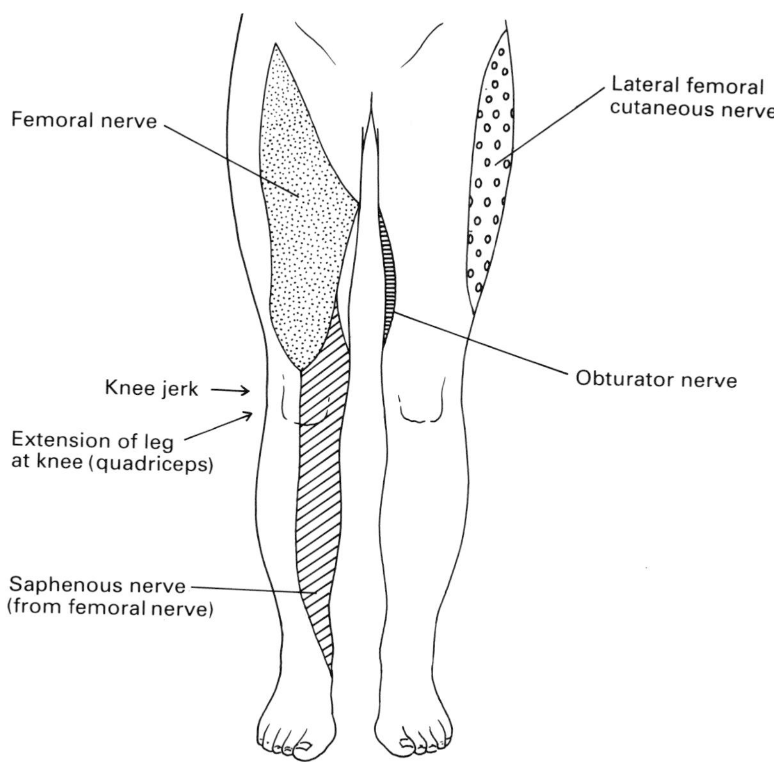

Fig. 16.6 Sensory territories of the femoral nerve vs. the lateral cutaneous nerve of the thigh. The femoral nerve territory in the thigh is mainly anterior; on the leg the distribution of the saphenous nerve (a large sensory branch of the femoral nerve) is medial and anterior. In contrast, a lesion of the lateral cutaneous nerve of the thigh (a purely sensory nerve, mainly from L2 root) causes a patch of sensory alteration on the lateral thigh (the syndrome of meralgia paresthetica). (For further distinction, test extension of the knee (quadriceps) and the knee jerk – both served by the femoral nerve.)

Nerve-oriented testing

Table 16.4 summarizes key muscles for screening tests of the major peripheral nerves (Figs 16.7, 16.8, 16.9, 16.10); which muscles are involved depends on the location of the lesion along the course of the nerve.

A STRATEGY FOR MOTOR DIAGNOSIS

Hypothesize a particular nerve

1 Based upon your initial muscle testing and review of the innervation of the weak muscles, postulate a lesion in a specific peripheral nerve (Table 16.5). As a rule, only one peripheral nerve innervates a single muscle in the limbs or limb girdles. But a given nerve root enters more than one peripheral nerve and, hence, innervates more than one muscle. For example, a failure of biceps function in the face of strong brachio-

Table 16.4 Key muscles for screening tests of the major peripheral nerves

Peripheral nerve	Key muscle and action	Root innervation
Median	Opponens (opposition of the thumb); short abductor of the thumb (abductor pollicis brevis, APB); flexor of distal phalanx, index finger	C8, T1
Ulnar	Abductor of the 5th finger (see Fig. 16.8); 1st dorsal interosseus – adduction of thumb and index finger	C7, C8, T1 C8, T1
Radial	Extensors of the thumb (see Fig. 16.9); radial extensors of the wrist; triceps (forearm extension)	C7, C8 C6, C7, C8 C7, C8
Musculocutaneous	Biceps (forearm flexion and supination)	C5, C6
Axillary	Deltoid (arm abduction, tested in abducted position)	C5, (C6)
Femoral	Quadriceps (extension of leg at knee)	(L2), L3, L4
Obturator	Adductor group (adduction of thigh)	L2, L3, L4
Sciatic:		
(posterior) tibial nerve	Gastrocnemius (plantar flexion of foot); posterior tibial muscle (inversion of foot)	L5, S1, S2 L5, S1
Common peroneal		
anterior tibial nerve (deep peroneal)	Anterior tibial muscle (dorsiflexion of foot) (see Fig. 16.10); extension of great toe	L4, (L5), (S1) L5, (S1)
superficial peroneal	Peroneal group (eversion of foot)	(L4), L5, S1

radialis contraction would suggest a lesion of the musculocutaneous nerve (C5, C6) which innervates the biceps but not the brachioradialis. A lesion in the radial nerve, which innervates the brachioradialis muscle (C5, C6), would be ruled out. Even a partial lesion in the C5 or C6 nerve roots themselves (before the lateral cord of the brachial plexus and musculocutaneous nerve), would be unlikely in the face of intact strength of the brachioradialis muscle.

Hypothesize a specific root

2 Postulate a lesion in one or more nerve roots. In the case of partial weakening of abduction of the arm, the lesion might be in the C5 anterior nerve root. This hypothesis would be supported if not only deltoid action were affected but also abduction in the first 30° from the side (supraspinatus muscle, C5, C6 from the superior trunk of the brachial plexus). (C5 also innervates the rhomboids and contributes to many other muscles.) Also, the proximal C5 nerve root innervates paraspinal muscles in the neck; denervation of these muscles can be detected by EMG

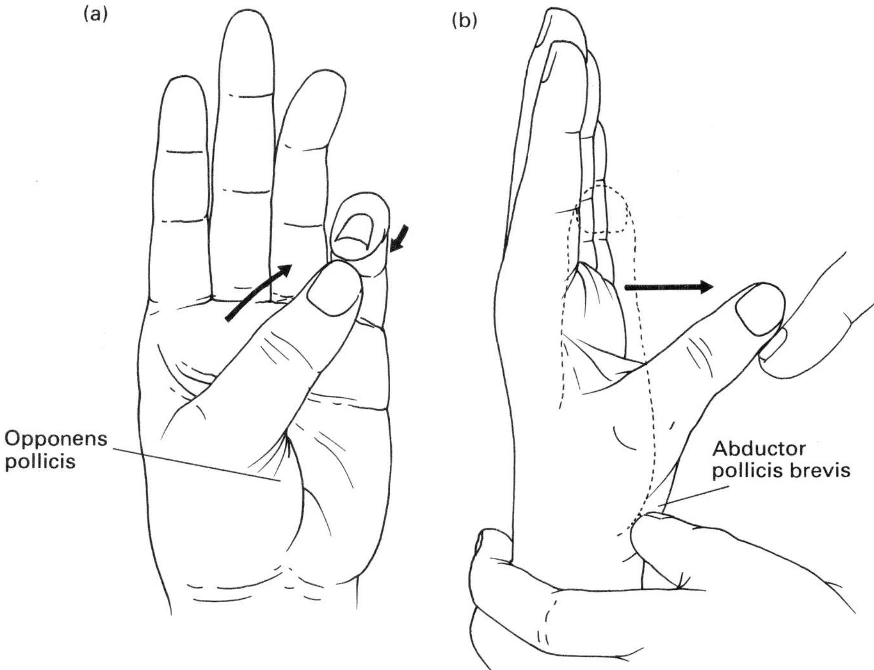

Fig. 16.7 Tests for median nerve motor function within the hand. (a) The thumb is shown in forceful opposition to 5th finger, mainly due to contraction of the opponens pollicis muscle. (b) Abduction of the thumb (out from the palm) is resisted by the examiner while the abductor pollicis brevis muscle (short abductor of the thumb) in the thenar eminence is palpated.

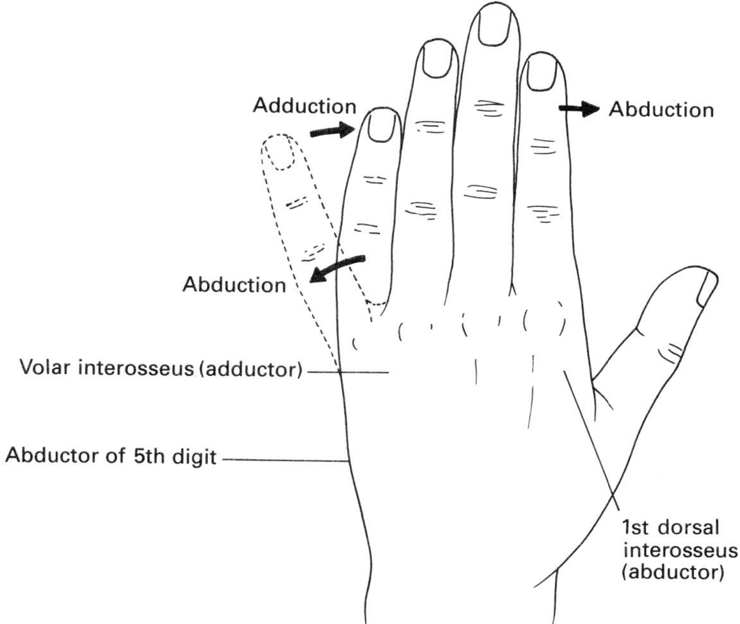

Fig. 16.8 Tests for ulnar motor function within the hand. Resistance against abduction of the 5th finger (abductor muscle of the 5th digit) or against adduction (volar interosseus) are good screening tests for distal ulnar motor function. In general, abduction and adduction are defined in relation to the middle finger, away from it or in, toward it, respectively.

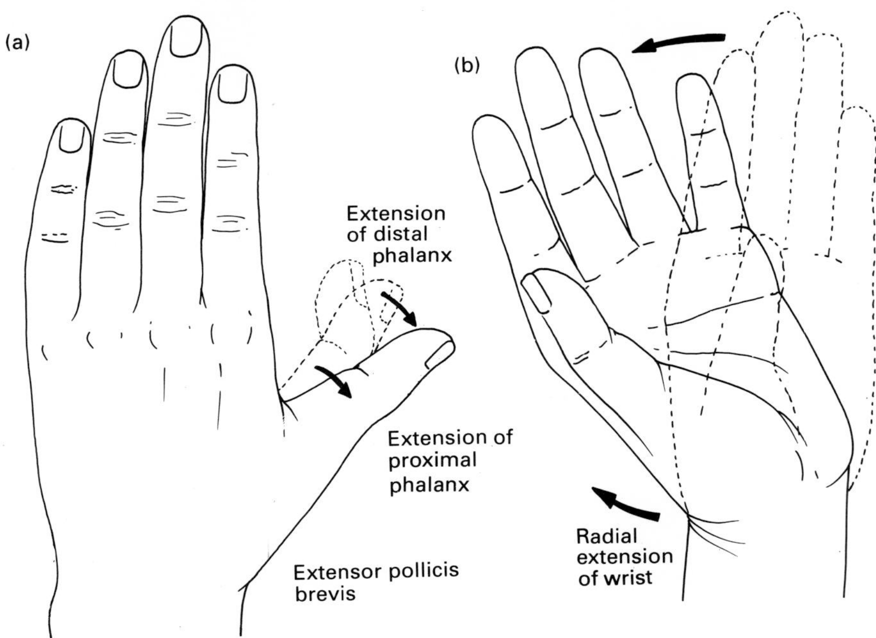

Fig. 16.9 Testing of radial nerve-innervated muscles acting on the thumb and hand. (a) The short and long extensors of the thumb (extensor pollicis brevis and longus) act on the proximal and distal phalanges of the thumb, respectively. (b) Radial extension (dorsiflexion) of the hand is accomplished mainly by extensor carpi radialis longus and brevis.

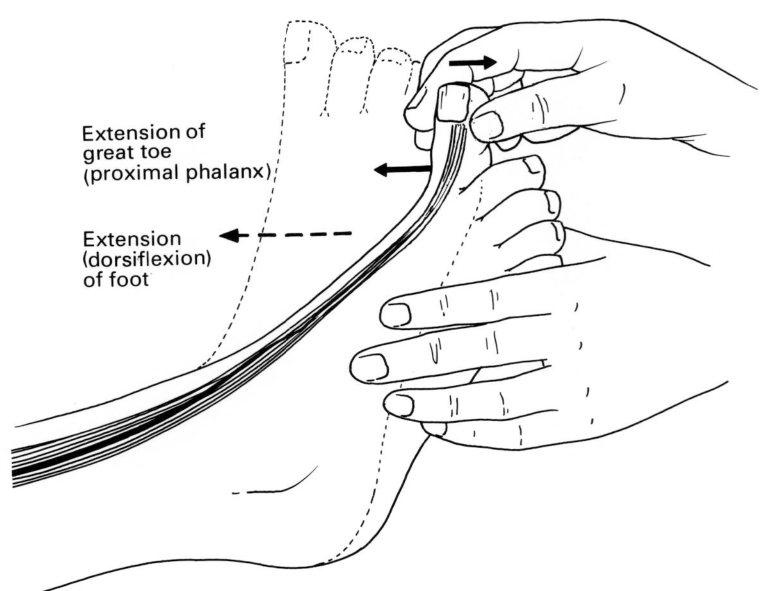

Fig. 16.10 Testing for extension (dorsiflexion) of the foot and great toe (proximal phalanx). Both these functions are innervated by the deep peroneal (anterior tibial) nerve from the common peroneal (see Table 16.4).

Table 16.5 Common mononeuropathies

Upper extremities	
Shoulder/arm	Radial neuropathy: the classic radial neuropathy is due to injury (such as fracture of the humerus) or compression. If damaged high enough on the arm, the triceps and brachioradialis muscles and triceps reflex may be affected. The most striking motor deficit is a "wrist drop" and inability to extend the fingers fully. Sensory loss occurs in the dorsal forearm and hand, including web area of the dorsal hand (deep radial nerve territory)
Elbow/forearm	Ulnar neuropathy: injury from fracture, bruising or chronic compression commonly occurs at the elbow ("funny bone"). Affected muscles controlling the fingers are "intrinsics" (muscles with origin and insertion within the hand itself). Sensory deficit in 5th digit, adjacent half of 4th digit, and ulnar (medial) aspect of hand (see Figs 16.3 and 16.4). Injury and compression also occur at the wrist
Wrist/hand	Median neuropathy (distal): most common site is the carpal tunnel (wrist): main weakness in thenar eminence (see Fig. 16.3); sensory loss mostly in palmar aspect of the first three and a half digits, and extending onto palm
Lower extremities	
Hip/thigh	Meralgia paresthetica: numbness in the distribution of the lateral cutaneous nerve of the thigh (L1, L2) (see Fig. 16.6)
	Sciatica: sciatic mononeuropathy results from trauma, compression, etc., but symptoms of "sciatica" usually signify a radiculopathy involving one of the roots of the sciatic nerve, most often L5 or S1 (see Fig. 19.1, regarding low back/leg pain)"
	Femoral neuropathy: occurs with trauma, hemorrhage into the femoral sheath (as in bleeding disorders), or in diabetes, etc. (see Fig. 16.6)
Knee/leg	Peroneal palsy: the common peroneal nerve, one of two main divisions of the sciatic nerve (see Fig. 16.5), is often compressed as it winds around the fibular head; sensory loss over lateral leg and dorsum of foot; foot drop and weak eversion. (Note that the common term "foot drop" – like "wrist drop" – does not imply total paralysis, and may be just the most obvious component of more extensive weakness)

testing. The axillary nerve, which carries fibers of C5 and C6 to the deltoid does not innervate the supraspinatus (or rhomboid muscles), and thus would not be the site of the lesion. Of course, the distribution and severity of sensory loss would also be a factor in differentiating a lesion of a mixed peripheral nerve vs. a lesion of one or more roots.

Segmental CNS vs. PNS

3 Establish whether the lesion is in the PNS or the CNS part of the segmental organization. In the example of biceps weakness, the lesion was in the peripheral nerve, and therefore obviously in the PNS. In contrast, if it had been possible only to localize the deficit to the C5 and C6 segments, but not to a particular peripheral nerve, the lesion could theoretically have been in the CNS component of segmental organization: the spinal cord gray matter at the C5 and C6 cord segments. Focal CNS segmental lesions occur rarely by comparison with PNS lesions. In segmental (lower motor neuron, LMN) disease or injury, fasciculations and neurogenic atrophy may appear, but will not be seen acutely.

Exclude suprasegmental patterns

4 After looking for positive evidence of a segmental lesion, you should also try to exclude any abnormality in the suprasegmental part of the CNS pathways. The biceps and brachioradialis muscles, mentioned in an example given above, mainly serve forearm flexion. An upper motor neuron (UMN) lesion would affect not only these muscles, but would also usually affect to some degree neighboring muscle groups innervated by several different root derivations and peripheral nerve trunks. Therefore, when motor testing identifies a weak muscular action, always examine other groups for signs of a more extensive distribution, even if more subtle in degree. Correlate with other UMN signs, such as hyperreflexia and increased tone.

Sensory, reflex, autonomic changes?

5 As will be elaborated subsequently, look for evidence of abnormality in other neural systems – sensory, reflex, and autonomic (skin temperature and color, sweating, skin wrinkling with prolonged submersion, etc.).

COMMON FEATURES OF PNS DISORDERS

PNS signs and symptoms come in diverse packages: focal or diffuse; root or nerve; single or multiple; partial or complete. Localization of these deficits may not be as obvious in patients as they are on paper. Nonetheless, the following common features (which are not criteria of PNS disease and not necessarily peripheral) should arouse strong suspicion of PNS pathology.

Well-demarcated, focal sensory deficits

1 Striking focality, as in a well-demarcated sensory deficit, on only one side of the body, involving no more than a small number of contiguous segments. To illustrate, an ulnar nerve lesion at the elbow causes a circumscribed sensory loss in the 5th digit and adjacent aspect of the 4th, and that side of the hand (see Fig. 16.4). Ulnar sensory fibers in the hand are mainly from C8 root, with some overlap from C7 and T1. In contrast, an extensive deficit involving arm and leg, or arm and face, is very unlikely to be due to peripheral lesions.

Dense, focal sensory loss

2 Severe sensory loss to pin and touch in a focal distribution. The dense deficit usually corresponds to the autonomous zone of a peripheral nerve territory in which there is no overlap from fibers of adjacent peripheral nerves.

3 Segmental motor signs (LMN signs) in a limited distribution on one side. Circumscribed weakness and neurogenic atrophy, with or without fasciculations, are quite likely to represent a PNS lesion, although focal disease of anterior horn cells on just one side does occasionally occur.

Focal lower motor neuron signs

4 An isolated decrease or absence of a deep tendon reflex (DTR). It may be hard to know whether a depressed reflex is the abnormal one or whether the reflex on the other side is abnormally increased. If only one reflex is decreased, it is likely to be abnormal. Two points of potential confusion: acute suprasegmental lesions (e.g. stroke) may be associated with decreased reflexes on the weak side of the body; a normal or decreased reflex, even chronically, never completely rules out a suprasegmental (UMN) process.

Isolated deep tendon reflex loss

5 Symmetric depression or loss of reflexes (DTRs). Especially if worse in the lower extremities and worse distally, this pattern suggests a polyneuropathy (or polyradiculopathy, see below).

Bilateral reflex loss

6 Persistent or recurrent limb pain that outweighs any mild tenderness or aggravation by gentle joint action. Radiculopathies involving a single root declare themselves more through symptoms than signs – more through pain than sensory loss. The pattern of pain and paresthesias is often so characteristic that it suffices for diagnosis, as illustrated in Chapter 19 for a lumbosacral radiculopathy. In some cases, the distribution remains ambiguous, thereby requiring clues from motor or reflex changes, if present, to pin down the exact root. From the standpoint of the usual conservative therapy, accurate root identification holds little importance, but is essential for establishing the relevance of imaged lesions. Radiculopathic or neuropathic pain is often burning, electric, or focally aching. Jolting or "electric-shock" radiation ("lancination") is characteristic, if present, but it need not be. Sources of visceral, bone, or joint pain should, of course, be excluded. In contrast, lesions limited to the CNS (except the thalamus) usually do not directly cause persistent pain, save for associated headache or spinal ache arising from vessels and meninges. Secondary discomfort from CNS lesions (resulting from spasticity, rigidity, immobility, and autonomic reactions) is rarely as well defined as radicular pain.

Limb pain

7 Bilateral symmetry of sensory, reflex and/or motor deficits in the lower extremities, with a distal (worse than) proximal gradient of severity. Since CNS lesions, especially of the spinal cord, can sometimes mimic this pattern, you should take pains to exclude any suprasegmental signs (see Chapter 14). Extension of any lower extremity PNS deficit onto the trunk is very unusual and should raise a red flag. Similarly, bladder, bowel, or sexual dysfunction rarely occurs with PNS lesions, except for diabetic autonomic neuropathy and the cauda equina syndrome of intraspinal, multiple lumbosacral root involvement.

Symmetric, distal deficits (polyneuropathic pattern)

NONFOCAL DEFICITS: POLYNEUROPATHY AND MULTIRADICULOPATHY

As you have seen, a distinction between focal and diffuse pathology divides PNS disorders. Focal or diffuse pathology should be distinguished from focal or diffuse deficits. Diffuse pathology, if fully expressed, always produces diffuse deficits (as in polyneuropathy). Focal pathology usually results in focal deficits. However, widespread symptoms and signs are occasionally encountered. This occurs only under special anatomic circumstances.

Focal pathology, multifocal deficits

The prime example of a focal PNS lesion causing widespread signs is the cauda equina syndrome. The multiple lumbosacral roots hang down within the lumbar meninges, each root descending to the appropriate level of "exit." This "horse's tail" (Fig. 13.9) of roots is vulnerable to compression, which produces extensive sensory, motor, and reflex impairment in the lower extremities and pelvic region. Focal pathology in a plexus, such as the brachial or lumbosacral plexus, also manifests a multifocal pattern of deficits. However, unlike the cauda equina syndrome, structural plexus lesions (as from tumor) are usually unilateral, because of the spatial separation between right and left. These deficits, are, in fact, multifocal rather than evenly symmetric, as is connoted by "diffuse."

Multifocal pathology and deficits

More often, multifocal signs result from multiple pathologic lesions that may share a common etiologic basis: for example, multiple root impingement (as from multiple intervertebral disc herniations) or multiple mononeuropathies (mononeuropathy multiplex). The net effect of multifocal lesions can, in the extreme, mimic a diffuse process like polyneuropathy.

Characteristics of polyneuropathies

Polyneuropathy: diffuse pathology and deficits

Whereas the defining characteristic of focal deficits is first of all anatomic, the basis of polyneuropathies is found in the pathogenesis: the development of disease depends upon a susceptibility of certain nerves, such as long nerves, myelinated nerves, etc. Thus, when a patient complains about diffuse symptoms such as numbness in the lower legs and feet on both sides, you may find a topographic pattern of neurologic signs that is quite distinct from the focal patterns caused by individual peripheral nerve or root lesions.

The following features characterize most polyneuropathies (so-called axonal polyneuropathies).

Shaded sensory boundaries

1 The sensory deficits in polyneuropathies (and diffuse polyradiculopathies) are harder to demarcate than in mononeuropathies. The area of sensory impairment does not conform to specific dermatomal or peripheral nerve distribution borders (Fig. 16.11).

Symmetric deficits

2 Since the deficits are bilaterally symmetric, you will not be able to rely

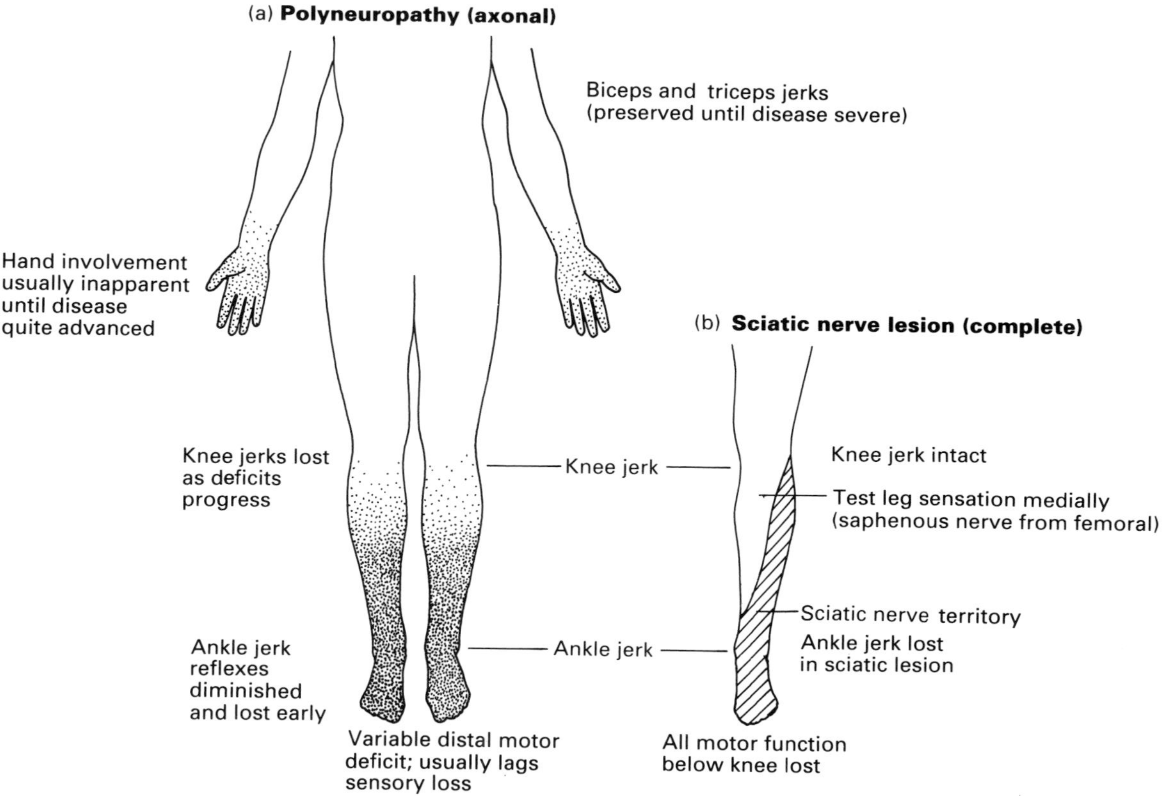

Fig. 16.11 Polyneuropathy vs. sciatic nerve lesion(s). (a) The common term "stocking and glove distribution" (for the sensory loss of axonal polyneuropathies) is memorable, but the actual boundaries proximally are shaded, not abrupt as in the articles of clothing. (b) Deficits due to a complete lesion of the sciatic nerve (shown on one side, but bilateral lesions also occur). From the anterior aspect, the main distinction from a "stocking" loss is on the anteromedial aspect of the leg (innervated by the saphenous nerve, a branch of the femoral nerve). Polyneuropathies are by definition bilateral and quite symmetric.

on the right–left comparisons which in other situations help to establish a subtle deficit (Fig. 16.11).

Multimodality (but variable effects)

3 Polyneuropathies (and polyradiculopathies) like mononeuropathies, usually involve multiple sensory modalities, but polyneuropathies commonly show marked disparities among them in degree of impairment. Different fiber sizes and degrees of myelination form the basis of selective vulnerability in some disease models. Many polyneuropathies are mainly sensory, at least until very severe, and a few are primarily motor. Some affect large fibers predominantly, so that decreased touch–position–vibration senses predominate over blunting of pain–temperature sensations. Polyneuropathies involving small, poorly myelinated fibers are also occasionally seen.

Distal–proximal gradient

4 Most polyneuropathies are of the axonal or "dying back" type: the ends of the longest nerves are affected first and foremost. Impaired axonal transport of needed constituents to the distal nerves probably accounts for this pattern. Therefore, deficits progress well up the legs before the hands become involved, and it is only in the most severe cases that intercostal and cranial nerves are clinically involved.

Distal sensory pattern

Sensory changes show a typical distal–proximal gradient (see Fig. 16.11). Note that the distal–proximal gradient does not correspond to the numeric order of dermatomes. While the S1 and L5 distributions are most distal, the progression of a deficit from distal to proximal reflects the length of the nerves, not the dermatomes, which are mainly oriented vertically on the extremities. Thus, the distal part of L4 territory is affected before the most proximal part of L5 territory. And the "lowest" sacral dermatomes of S3, S4, S5 are served by very short nerves to the perineum – which is therefore rarely affected in a polyneuropathy.

Distal areas, not lowest dermatomal numbers

Distal weakness (if any)

Motor involvement, if present, does not adhere to particular root or nerve innervations. Weakness tends to follow a distal–proximal gradient without extreme differences among muscles that are equally large and equally distal.

DTRs sensitive to afferent pathology

5 Because of the distal to proximal gradient that is characteristic of axonal polyneuropathies, DTRs are affected along the same gradient, but not paralleling sensory or motor signs in degree of change. Most polyneuropathies involve fibers serving the afferent segment of the reflex arc. Polyneuropathies may be manifest by loss of ankle jerks, knee jerks, or even all DTRs – despite only modest distal sensory loss and possibly no overt weakness at all.

Focal neuropathy, focal reflex loss

In contrast, focal damage to a root or nerve only affects a reflex if that particular root or nerve serves the reflex. A focal lesion of the sciatic nerve or of the S1 root may depress or abolish the ankle jerk, but will leave the contralateral ankle jerk and both knee jerks intact. A lesion of the L5 nerve root, which is not a major contributor to the ankle jerk (or to the knee jerk), typically remains "silent" from the point of view of these standard reflex tests.

MUSCLE DISORDERS

Muscles constitute the end-organs of the entire LMN system. Since they enable all movement, they express all active behavior. In terms of the suprasegmental/segmental concept of neural organization, muscles obviously fall on the segmental side of the divide. They are activated by LMNs and dependent on neurotrophic factors, but survive (albeit in a state of disuse atrophy) without neural stimulation.

Neurogenic vs. myopathic

Disorders of muscles have traditionally been divided into those that are neurogenic, deriving from impaired LMN innervation, and those that are non-neurogenic, i.e. myopathic (see Table 16.1). Some of these myopathies develop as a manifestation of a systemic disease acting on muscles without affecting their nerve supply. Others, like the inherited muscular dystrophies, are truly primary to muscle. Refer to Chapter 6 regarding the inspection and palpation of muscles.

LMN (anterior horn cell, root, nerve) disorders declare themselves through several aspects of muscular function and structure: weakness, neurogenic atrophy, and often fasciculations. In contrast, through much of the course of disease, non-neurogenic muscle pathology is revealed almost exclusively through weakness. Non-neurogenic atrophy and reflex changes tend to lag behind the development of weakness, and thus are typically not profound until relatively late in the course of a muscle disease. Most myopathies, as well as syndromes of the neuromuscular junction (NMJ), manifest symmetric weakness that affects neck or cranial musculature and proximal limb muscles more than distal muscles (one of the exceptions being myotonic dystrophy). Thus, a clinical profile of the prototypic myopathy includes the following: lack of sensory loss, no atrophy or depression of reflex activity early on, and weakness (without neurogenic features) that is generally symmetric and usually predominant proximally. EMG testing confirms the differentiation from neurogenic muscle disorders.

ELECTROPHYSIOLOGIC DIAGNOSIS OF NERVE AND MUSCLE DISORDERS

In the Further reading section of the last chapter, references are given to summaries of nerve conduction and EMG testing. New techniques of magnetic stimulation have thus far been applied mainly to the brain. However, proximal motor roots can also be evaluated by stimulation over spinal cord segments. The common factor among these tests is that they are functional rather than structural. Even the rapidly developing field of magnetic resonance imaging and spectroscopy (not to be confused with magnetic stimulation) has not as yet achieved major clinical impact in extraspinal problems of the PNS. The goal of obtaining integrated structural and physiologic data on peripheral nerve disorders remains to be fulfilled.

In summary, it is fair to say that electrophysiologic testing is sometimes ordered excessively and poorly planned, but such investigation in the appropriate case can make a decisive contribution. It has the capability of revealing or confirming the location and category of PNS, NMJ, and myopathic disorders, including the following:

1 localizing focal peripheral nerve and root lesions, such as those resulting from trauma, entrapment, or disc compression (of spinal roots);

2 detecting or confirming a polyneuropathy;

3 distinguishing axonal neuropathies from demyelinating neuropathies (in which marked slowing of nerve conduction velocities is a hallmark);

4 differentiating neurogenic muscle disorders from primary myopathies;
5 characterizing certain types of neuromuscular junction (NMJ) or muscle disorders (such as myasthenia gravis and polymyositis, respectively) which are medically treatable;
6 providing confirmation of acute polyradiculopathy/polyneuritis (such as the Guillain–Barré syndrome, which represents a life-threatening but treatable emergency).

PROBLEMS FOR SELF-STUDY

Problems

1 Numbness in the thumb of the right hand, as well as intermittent shooting pains in the forearm, represent the presenting symptoms. What additional data would you want in order to evaluate the initial diagnosis of a right C6 radiculopathy?
2 A diabetic patient is said to have no motion, feeling, or reflexes below the knee on the right. Since that distribution is presumed to be nonanatomic, the diagnosis of hysteria is entertained. What particular aspect(s) of the examination would you like to check?
3 A 33-year-old alcoholic male is said to have a "stocking–glove" sensory loss. Is this term a misnomer or a good descriptor of the sensory deficit in a polyneuropathy?

Comments

1 A C6 radiculopathy in the neck may cause pain shooting through the arm or forearm and numbness in the thumb. If C6 is sufficiently affected, the biceps or brachioradialis reflexes might be diminished, and C6-innervated musculature might be weakened. However, an alternative explanation would be a partial carpal tunnel syndrome involving the median nerve. Although sensory and motor deficits are entirely in the hand, pain may be experienced more proximally. A careful review of sensory symptoms and testing might show involvement of more of the typical territory – the first three and a half digits. Any weakness will be limited to intrinsic muscles of the hand, such as the opponens (opposition of the thumb) and abductor pollicis brevis (see Fig. 16.7). If necessary, EMG/nerve conduction studies will settle the issue.
2 Since a severe lesion of the sciatic nerve trunk does cause paralysis below the knee (i.e. at the ankle and foot) and loss of the ankle jerk and plantar response, the sensory distribution is critical. The medial aspect of the leg is innervated by the saphenous nerve, the long, terminal sensory branch of the femoral nerve (Fig. 16.6). If the original examiner missed the sensory sparing of this area, then the findings are consistent with a sciatic trunk lesion (given some variability in the demarcation of the sciatic territory just below the knee). In a diabetic patient, ankle jerks are often absent (bilaterally) due to polyneuro-

pathy, so there might not be a left ankle jerk to contrast with the right one. Beware of facile presumptions of "nonanatomic" deficits!

3 Patients with axonal polyneuropathies that involve the longest nerves first and foremost do manifest a distal-worse-than-proximal sensory loss (see Fig. 16.11). As the deficit worsens, rising up the legs, it appears in the fingers and hands. The area of sensory impairment might suggest long stockings and short gloves at this point. The misleading aspect of the vivid "stocking–glove" image is the demarcation of abnormal from normal: in a polyneuropathy, this transition is shaded, not occurring suddenly, as the top of a stocking or glove implies.

FURTHER READING

Appenzeller, O. *The Autonomic Nervous System*. 4th edn. Elsevier, Amsterdam, 1990. A comprehensive reference source with enough information to put the serious reader in a sweat.

Bannister, R., Mathias, C.J. *Autonomic Failure*. 3rd edn. Oxford Medical Publishers, London, 1992. Another valuable, exhaustive reference text.

Brooke, M.H. *A Clinician's View of Neuromuscular Disease*. 2nd edn. Williams and Wilkins, Baltimore (MD), 1986. A practical and accessible approach to segmental neurologic and primary muscular disorders.

Dawson, D.M., Hallett, M., Millender, L.H. *Entrapment Neuropathies*. 2nd edn. Little, Brown, and Company, Boston (MA), 1990. Carpal tunnel and other entrapment or compression neuropathies qualify as neurologic disorders that virtually every practicing physician should know something about.

Dyck, P.J., Dyck, P.J.B., Chalk, C.H. The 10 P's: A mnemonic helpful in characterization and differential diagnosis of peripheral neuropathy. *Neurology* 1992; 42:14–18. Preferred points to promote probing of puzzling peripheral problems.

Dyck, P.J., Thomas, P.K., Griffin, J.W. *et al.* (eds) *Peripheral Neuropathy*. 3rd edn. WB Saunders, Philadelphia (PA), 1992. The most comprehensive general text on neuropathies.

Katz, J.N., Larson, M.G., Sabra, A., *et al*. The carpal tunnel syndrome: diagnostic utility of the history and physical examination findings. *Ann Int Med* 1990; 112: 321–7. Can symptoms and signs "make the diagnosis" or guide test-ordering decisions?

Medical Research Council of the UK. Aids to the examination of the peripheral nervous system. Memorandum 45. Pendragon House in North America, Palo Alto (CA). Reprinted by permission, Her Majesty's Stationery Office, 1976. An illustrated pamphlet on muscle and nerve testing for ready reference; I still keep my student copy in my medical bag.

McLeod, J.G., Tuck, R.R. Disorders of the autonomic nervous system. *Ann Neurol* 1987; 21:419–30, 519–29. A brief and understandable survey of this often intimidating subject.

Ropper, A.H. The Guillain–Barré syndrome. *N Engl J Med* 1992; 326:1130–6. Acute demyelinating polyneuropathy is a "don't miss" diagnosis.

Schaumburg, H.H., Berger, A.R., Thomas, P.K. *Disorders of Peripheral Nerves*. 2nd edn. F.A. Davis, Philadelphia (PA), 1992. A readable, informative, and updated shorter text.

Spinner, R.J., Bachman, J.W., Amadio P.C. The many faces of carpal tunnel syndrome. *Mayo Clin Proc* 1989; 64:829–36. A common and important syndrome viewed from the perspective of less common and atypical manifestations.

chapter

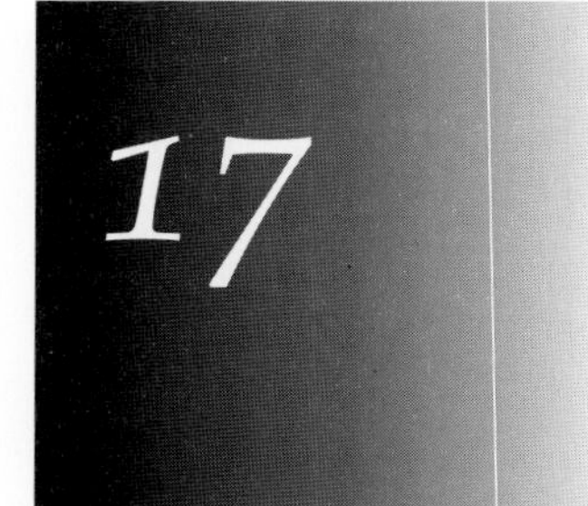

Eye Movements: Examining and Interpreting Abnormal Gaze

Introduction

A neurologist examining a patient who is stuporous, comatose, having a seizure, or showing signs of a stroke, usually looks at the eyes as soon as vital functions are assured. The assessment will include the position of the eyelids (are the eyes open, is there wakefulness), the pupils (their size, shape, and reactivity), and the position and movement of the eyes. The following sections of this chapter offer a guide to the examination of eye movements with emphasis on abnormal gaze, utilizing a simplified, practical schema that you should be able to reconstruct when you need to use it. (For pupillary function, see Chapter 5, section on CN 3, and Tables 5.5 and 5.6.)

Definitions

Gaze

Gaze is the position or direction of movement of the eyes as a unit. (If the patient cannot look up, we speak of a palsy of upward gaze. If the eyes remain pointed to the left, this is a left gaze deviation.) Gaze is organized as a conjugate activity of the eyes; their movement is yoked together, so that the eyes act in concert, whether or not they are looking at something. Gaze can be analyzed as an important clue to neurologic function, even when individual eye movements may be restricted. Thus, you should distinguish specific movement (or failure of movement) of an eye from the direction of gaze or attempted gaze. Horizontal gaze denotes gaze to one side or the other – in the horizontal plane. This is sometimes called lateral gaze to distinguish it from vertical gaze. However, lateral gaze should not be confused with simple abduction of one eye accomplished by action of one lateral rectus muscle.

Horizontal gaze

Lateral gaze

Individual eye movements

The mechanisms of individual eye movements – which nerves and muscles move an eye in a given direction – will be important for you to learn, but are not necessary for understanding gaze abnormalities. For the present purpose of analyzing horizontal gaze, just think of the lateral rectus muscle of one side and medial rectus of the other side as working in concert to achieve conjugate horizontal gaze to the right or left. (Refer back to Chapter 5 for a summary of individual eye movements.)

Overview of eye movement examination

There are three important steps in the initial approach to eye movements.

1 Articulate the goal of each component of the examination.

2 Make simple empirical observations. Do not be intimidated by potential problems of interpretation.

3 Start your analysis with simple rules that you can reconstruct from basic principles (see schema below). Do not depend on rote memory of mystifying correlations: "Let's see now, do the eyes look towards the lesion, or towards the hemiparesis?"

Sequence of evaluation

The objectives of the eye movement examination are to observe alignment, position, and movement. The following sequence of more specific questions should be asked and should guide the examination.

Alignment

1 Are the two eyes aligned at rest and with movement (conjugate)?

Position

2 What is their position (direction) of gaze at rest? Is there any deviation to one side?

Movement

3 Do the eyes move fully, in alignment, and without any adventitious (extraneous) movements superimposed? Do they move preferentially to one side?

Testing

1 Observe:

(a) the position of each eye and the direction of gaze at rest;

(b) spontaneous movements.

2 Instruct the patient to follow visually your finger or a light stimulus fully to right, left, up, down, and diagonally.

3 If you encounter any difficulty with following movements, request the patient to look in each direction: "look way over to the right," etc. (In this way you can confirm full eye movements even when vision is poor or absent.)

Abnormalities of horizontal gaze

In the course of these observations and maneuvers you will have determined whether the eyes are aligned at rest and move conjugately and whether there are any abnormal movements, such as nystagmus (see Chapter 5, sections on CNs 3, 4, 6, and 8). But for present purposes the main questions are whether there is a gaze deviation, a gaze preference, and/or difficulty in moving the eyes fully in any direction. Often these problems occur together: for example, a patient's eyes deviate slightly to the left at rest, they move more often to the left than to the right, and there is failure of complete gaze to the right. A gaze preference may occur for various reasons, including purely visual receptive ones: the visual environment on one side may be more interesting, as when you stand at one side of the patient's bed! The patient with a hemianopsia will gaze preferentially toward the other, intact field. When the patient has a gaze palsy, or a preference or deviation independent of visual stimulation, then the following schema will assist your analysis.

SCHEMA FOR ANALYSIS OF HORIZONTAL GAZE

Hemisphere vs. brainstem

When there is a tonic gaze deviation to one side and/or inability to turn the eyes conjugately and fully to the other side (gaze paresis or palsy), what is the localization of the responsible lesion? Is the lesion in the cerebral hemisphere or in the brainstem? The most simplified schema (Fig. 17.1) includes two levels: a right and a left hemispheric (suprasegmental, supranuclear) center for conjugate horizontal gaze (the hemispheric centers) and a segmental brainstem horizontal gaze center in the right and left pons (the "pontine gaze centers"). (A hemispheric lesion causing gaze deviation need not be strictly localized to the "frontal gaze center" which is only part of the hemispheric control system.)

The schema is founded upon several principles that you will be able to retain, because they should make sense in terms of what you already know about the nervous system (see Table 17.1).

Note that a lesion need not involve tissue destruction (like an infarct or hemorrhage) to inhibit a gaze center. After a seizure has ended, the region of the seizure focus is physiologically depressed: it functions as if a destructive lesion were present. The eyes, therefore, often exhibit a transient deviation opposite to the direction of the earlier "driving" of the active seizure discharge. This postictal (postseizure) deviation is towards the side of the hemispheric focus.

The deviation (and paresis) caused by a destructive hemispheric lesion (damaging suprasegmental control, but not brainstem segmental control) is temporary and not absolute. As you might predict, this deviation can be overcome by other influences acting independently upon the pontine gaze center, namely, vestibular inputs from the medulla. In contrast, a complete destruction of the pontine center would be expected to cause permanent gaze palsy to that side, and should not be overcome by any stimulus input. This ability to overcome a gaze deviation or gaze palsy is the basis for interpretation of the Doll's Head (oculocephalic) maneuver and ice water caloric test (see below).

Localization of the lesion

Since a tonic gaze deviation to the right may result from either a right hemispheric lesion or a left pontine lesion, how would you know where the lesion is? There are two main methods:

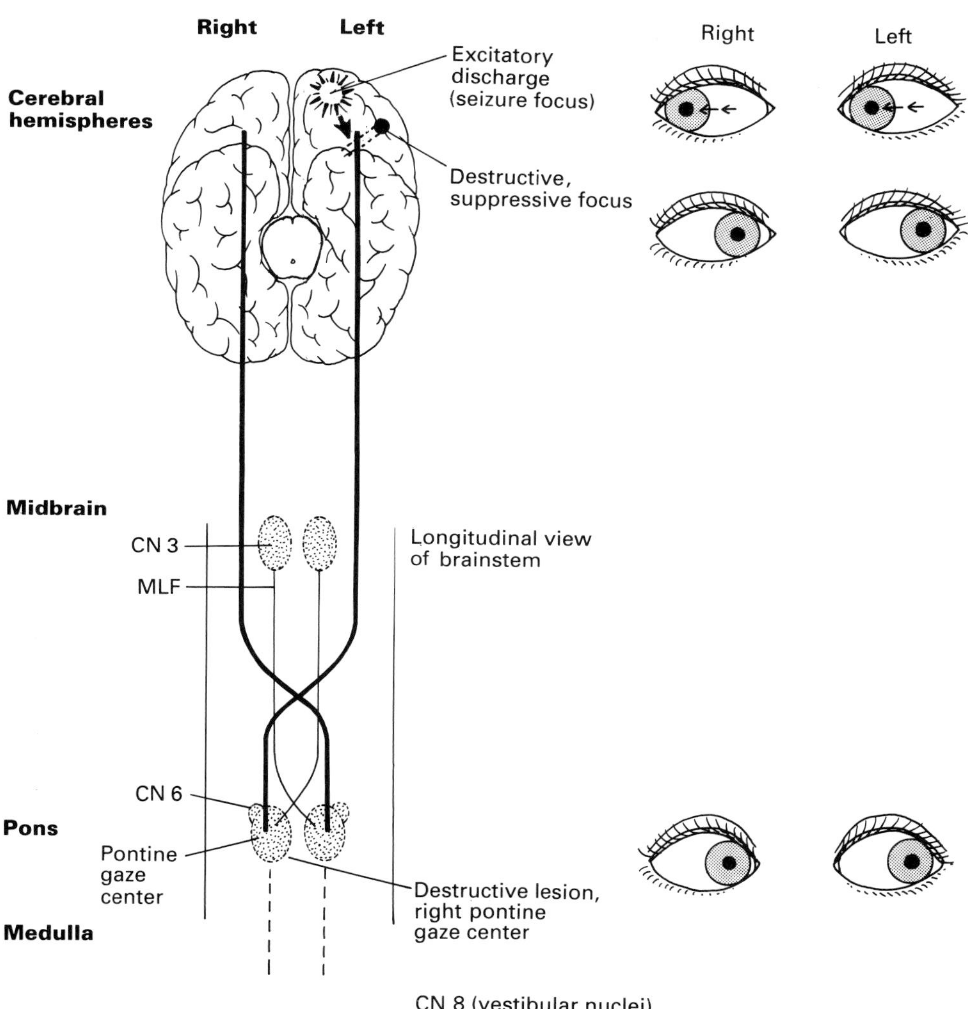

Fig. 17.1 Simplified schema for control of conjugate horizontal gaze. The suprasegmental control descending from the cerebral hemispheres crosses in the brainstem, thus acting on the contralateral pontine horizontal gaze center (in the paramedian reticular formation). The pontine gaze center then activates the adjacent CN 6 nucleus and, by means of the crossing medial longitudinal fasciculus (MLF), the contralateral CN 3 nucleus to achieve conjugate horizontal gaze. Excitatory and suppressive (destructive) hemispheric lesions and destructive pontine lesions are represented in this and subsequent Figures 17.2–17.4. In all of these figures, the hemispheres are viewed from the ventral aspect (to maintain right–left relationships), but this does not mean that the gaze centers are ventrally located.

1 compare the side of gaze deviation with the side of the hemiparesis;
2 assess whether the gaze deviation (or palsy) can be overcome (see Doll's Head maneuver and ice water caloric stimulation, below).

Compare side of hemiparesis with gaze deviation

Most often when you encounter a tonic gaze deviation, you will also note a hemiparesis. If you find a left arm and leg weakness, then the

Table 17.1 Schema for analysis of the horizontal gaze

Basic principles	Gaze schema
1 Long tracts (suprasegmental, supranuclear) mainly cross, and thus act to influence the opposite side	The supranuclear tracts from the "hemispheric gaze centers" to "pontine gaze centers" cross (in the brainstem)
2 Cranial nerves generally do not cross and thus influence functions on the same side. Lateralized control centers in the brainstem similarly exercise their influence ipsilaterally	The pontine gaze centers (that coordinate individual cranial nerve) control conjugate horizontal gaze to the same side
3 An excitatory stimulus produces an excess of the usual neurologic response, i.e. "overpowers" the tonic influence from the other side. (Abnormal discharging lesions do not occur in the brain stem)	An abnormal excitatory hemispheric discharge overstimulates the contralateral pontine center, e.g. right frontal discharge increases the input to the left pontine gaze center, causing the eyes to "drive" to the left (often with some intermittency due to the discontinuous discharges)
4 A destructive lesion inhibits the normal tonic influence arising from that side, thus allowing the tonic influence from the other side to act unopposed	The effect of a destructive lesion (inhibitory influence) at each of the four sites (right and left hemispheric centers and right and left pontine centers) can thus be determined. For example, a right frontal destructive lesion decreases the tonic input to the left pontine gaze center. The eyes deviate to the right because of the unopposed influence of the right pontine center (receiving continuing supranuclear input from the normal left hemisphere). In contrast, a right pontine lesion allows the left pontine gaze center to act unopposed, deviating gaze to the left

(Note: tracts linking structures on opposite sides must be crossed. e.g. connections between nuclei of CN 6 and CN 3 in the brainstem. This enables the coordination of both eyes to achieve conjugate horizontal gaze. Lesions of these tracts (the medial longitudinal fasciculi) do not affect the organization of horizontal gaze but do interrupt the execution of conjugate movement. See Fig. 5.7g)

lesion is in the right brainstem or the right hemisphere (because the corticospinal motor tracts cross at the medullary–cervical junction). But which is correct, hemisphere or brainstem? Look at the gaze deviation. A right gaze deviation must be due either to a left brainstem lesion or a right hemispheric (frontal) lesion, as explained above. Therefore, putting the two pieces of data together, you will deduce that the lesion is right frontal. With left gaze deviation, the lesion would be in the right pons (see Table 17.2). Note: a tonic gaze deviation is linked to a gaze paresis to the other side.

Table 17.2 Diagnostic use of horizontal conjugate gaze deviation

	Comparing the side of gaze deviation to the side of a hemiparesis	
	Gaze deviation to the left	Gaze deviation to the right
Right hemiparesis	Lesion (dysfunction) in left hemisphere (deviation can be overcome by Doll's Head maneuver or ice water calorics; usually transient, hour or days to weeks)	Lesion in left brainstem (pontine gaze center); (paralysis of left gaze cannot be overcome by any stimulus)
Left hemiparesis	Lesion in right brainstem	Lesion (dysfunction) in right hemisphere

DOLL'S HEAD MANEUVER (OCULOCEPHALIC REFLEX)

Objective

The purpose of this maneuver in the stuporous or comatose patient is to demonstrate that the right and left conjugate gaze centers in the pontine tegmentum are working. Since horizontal gaze to each side is the issue, how can such movement be demonstrated? If the patient is awake and comprehending, simply request gaze to the right and left, or following a stimulus to each side. If the patient does not understand or is stuporous, watch the eyes for spontaneous side-to-side movements. The presence of full horizontal gaze in both directions answers your question: the pontine centers must be working. In that case, there is no need to supply any other stimulus, but when full horizontal gaze is not demonstrated by these methods you will need to stimulate the eyes to move horizontally by other means. The simplest way is the Doll's Head maneuver.

Testing

First, ascertain that there is no contraindication to vigorous head rotation (such as neck trauma or severe cervical spine or vascular disease). Then turn (rotate) the head quickly to one side, watching what the eyes do; then rotate to the other side. (The object of rotation is to stimulate the labyrinths, activating the vestibular inputs to the central gaze mechanism.) You do not need to remember which way to turn the head. Just turn it either way and observe the result.

Response

1 If you were to rotate the head rapidly in the alert person (which is not indicated for this purpose), the eyes would move more or less with the head – they would not swing smoothly in the opposite direction.

2 In the stuporous or comatose patient (in whom you cannot observe or demonstrate eye movements), you will see that the eyes either maintain their position relative to the head (move with the head), or move in a direction opposite to head turning. (In the latter case the movement is relative: if you rotate the head to the left, the eyes end up at the right side of the orbits). This is the Doll's eyes phenomenon – the free floating effect of the eyeballs, such that when the head is turned one way, the eyes do not move with the head, but deviate in the opposite direction.

Doll's eyes

Interpretation

1 When the eyes move with the head and do not change their position, you will not have been able to demonstrate that the brainstem horizontal eye movement mechanism is working. Consider the reasons listed below.

(a) The pontine gaze center (or each of its effector pathways) is not operational. The faulty gaze center is the one on the side to which the eyes should have turned, but did not. The cause might be either structural damage or toxic–metabolic dysfunction (like severe barbiturate intoxication) which would cause bilateral effects.

(b) Your vestibular stimulation was ineffective because of too weak a rotation or, rarely, because of labyrinthine or other peripheral vestibular abnormality.

(c) Of particular importance, sometimes a hemispheric gaze deviation is so strong initially that the Doll's Head (oculocephalic) maneuver is simply insufficient to overcome it, in which case you need to supply a stronger stimulus: ice water calorics (see below).

(d) The patient whom you have assumed to be comatose may in fact be alert, but unable to communicate this to you.

2 When full horizontal eye movements are demonstrated, you can then say that the brainstem mechanism for these movements, from the medullary vestibular input, to the pontine gaze centers, to the connections with and output of CN 6 and CN 3, are working. This does not mean that the brainstem is "intact": other structures may be damaged.

3 You may see a partial response: e.g. when the head is turned to the right the eyes cross the midline to the left but do not move fully to that side. This usually indicates that the brainstem mechanism is working and that the lesion is suprasegmental (partial brainstem lesions are possible).

4 Another type of response consists of disconjugate movement – one eye moving fully and the other eye not moving. In this case, the pontine gaze center itself must be working, because one eye is activated. However, there must be a lesion further along the chain of function to account for the lack of response of the other eye.

Summary of "Doll's eyes"

1 The purpose of the Doll's Head maneuver in the stuporous or comatose patient is to determine whether the brainstem mechanism for conjugate horizontal gaze is functioning. Use this maneuver when you cannot document gaze to the right and left by other, simpler means such as observation of spontaneous eye movements following a stimulus, or response to a command.

2 If, in the stuporous or comatose patient, the eyes swing to each side as you rotate the head in the opposite direction, then this brainstem mechanism is working as it should be. A more powerful stimulus (ice water calorics) is sometimes required to demonstrate this function.

3 Describe what you observe. ("With head turning to the right, the eyes moved fully and conjugately to the left.") Do not use normal or abnormal, positive or negative: what is normally expected in the comatose patient with an intact brainstem is not normal for the alert, asymptomatic patient, and vice versa.

ICE WATER CALORICS

Objective

The goal of ice water caloric testing at the bedside is the same as for the Doll's Head maneuver. Ice water irrigation of the ears provides maximum stimulation to the brainstem mechanism subserving horizontal eye movements. Perform ice water calorics only if you have been unable to demonstrate by other means that the horizontal gaze mechanism is working. Distinguish gross (large volume) ice water irrigation of the ears at the bedside – used in stuporous and comatose patients – from the microirrigation that is done in quantitative and controlled fashion for the evaluation of dizziness and other problems in an otoneurologic laboratory. Do not flush ice water into the ears of alert and responsive patients at the bedside!

Testing

Check ears to insure that perforation of the tympanic membranes is not present. With the patient supine and with pads and kidney basin under the ear to catch the irrigant, proceed to flush 30 cc or more of ice water into the ear canal. Draw the ice water up into a large syringe, preferably with a long bevelled spout that can be directed well into the ear canal; alternatively, one can attach a scalp vein needle to the syringe, then cut off the needle, leaving the tubing that can be directed into the ear canal. Beware: sharp tubing can lacerate the ear canal or even perforate the eardrum.

Responses

The eyes are expected to deviate slowly towards the irrigated ear, usually after a latency that may be as much as 30 seconds. (Wait a couple of minutes before doing the other side.) You do not need to remember which way the eyes are supposed to turn; simply observe whether they do in fact deviate with irrigation of each ear.

Interpretation

Failure of the eyes to deviate may mean:

1 a brainstem lesion on that side;
2 a "dead" (unresponsive) labyrinth;
3 an awake patient in pseudocoma (in which case there should be marked nystagmus with the fast component away from the irrigated ear).

The mnemonic COWS – cold opposite, warm same – refers to the direction of nystagmus, which is designated by the direction of its fast component, produced by cold or warm irrigation. In the comatose patient, the slow deviation towards the side of the ice water irrigation corresponds to the slow phase of the nystagmus. If you like mnemonics, such as COWS, beware of this confusion.

Case illustrations

Case 17A
Stroke localization

Margie Akers, a 74-year-old right-handed woman with atrial fibrillation, suddenly slumped in her chair, unable to move her right side. In the emergency room a severe right hemiparesis was noted, along with a right homonymous hemianopia, lack of speech, and a right-sided sensory deficit. Her eyes were conjugately deviated strongly to the left, and did not rove spontaneously past midline towards the right. (Where do you think the lesion is?)

Analysis

The attending doctor deduced that a lesion producing a strong left gaze deviation should be either in the left hemisphere (decreased tonic activity in the crossed frontopontine pathway to the right pontine gaze center) or in the right pontine gaze center itself. In either case there would be unopposed activity of the left pontine gaze center (resulting in a leftward gaze deviation) and a deficit in right lateral gaze. But which is correct, left hemisphere or right pons? Possible localization of the gaze "palsy" was compared with that of the hemiparesis: a right hemiparesis could result from a left-sided brain lesion, either in the pons or in the hemisphere. Thus, a left hemispheric localization (Fig. 17.2) is the only one that explains both the right hemiparesis and the left gaze deviation (right gaze palsy).

Two other pieces of corroborative data were also noted: first, Doll's Head maneuver succeeded in swinging the eyes across the midline to the right, indicating that the right pontine gaze center was capable of function, but was simply understimulated by the left hemisphere. Secondly, Ms Akers' speech problem was shown to represent an aphasia, which would be localizable to the left hemisphere in this right-handed patient. The pathogenesis of the lesion was an embolic stroke in the territory of the left middle cerebral artery.

Case 17B
Seizure focus

Sandy Jamieson, a 19-year-old right-handed man, collapsed on a sidewalk with a convulsion. An emergency medical technician, who arrived after the convulsion had subsided, noted that the eyes were conjugately deviated to the right. Shortly, jerking movements began again in the left arm and the eyes were observed to be darting rhythmically to the left. (Where was the focus of dysfunction causing the eye signs?)

Analysis

At the local hospital the emergency physician hypothesized that the lesion causing the seizures and the eye signs was very probably in the right hemisphere. On the basis of the initial (postictal) conjugate deviation to the right, the lesion could have been either in the right hemisphere or the left brainstem. (No lateralizing signs, such as a hemiparesis, were available for comparison to help distinguish between these two localizations.) However, the subsequent "driving" of the eyes from right to left during the second seizure indicated an excitatory phenomenon in the right hemisphere (Fig. 17.3). Increased activity in the right frontal to left pontine pathway was causing the left pontine gaze center to drive the eyes to the left in rhythmic fashion. Moreover, the focal onset of clonic (jerking) activity in the left arm signified activation of the corticospinal tract descending from the right frontal region.

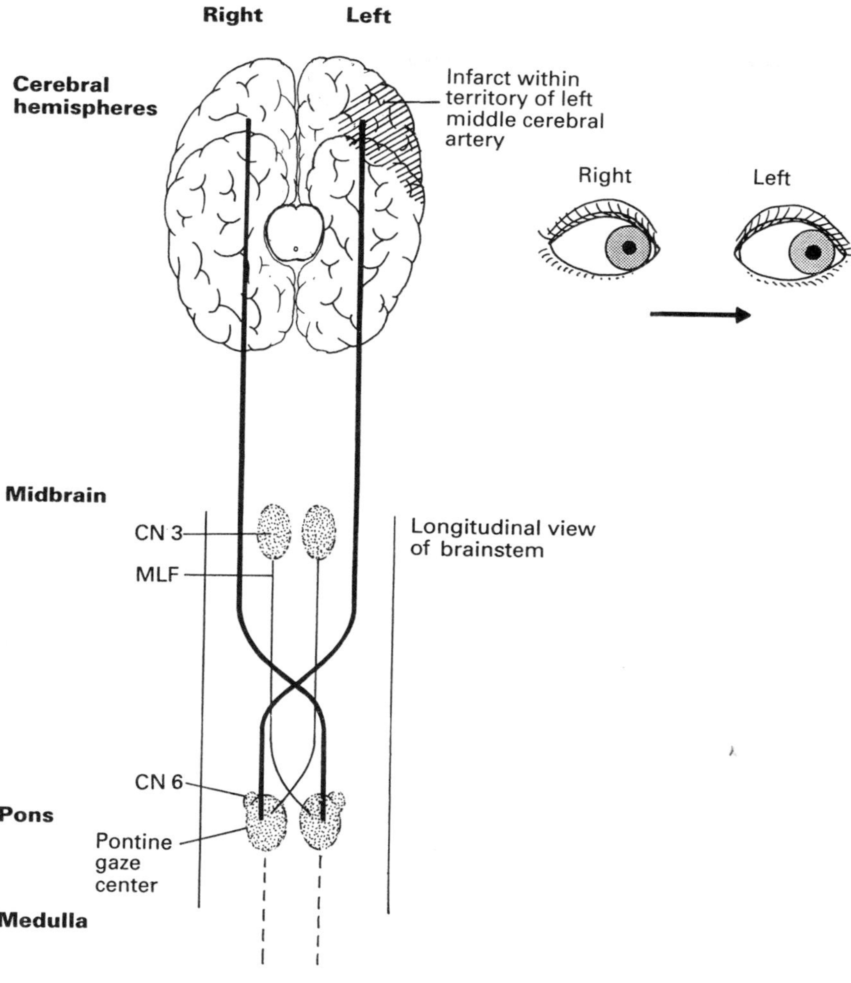

Fig. 17.2 Gaze deviation in Case 17A. The left gaze deviation is due to a destructive left hemispheric lesion. The lack of left hemispheric stimulation to the right pontine horizontal gaze center leads to the unopposed action of the left pontine center, resulting in gaze deviation to the left and paresis of gaze to the right (which can usually be overcome by Doll's Head maneuver).

Follow-up

As the patient regained consciousness and became more fully testable, he was found to have a mild left-sided weakness (a Todd's paralysis or temporary postictal weakness). When further history became available the doctor learned that Mr Jamieson had suffered a right frontal contusion in a motorcycle accident 2 years previously.

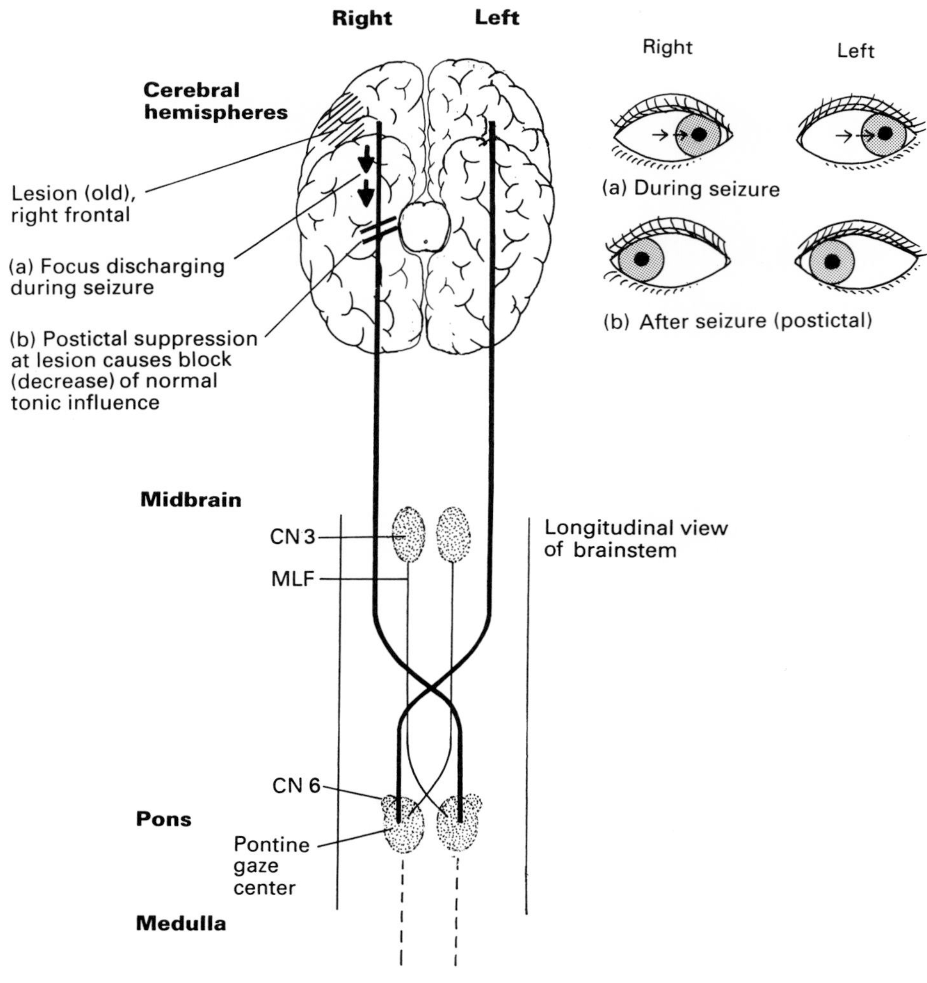

Fig. 17.3 Abnormalities of gaze in Case 17B. (a) The eyes "drive" to the left during the seizure, which originates from the right frontal lobe, stimulating the suprasegmental pathway to the left pontine center. (b) In the "suppressive," postictal phase, with decreased stimulus from the right frontal lobe to the left pontine center, the eyes are deviated to the right, due to unopposed influence from the right pontine center (and left hemisphere).

Case 17C
Gaze palsy in a comatose patient

Margaret Trujillo, an 86-year-old right-handed woman with longstanding, severe hypertension, collapsed while seated on her sofa at home. She was brought to the emergency department in a coma. Her left pupil was pinpoint, the right small, and she moved only her left arm slightly. Both plantar responses were upgoing. Her eyes were conjugately deviated to the right. Neither Doll's Head maneuver nor ice water calorics succeeded in eliciting gaze across the midline to the left, but

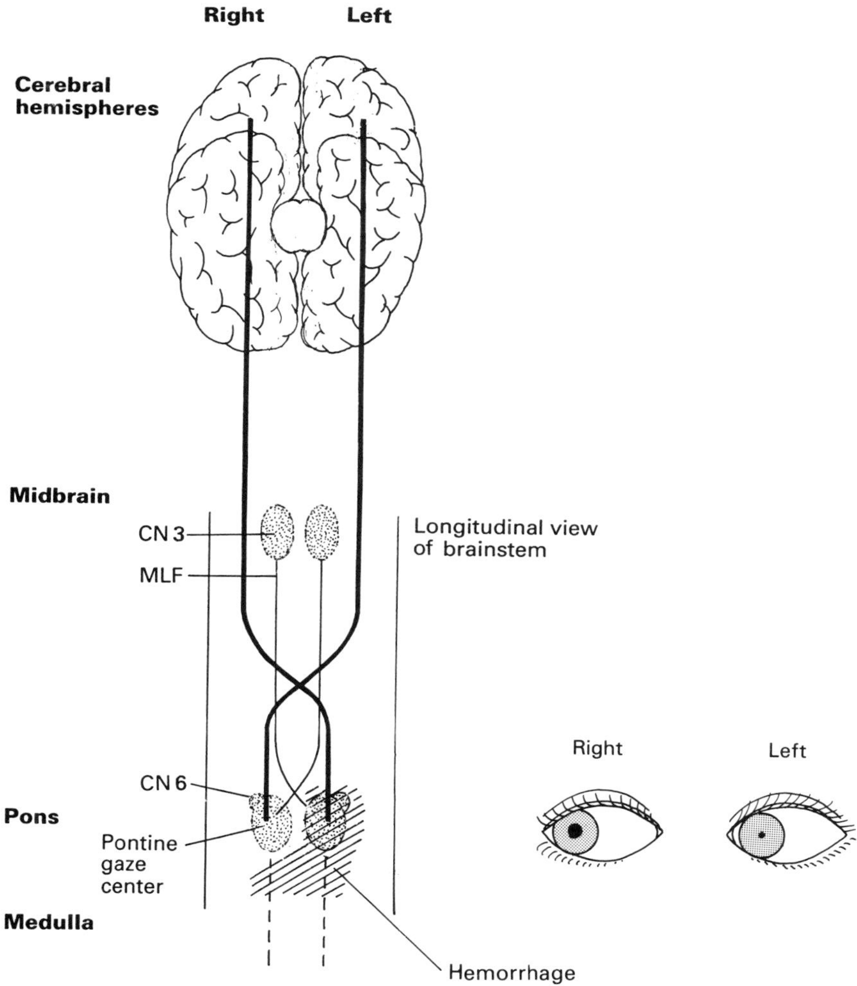

Fig. 17.4 Right gaze deviation (and left gaze palsy) in Case 17C. The rightward conjugate gaze deviation is due to a destructive lesion in the left side of the pontine tegmentum, affecting the left pontine horizontal gaze center. (The palsy of left horizontal gaze cannot be overcome by any stimulus, including ice water calorics.) Note also that the left pupil is pin-point and the right pupil will soon constrict further, due to interruption of the descending sympathetic pathways in the pons; a hemorrhage affects much of the left side of the pons and extends towards the right more ventrally, affecting descending tracts in the basis pontis.

did elicit further rightward gaze. (Was the lesion in the brainstem or in the cerebral hemisphere?)

Analysis

As reasoned in the previous cases, the lesion causing a gaze palsy to the left and a gaze deviation to the right would be in the left side of the pons or the right hemisphere. The patient appeared to have a bilateral hemiparesis, but the slight movement of the left arm suggested that the brunt of the lesion might be on the left, with slight sparing of the descending corticospinal tract on the right side of the brainstem. If so, then the lesion should be centered in the left pons, causing the gaze palsy and the worse weakness in the right limbs (see Fig. 17.4). The Doll's Head and ice water caloric responses supported the hypothesis of a left pontine lesion, since neither maneuver stimulated leftward gaze (as might have occurred typically with a supranuclear, hemispheric lesion). A computerized tomography scan revealed a pontine hemorrhage affecting the left tegmentum and basis pontis, but extending into the right base of the pons as well.

Follow-up

Ms Trujillo briefly regained minimal responsiveness to voice, but then worsened and died several days later from medical complications.

Use of the schema

These illustrative cases are quite typical of the kinds of gaze deviations or palsies which are seen in clinical practice. By reconstructing the basic anatomic schema, you will be able to deduce the two chief possibilities for the localization of the gaze disorder – one hemispheric, one brainstem. Then, by applying other evidence, such as the side of a hemiparesis, the direction of "driving" of the eyes during a seizure, and the responses to Doll's Head and ice water calorics, you will usually be able to achieve the desired "big picture" localization: (a) whether the lesion is in the brainstem or cerebral hemisphere; and (b) the side of the lesion.

As with any clinical rules, there are exceptions: sometimes in seizures the head and/or eyes turn towards, rather than away from, the discharging epileptogenic focus. Occasionally, in hemorrhage into the thalamus and 3rd ventricle, the eyes deviate in a direction contrary to what would be expected for a hemispheric lesion.

CONJUGATE VERTICAL GAZE

Testing

In observing vertical gaze look for position, alignment, and movement, as you do for horizontal gaze. If you cannot document vertical eye movements by command or following because, the patient is stuporous or comatose, try the vertical head tilt maneuver ("vertical Doll's eyes"). With downward tilt, the eyes will tend to roll up if the midbrain vertical gaze mechanism is working, and similarly a quick tilt upward would produce a downward deviation of the eyes relative to the orbits. (As with the Doll's Head maneuver, be sure there is no traumatic or other condition of the neck that would contraindicate vigorous flexion or extension of the neck.) It is possible to produce vertical eye movements by simultaneous ice water irrigation of both ears, but the results of this procedure are variable and it is not often used.

Clinical correlation

Clinically significant abnormalities of conjugate vertical gaze occur much less commonly than horizontal gaze deviations or preferences. Partial limitations of upward gaze occur commonly as isolated findings in older patients; they are of no clinical importance. Thus, to employ an upward gaze limitation as an acute, localizing sign, you must know the baseline status of upward eye movements or identify other signs suggesting midbrain or thalamic lesions. Control of upward and downward gaze is localized in the midbrain/pretectal area, rostral to the CN 3 nuclei and superior colliculi. In addition to acute midbrain lesions (such as infarction) which may alter vertical gaze, pressure effects on the midbrain can produce downward deviation of the eyes, limitation of upward gaze, alterations in pupillary size and reactivity, and impairment of accommodation and the near reaction – all upper midbrain-mediated functions.

SUMMARY

Priorities

1 Be able to describe the position and movements of the eyes with respect to any gaze deviation, misalignment, or impairment of conjugate action (gaze paresis or palsy).
2 If you observe a deviation or limitation of conjugate gaze, use the schema described in this chapter to establish the site of the responsible lesion, i.e. brainstem vs. hemisphere.
   (a) Determine the two possible options for a tonic gaze deviation or palsy – one hemisphere or the contralateral brainstem.
   (b) Decide between hemisphere or brainstem by correlating with a hemiparesis (or other sign), if present.
   (c) If there is no deviation or hemiparesis to correlate, but there is a gaze palsy in a comatose patient, consider vestibular stimulation (Doll's Head or ice water calorics) to overcome the gaze palsy. As a rule, a hemispheric mechanism of gaze palsy can be overcome.

Pitfalls

1 Not articulating the question being asked when doing the Doll's Head maneuver (or ice water calorics), namely: is the brainstem mechanism for horizontal conjugate gaze working? If the eyes move fully – spontaneously, by following, or on command – then the question is answered and Doll's Head need not be done. In the stuporous or comatose patient, full gaze elicited by Doll's Head (or ice water) shows that the brainstem mechanism is working and the lesion responsible for the gaze abnormality is above the pons, and usually hemispheric. Record what happens, not "positive," "negative," "normal," or "abnormal."
2 Not remembering that a tonic gaze deviation to one side is usually linked to a gaze paresis (weakness) or palsy (paralysis) to the other side. In the schema comparing gaze deviation and hemiparesis, a gaze palsy to the right is analyzed like a gaze deviation to the left, which usually coexists. (As with a hemiparesis or palsy on a suprasegmental

basis is not absolute, since movement can be achieved by appropriate stimuli.)

PROBLEMS FOR SELF-STUDY

Problems

1 A patient is asked to look to the right. In doing so, the left eye adducts, moving fully to the right, but the right eye does not abduct, i.e. does not move laterally to the right. How would you evaluate this finding reported as a "right lateral gaze palsy"?

2 A hospitalized patient is noted to be "always looking towards the right." How would you analyze this observation and what might be the basis for it?

Comments

1 This is not a gaze palsy, because the stimulus to look to the right is translated into action: the left eye does move fully to the right. However, the right eye does not achieve abduction, due (in this particular case) to a peripheral lesion of the right CN 6. (In addition, the right eye would be adducted at rest.) Do not confuse dysfunction of the lateral rectus muscle (or of abduction mediated by the abducens) with a problem in the conjugate control mechanism for horizontal (lateral) gaze.

2 Consider several possible interpretations: first, is this a gaze preference to the right because of a left homonymous hemianopia? (Gaze to the right and left on command should be full.) Second, this might be a gaze preference to the right due to a more general inattention to the left (with only a partial field cut or none at all), resulting from a right (nondominant) parietal lobe lesion. Finally, the rightward gaze might represent a tonic gaze deviation to the right (with a gaze palsy to the left); the responsible lesion would be in the right hemisphere or left brainstem (pons).

FURTHER READING

Brazis, P.W., Masdeu, J.C., Biller, J. *Localization in Clinical Neurology*. 2nd edn. Little, Brown, and Company, Boston (MA), 1990. A detailed summary (Chapter 7) of the complex suprasegmental gaze control systems, revealing the gap between the simple clinical construct and the level of current scientific knowledge.

Leigh, R.J., Zee, D.S. *The Neurology of Eye Movements*. 2nd edn. F.A. Davis, Philadelphia (PA), 1991. Exhaustive survey, for the serious student of the subject.

Tijssen, C.C., van Gisbergen, J.A.M., Shulte, B.P.M. Conjugate eye deviation: side, site and size of the hemispheric lesion. *Neurology* 1991; 41:846–50. Conjugate eye deviation varies with location and size of the hemispheric lesion, which need not (and usually does not) involve the frontal cortical eye fields themselves.

chapter 18

Patients who are Difficult to Examine

The neurologic examination requires special effort and patience on your part in four general situations, based on the patient's behavior:

1 the agitated patient;

2 the poorly responsive patient;

3 the "unreliable" patient;

4 the patient suspected of hysteric conversion.

These patients will tax not only your powers of observation, tenacity, and ingenuity, but also your own attitude. At times you will probably experience a sense of repugnance, a strong urge to retreat, to put a distance between yourself and the delirious or "unresponsive" patient. There may be a handy rationale: "He is too agitated to be examined," or "She can't cooperate with testing." Whatever limitations may actually apply, the need for gathering appropriate neurologic data is not diminished. Often the real reason for backing off is the discomfort of confronting a frightening situation in which your own vulnerability or inexperience may be exposed. At other times, certain perfectly harmless, but initially disconcerting manifestations of disease (such as severe choreoathetotic involuntary movements) may make you reluctant to approach the patient and lay on hands for close examination. This is an understandable response, but one that you can overcome (see Case 3A).

THE AGITATED PATIENT

The very agitated patient is hyperactive, distractable, and sometimes threatening or violent. Such patients frequently evidence confusion (being inattentive and disoriented) and irrationality. From the standpoint of the examination, the failure of such patients to hold still, pay attention, and follow commands quickly and consistently represents the main problem. In short, it is hard to control their behavior.

Testing

As in all patients who are difficult to examine, you will learn primarily from simple observation rather than from the controlled type of testing that fills up much of your ordinary examination. In fact, your first reaction may be that this patient is "unexaminable," but when you run down the list of items on the neurologic examination, you will probably be surprised to discover what an extensive array of data you can assemble on a patient with "high-output" behavior, disordered as it may be.

CASE 18A
Kicks and curses

Hamilton Green, a 53-year-old alcoholic with an epileptic seizure disorder, had been well known to the emergency department for years. On this occasion he was brought in by police who had found him sitting on the sidewalk with a gash on his forehead. He permitted the staff to suture and dress his wound, but then insisted on leaving. On his way out he staggered and would have fallen if he had not been caught by a nurse. He screamed "Let me go," kicked her, and again started to weave towards the door, but was restrained, to which he responded with long strings of obscenities.

The staff were concerned about the possibility of more serious head injury and asked for a neurologic evaluation. His foul behavior was "nothing new," but was he more ataxic than could be accounted for by his inebriation? Imagine yourself as the one called upon to assess his neurologic condition. What would you have been able to observe?

You find Mr Green seated on a chair in a room by himself. As you enter and approach him, he curses and flails at you. You retreat to the entrance to see what you can observe from a short distance.

Mental status and behavior

You have already noted Mr Green's disheveled, unshaven appearance and violent expression of his antagonism. He obviously speaks in fluent prose. He is alert but rather easily distracted. The less stimulation you provide, the less agitated he acts. When aroused, he vents his angry mood again. He shows strong affect within a restricted range, from anger to sullen dejection. He understands what you say, judging from the content of the eruptions that follow, but does not identify himself or answer any substantive questions directly. When you mention the name of a well-known local politician, he makes a barbed comment, indicating that he recognizes the name, but he does not engage in further conversation on this or other topics that you introduce.

Head and neck

Aside from the dressed laceration and nearby abrasion, you notice that he moves his neck freely and without evident pain and that his front teeth are missing. The eyes do not look jaundiced.

Cranial nerve functions

CN 1	Not tested
CN 2	He attends to visual stimuli from both sides and does not selectively bump into the chair or walls on his right or left, as he intermittently storms around the room. He quickly spots you making a note on a file card (so his vision in one or both eyes must be at least fairly good). He also reaches to touch a point on the wall, as if there were a little spot there; you cannot see it from where you are (so you are unsure if he has the acuity to spot a tiny mark or whether he might be visually hallucinating). You try writing "Are you hungry?" on a card, but as you hold it up he just scowls and kicks at it, not revealing whether he has actually read the message.
CNs 3, 4, 6	You cannot see his pupils well enough to assess their size accurately, but they do not appear very large or small or grossly asymmetric. His eyes move conjugately and fully to right and left; up and down gaze is also present, but you cannot be sure it is full. There is no lid droop.
CN 5	His jaw seems tireless!
CN 7	You note that he knits and furrows his forehead symmetrically, has symmetric palpebral fissures, closes both eyes (lightly), has no droop of either side of the mouth or flattening of the nasolabial fold, and grimaces and scowls symmetrically.
CN 8	He picks up comments in moderate conversational tones (so he is not very deaf); he does not turn either ear preferentially toward you. He does not behave as though he is vertiginous (such as holding on to his chair after turning his head quickly).
CNs 9, 10	He phonates very well! His speech is slightly slurred, but easily understandable. He spits occasionally, but otherwise seems to swallow his saliva without coughing.

You offer him a drink of water in a paper cup, but he knocks it out of your hand with a well-directed swat.

CN 11 There is no obvious droop of either shoulder or asymmetry of the profile of the lower neck as you face him, but you do not observe any shrugging movements.

CN 12 At one point he actually sticks his tongue out at you – it protrudes in the midline! His lingual articulation is quite good ("d" and "t" sounds).

Motor

You might well experience the power of his kick if you moved too close, or the strength of his arms if you tried to restrain him bodily, but instead you settle for the observation that he moves all four limbs vigorously. He supports his weight, and when he loses balance he is able to brace himself. He does not seem to favor one arm as he gesticulates, but he shakes his right fist preferentially, making you wonder whether he is right-handed. No tremor is evident.

Sensory

While it is not wise to approach for pin, vibratory, or other direct sensory testing just now, you hope to get some idea of his proprioception from observing his limb placement. He staggers at times, but otherwise places his feet well, without striking the floor too hard (as might occur if he had impaired feedback on the position of his feet).

Coordination

His gait is characterized by intermittent staggering and weaving. When he takes a swipe at the cup of water with his right hand the movement is quite smooth and well directed. There is some slurring of speech, but no marked decomposition of rhythm. When you attract his attention, his eyes dart towards you quickly and accurately, making steady eye contact.

Reflexes

These require direct testing which you do not try at the present time. (Note incomplete data base.)

Synthesis and plan

In summary, in addition to his major behavioral abnormalities, you can only identify slurred speech and poor balance. Horizontal eye movements, vision, limb and facial movements, and limb coordination are either normal or at least quite good, and alertness is maintained. To obtain further data it will be necessary either to restrain him or to await an improvement in his behavior, while watching for deterioration. In some cases further examination and diagnostic procedures, such as a computerized tomography (CT) scan or lumbar puncture, might be required immediately, but in this case a course of continued observation seems more prudent. You and the nursing staff will watch for a declining state of consciousness, for worsening of stance and gait, for alteration in breathing pattern, etc. At the same time, attempts will be made to cajole him into more cooperation with testing, acceptance of vitamins including thiamine, and planning for subsequent care.

This strategy ultimately proves successful. He sobers up, becomes more compliant, much steadier on his feet, and the principal physical abnormalities evident on further examination are the absent ankle jerks and decreased sensation in the feet that bespeak an alcoholic–nutritional polyneuropathy. He still will not submit to more specific mental status testing, but appears competent and is released when he refuses additional care.

THE POORLY RESPONSIVE PATIENT

Overview

The "low-output" patient poses more of a challenge to the neurologic examination than the agitated patient. It is beyond the scope of this chapter to discuss the differential diagnosis of patients who are mentally or physically inactive and respond little or not at all. However, the following are some general categories to be considered:

1 decreased level of consciousness – stupor and coma;

2 akinesia, as in parkinsonism; akinetic mutism; catatonia; locked-in syndrome;

3 depression with psychomotor retardation;

4 abulia (a state marked by slowness and lack of spontaneity, usually associated with frontal disease).

In contrast to the agitated patient, these patients are usually passively compliant with testing, but fail to participate. You can usually check vital signs and temperature, visualize the fundi, auscultate the neck, assess the pupils, test reflexes, evaluate tone, etc. – in short, succeed with many parts of the evaluation that you could not accomplish on Mr Green because of his violence. However, you still would have more or less difficulty testing resistive strength and all but the crudest responses to sensory stimulation. Typically, you would have an even harder time in evaluating visual fields, movement of face and limbs, stance and gait, and higher cortical functions. The following case illustrates the kinds of information obtainable from a comatose patient (to take an extreme example).

CASE 18B
The man with "nothing working"

A 27-year-old man, Jun Kim, was resuscitated following cardiopulmonary arrest due to an electric shock (received while using a hair dryer with wet hands while still standing in a tub after his bath). After stabilization of his circulatory status, his neurologic condition needed to be evaluated in order to establish a prognosis. His breathing was controlled on a ventilator and it was believed that there would not be much to examine, because "nothing was working" neurologically.

General appearance

A well-developed, healthy-appearing man was lying in bed with an endotracheal breathing tube, several lines (intravenous and intraarterial) and a Foley catheter (to drain the bladder) in place. His eyes were lightly shut, and he did not respond to voice; with his eyelids held open, he still did not shift his eyes when addressed.

Head and neck

No sign of cranial or neck trauma; neck supple with the range of motion in all planes only limited by attached tubes and lines. Carotid pulses 3+, without bruits. Eyes moist, corneas clear by flashlight inspection; conjunctivae suffused (injected, reddened). Funduscopic examination normal: flat, sharp discs, venous pulsations present bilaterally; no hemorrhages; normal vessels.

Cranial nerve functions

CN 1	Not tested
CN 2	No visual fixing or following in any field; no change in facial expression when the doctor (or his wife, who had asked to see him) looked at him head-on, with his eyes held open.
CNs 3, 4, 6	Pupils both 3 mm; when the eyelids were opened and on each side, in turn, brightly illuminated, a slight but definite direct and consensual pupillary light reaction could be seen. The eyes were not deviated to either side and were very slightly divergent. They did not move at all when he was asked to look up, down, to the right, left, or any way that he could. With Doll's Head maneuver (see Chapter 17) the eyes moved 2–3 mm in the direction opposite to the way the head was moved.
CN 5	When his endotracheal tube was suctioned he clamped down with his teeth, the contraction of the masseter and temporalis muscles being visible and palpable. With a heavy strand of cotton swab, but not with the usual wisp, corneal stimulation produced a slight ipsilateral contraction of the medial parts of the eyelids, as the lids were held open. Pin stimulation on the face produced no grimace.
CN 7	The eyelids were lightly closed (and the movement with corneal stimulation was noted above).
CN 8	No response to sound; no nystagmus.
CNs 9, 10	Suctioning through the endotracheal tube stimulated some contraction of the pharyngeal and laryngeal musculature, evident from observing the neck and noting some movement of the tube.
CN 11	No atrophy of trapezius or sternocleidomastoids.
CN 12	No atrophy in visible parts of the tongue.

Motor, sensory, and coordination

No spontaneous limb or trunk movements were evident except for occasional shivering-like activity seen mainly in the legs. At rest there was a moderate increase in tone with passive movement of the limbs, more in the legs than arms. Suctioning produced slight plantar flexion of the feet and extension and internal rotation of the legs more than the arms. Although small in amplitude, these movements were very forceful. With a firm pinch to the inner arms or thighs similar movements occurred. Coordination was not tested.

Reflexes

Biceps, triceps, knee, and ankle jerks all were 3+ (on a scale of 4+). Unsustained ankle clonus bilaterally. Plantar responses extensor bilaterally; no other pathologic reflexes. Superficial abdominals absent.

Just after this examination was completed, Mr Kim had a generalized seizure in which the eyes rolled up (no lateral deviation), his face, limbs, and trunk tensed in a tonic contraction, and then the limbs jerked symmetrically in low-amplitude, rhythmic contractions in the plane of flexion/extension. This ceased spontaneously after 15–20 seconds.

Interpretation

Following electric shock and cardiopulmonary arrest, Mr Kim presented in coma. He scored only 4 on the Glasgow coma scale (Table 18.1). He demonstrated no eye opening or verbal response, and only extensor responses to pain.

He showed no sign of chronic disease or other prior ill-health (not surprising here, but a factor in prognosis). More importantly, there was no indication of secondary injury to his head or neck from his fall onto the bathroom floor. No focal or lateralizing signs were present to suggest either any major traumatic effects or electric current injury. The reactive pupils and horizontal eye movements (although incomplete) indicated

Table 18.1 Glasgow coma scale

Test	Response	Score
Eye opening	Spontaneous	4
	To speech	3
	To pain	2
	None	1
Best verbal response	Oriented	5
	Confused	4
	Inappropriate	3
	Incomprehensible	2
	None	1
Best motor response (arm)	Obedience to commands	6
	Localization of pain	5
	Withdrawal response to pain	4
	Flexion response to pain	3
	Extension response to pain	2
	None	1

function of these brainstem mechanisms. The reflexive motor movements demonstrated that at least segmental motor (and pain) pathways were operative at the level of the head, arms, and legs. Moreover, the observed seizure revealed that upper motor neuron (corticospinal) pathways were operative, albeit with abnormal discharges. A slight divergence of the eyes (from the visual axis towards the anatomic axis of the orbits) is considered normal in coma.

Follow-up

Over subsequent days and weeks, Mr Kim went on to regain alertness and full neurologic function except for some impairment of memory and other cognitive functions that were showing a more gradual improvement.

The next case is presented for comparison, since the patients appeared similar in many ways, but with major underlying differences.

CASE 18C
The flick of a thumb

Sam Emerson, a 23-year-old right-handed man, was examined in a chronic hospital to help establish his neurologic prognosis. He had suffered a severe head injury in a vehicular accident 6 months before and had remained in what was described as a vegetative state. The examination was much like that of Mr Kim, except that Mr Emerson's eyelids would partially open; both eyes abducted fully and adducted partially; no visual fixing was apparent. He was breathing on his own through a tracheostomy.

The limbs were contracted and only minimal movements seen. No posturing was evident. No signs of emotional expression could be observed (although the family thought they had).

In sum, it had been impossible thus far to establish any evidence of cognizance. However, when a standard test was tried to see whether the patient might be cognizant but unable to communicate it in the usual ways – he was asked to look up or down and to signal that he understood what was being asked – the eyes moved, but not reproducibly. However, at this time the medical student noticed a slight flick of the right thumb. Mr Emerson was asked to move his thumb again; it moved. Before long he was using his thumb signals to communicate, including "yes" (thumb moved) or "no" (thumb still) to answer complex questions correctly. He was alert and cerebrating at a high level, but had heretofore not succeeded in letting anyone know it, because he was "locked-in" by his severe motor deficits. A computer-assisted keyboard communications system was established.

This is an unusually dramatic example of the benefit of observing and reexamining patients with "complete unresponsiveness."

In the next case, the ability of the examiner to measure the patient's behavioral output over time, and thus to achieve a better neurologic data base, is illustrated.

CASE 18D
Decline and fall

Annette Wilkinson, a 65-year-old woman with a history of depression, had been functioning well until about 3 months before being hospitalized for evaluation and treatment of "failure to thrive." According to her sister, with whom she lived, she began to show signs of confusion and apparent forgetfulness on a trip that they took together. While traveling on a bus she fell, banging her head but apparently not hurting herself. Over the ensuing months she steadily declined in her interest in and ability to manage everyday activities. She offered no pressing complaints.

General examination was unrevealing. The neurologic examination was as follows: she lay on her bed with her eyes closed and did not answer at all when addressed. With persistent verbal stimulation her lips moved a little, forming the word "no" when asked whether she was asleep. She then opened her eyes but did not have the look of someone who had just awakened – no yawning, rubbing her eyes, or turning over. She submitted passively to the examination: head and neck examination were normal, including the funduscopic examination. No attention was paid to visual stimuli presented from either side. Her facial and limb movements were languid, without real exertion. Tone was normal. She did not attempt any coordinated movements and simply moved her limbs slightly when tested with a pin. Reflexes were 2+, symmetric, and plantar responses flexor; no grasp, sucking, rooting, snout, or jaw jerk reflex was present. When asked if she would sit and stand up, she lay still and shut her eyes again. When asked her name she whispered it, but not her correct address, the name of the hospital, or the name of her doctor. She shrugged her shoulders at inquiries as to the year, month, or season.

This first attempt at an examination garnered a few clues to the nature of her problem, but did not go very far in defining her best physical and cognitive capacities. What would you think about her condition, and how might more information be gained? Was she mainly depressed or was she suffering from an intracranial sequel (such as subdural hematomas) to her seemingly minor head injury? Was she possibly becoming demented, the fall serving to direct attention to a decline that was already in progress?

Further examination

A diagnostic decision was made to obtain a CT scan, but in the meantime the examiner returned to see whether better bedside data could be obtained. Despite Ms Wilkinson's listless and apathetic response earlier, the physician greeted her with quiet warmth and sat with her for several minutes before making any requests. He mentioned that he would like to meet her children and grandchildren if they came in to visit. The patient responded to this unhurried show of interest and concern by whispering a brief "Thank you." To fill out the examination, he asked her to nod if she saw his wiggling finger out of the corners of her eyes. She complied. Much better motor and sensory examinations were now accomplished as a result of more vigorous physical output and "yes and no" indication of sensory perception. She whispered correct answers to the month and year before indicating that she was tired and wished to stop the testing. When the physician left, she thanked him by name.

Assessment

The cranial CT scan was within normal limits for age. The question of simple depression vs. dementia with superimposed depression remained. Metabolic screening being normal, her physician decided to offer a therapeutic trial of an antidepressant medication and to follow her neurologic status closely with the consulting neurologist. Five weeks later she appeared much livelier. A detailed neurologic physical examination was normal. Her spontaneity and vigor were still impaired, but her recent memory capacity was quite good, as were a variety of other cognitive functions. It remained to be seen whether, with further lifting of her depression, her mental acuity could be documented as entirely normal. Nevertheless, her course had left virtually no doubt that her decline and "pseudodementia" had been due to depression. The physician's approach, including a "second effort" had mobilized additional psychic energy that substantially increased the quality of examination data. With pharmacotherapy her further progress towards normal responsiveness and cognition clarified the diagnostic issues.

THE "UNRELIABLE" EXAMINATION

Patients who are inattentive and confused, preoccupied, or very suggestible cause examiners great frustration because of difficulty in reproducing neurologic findings. (However, there are other possible reasons for such discrepancies: is the patient's neurologic condition changing? Might your testing technique be the source of variation, due to lack of uniformity of the stimulus?) Only after you have tried to account for changing signs in these ways should you focus on the personality as the source of variation. The following approach may prove helpful.

Motivation

1 Assume, until shown otherwise, that the patient is well-motivated and trying to cooperate. Rarely, a manipulative patient will "make a fool" of you, but far better that than to disbelieve or discount your findings in the vast majority of patients who are doing the best they can.

Effort

2 Assess physical effort. In strength testing, demonstration of full strength (as discussed in Chapter 6) depends upon an ability to elicit a full effort, which is subject to fatigue, pain, etc. You can usually assume that the patient (if not guarding because of local pain) is exerting full effort if full effort is evident elsewhere in the body. That is, normal resistive strength in shutting the eyes or gripping with the right hand usually means that decreased effort (as from fatigue or systemic illness) is not the cause of a weak grip on the left.

Indirect and functional evaluations

3 When direct testing leads to results that are hard to reproduce, try observation and indirect methods of testing. Deduce what you can about leg strength from observing walking and stair climbing. For coordination, watch how the patient manipulates buttons, handles eating utensils, etc. Such clues may not tell the whole story, but they will at least demonstrate a minimum level of capability.

Patient as ally

4 Try enlisting the patient as an ally in what is openly acknowledged as a difficult process. If the problem is one of sensory mapping, some patients can define the abnormal area better by testing themselves than by responding to your stimuli (see Chapter 7).

These approaches will not necessarily uncover the malingerer or the unusual patient with full-blown conversion hysteria (see next section). Much more common are patients who are anxious, tense, frightened by their symptoms, or upset by the process of examination. With these patients, you can make a good start by simply being human. Acknowledge, at least to yourself, your frustration, but avoid projecting this onto the patient. The next section will explore some of these issues more fully in the context of a highly charged topic, hysteric conversion.

THE PATIENT SUSPECTED OF HYSTERIC CONVERSION

The issue of hysteric conversion challenges the clinician's cognitive examination skills in a unique way. Although theories abound, we do not truly know how it is that the nervous system, at whatever level of the subconscious, can produce symptoms and signs that masquerade as neurologic deficits – for example, a sensory loss so profound that no pain is reported with "painful stimuli." Because of our ignorance of the underlying psychophysical mechanisms, the best approach to diagnosis and management is a very practical one. Unlike poorly responsive or highly agitated subjects, the patient suspected of hysteric conversion poses no barrier to the simple mechanics of the examination. How to weigh the findings, how to elicit contradictions, and how to induce a return to normal performance are the vexing problems.

CASE 18E
Paralysis

Pain

Alfredo Correia, a 48-year-old right-handed man, was admitted because of pain in the left shoulder and arm, as well as slight left chest discomfort. On examination, no cardiac, cervical spine, or carotid vascular abnormalities were found, but the left arm was moderately and diffusely weak on resistive strength testing. No sensory, reflex, or other abnormal signs were found in the arm, nor were there any deficits in the face, trunk, or leg. Myocardial infarction was ruled out.

Arm weakness

Arm and leg paralysis

A follow-up examination by the medical resident revealed severe weakness in the left lower extremity as well, but no weakness above the neck. The neurologic consultant observed that the patient exhibited no spontaneous movement of the left upper and lower extremities, as he lay in bed. He said he could not walk, but when helped to his feet he actually bore his own weight. With encouragement he walked, favoring the left leg as if it were painful to bear weight (although he denied pain). On testing strength in the arms, both hands and forearms were tested simultaneously, although all the visual attention and instructions were directed to the right arm. As he was rapidly tested in pushing, pulling the right forearm, dorsiflexing the fist, etc., it became apparent that he was simultaneously exerting resistance with the left arm and hand. In fact, when the examiner let go of the left hand while continuing to test the right, posture in the left forearm was maintained – it did not drop limply.

Able to walk

Explanation to patient

His symptoms were interpreted to him in the following way: "I understand that you have been experiencing pain in your left shoulder, arm, and chest that has been very worrisome to you. As you can see, your strength is improving. With more physical therapy of the sort I have just been using to treat you, I anticipate that your strength will soon be normal, but I am not sure whether the pain will respond as quickly. I will be back later today, because I want to understand better what you have been going through. In the meantime, you can be working on these exercises. . . ."

Observation of activity

Although it appeared that the neurologic deficit was not due to any neurologic lesion that could be identified, but rather had a psychologic origin, it was decided to continue neurologic observation of his function in ordinary activities (eating, walking to the bathroom, etc.) Also, since little was known of his psychosocial background or current status, more history would be obtained from his family, from him, and from old medical records, etc. The medical team would discuss the issues with the liaison psychiatrist, but would not request a formal consultation just yet. With regard to further neurodiagnostic testing, neck and shoulder X-rays would be obtained as a screen for coexistent disease that might have instigated the initial symptoms. Other tests, such as cervical magnetic resonance imaging would be deferred, as clinical improvement was occurring.

Work-up

Psychosocial inquiry uncovered no exceptional stresses or psychodynamic issues, but further probing was planned. Over a couple of days Mr Correia regained normal strength and full use of the limbs, but continued to complain of some shoulder and arm pain. Despite the lack of definite signs of cervical radiculopathy (or X-ray evidence of cervical spine abnormalities), the working formulation postulated a cervical root origin for the pain. In addition, he probably harbored some cardiac anxiety. There had been an elaboration of symptoms and deficits into an apparent paralysis.

Psychosocial assessment

Some cautionary notes

In approaching this kind of case, the first objective is to put aside biases and facile assumptions. Consider the following cautions and pitfalls.

Misdiagnosis

1 The distinction of neurologic problems from those that are of psychologic origin is notoriously difficult, even for experienced neurologists and psychiatrists.

"Nonanatomic" deficits

2 Beware of an assertion that a deficit is "nonanatomic." Some depth of knowledge is necessary to be quite sure of an anatomically impossible deficit, and even then (as emphasized in Chapter 14), our working constructs of clinical anatomy fall far short of reflecting CNS complexity. Moreover, the nonanatomic features of a deficit may obscure a smaller, more credible finding.

Bizarre symptoms

3 Just because neurologic symptoms and signs are "bizarre," do not presume that they are in some sense psychologic. For a general clinician, especially an inexperienced one, to say, "I've never seen anything like that – it isn't neurologic" is thoughtless and arrogant, but even the most seasoned specialist has not "seen it all."

Psychodynamic seduction

4 Psychodynamic explanations can be not only plausible, but amazingly seductive. They are often wrong. In almost any patient's history, you can find stress, conflict, and deeper, unresolved psychologic issues, as well as atypical behaviors. This does not mean that the tantalizing psychodynamic tidbit is the key to conversion. At the same time, do not ignore psychodynamic information. If not the answer, it may still be relevant to the care of the patient.

Ruling out organic lesions, identifying psychiatric issues

5 A diagnosis of hysteric conversion should not be just a matter of exclusion. Ruling out identifiable neurologic processes is important but never absolutely establishes a diagnosis of conversion. To be as certain as possible, put this evidence together with psychiatric evaluation and the response of the patient to intervention.

Patient's affect

6 Do not diagnose hysteric conversion based upon your impression of the patient's affect. Many errors arise from presumptions as to what affect or behavior a person with a deficit should display. Individuals vary greatly in their response to illness and in their ability to adapt emotionally over time. "Indifference" (an attitude traditionally attributed to conversion hysterics) may be very difficult to judge, in the present day, given prevalent cultural differences.

Open-mindedness

7 Resist premature closure on a diagnosis of hysteric conversion. An erroneous diagnosis of conversion will distract you from a proper work-up and, at the least, may spoil the doctor–patient relationship. The physician caring for a case of suspected conversion strives not to miss a treatable condition, but also must protect the patient from iatrogenic injury, due to unnecessary or excessive medications or invasive procedures.

Interpreting inconsistencies

8 Beware of overreliance on minor inconsistencies as a criterion of conversion. Symptoms are often hard to convey, and there may be an evolution in the patient's attempt to do so. Subjectively based findings, such as the demarcation of sensory deficits, are often hard to "pin down" for both patient and examiner. Exertion is frequently affected by fatigue and discomfort, both of which vary. Rapid or prolonged testing can introduce a fluster-factor. Some neurologic processes are intrinsically unstable, leading to fluctuating deficits.

Some "tricks" of examination

There are many so-called tricks used to demonstrate that a neurologic deficit is either nonanatomic or inconsistent. Insofar as possible, avoid the appearance of trying to trick or expose the patient. (If the patient confronts you, which is rare in conversion, but may occur in malingering, you can honestly say that he or she has "some confusion in the nervous system" which you are trying to understand.) In any case, the search for contradictions does play a central role in the exclusion of credible deficits. A few of the commonly used "tricks" include the following, and additional material on this subject will be found in the Further reading section.

Side-to-side transmission of vibration

1 Assess a hemisensory loss by placing the vibrating fork first on one side of the head, then the other. The stimuli can be either well separated or just to the right or left of the midline. Since vibration is so well transmitted through bone, there will never be a purely one-sided loss of vibration on the head (or sternum or sacrum). (In case of an abrupt sensory loss on a limb, this principle can also be employed. Strong vibration applied to the end of a bone in the anesthetic area should be transmitted proximally to the region of normal sensation.)

"Fooling" right–left distinctions

2 Although somewhat transparent, you can utilize the ploy of crossed hands and fingers to test one-sided lack of touch or pin sensation. Rapid testing with insistence on rapid responses may reveal "lack of sensation" scattered among fingers of both hands when tested in this way.

Slanting dermatomes

3 In mapping a segmental sensory loss on the trunk, remember that the dermatomes on the back slant downward from the midline to the lateral thorax and abdomen. One patient presented with a painful "shingles rash" that did not show this anatomic distribution (or other true characteristics of the dermatomal pattern seen in herpes zoster). Other anatomic sensory patterns that are unknown to most patients can be helpful in a similar way. Medically knowledgeable patients are difficult!

Head turning

4 In cranial nerve motor testing, examination of head turning is a useful maneuver. The contraction of the right sternocleidomastoid muscle (SCM) pulls the mastoid process forward, turning the head to the left, since the mastoid is behind the axis of rotation. In a left hemiplegic conversion, the patient will typically not turn the head to the left against resistance, but will do so to the right (utilizing the left SCM).

Synergisms

5 The Hoover test capitalizes upon the employment of synergistic, "fixing" muscles when exerting a limb. A normal patient lying supine will press the left heel downward into the bed for stabilization while trying to raise the right lower limb, especially against firm resistance. If you put your hand under the left heel, you will feel no increased downward pressure if the patient is not exerting the right limb in flexion at the hip.

Misdirecting attention

6 Try misdirecting the patient's attention to one aspect of a test while observing another. For example, in a case of hand weakness, direct the patient to feel a coin and state its denomination (with eyes closed). Emphasizing verbally that he or she has good sensation and should be able to feel the coin well, observe the fine motor control involved in manipulating the coin in the hand. If well handled (even though the patient reports not feeling the surface characteristics), major weakness of distal muscles would be doubtful.

Positive guidelines for assessment

The clinical evaluation of suspected neurologic conversion should always extend beyond mere "tricks."

Mismatch: direct testing vs. function

1 Observe for a mismatch between the results of direct testing and functional performance. (Note that "functional" as employed here refers to use in practical operations, such as activities of daily living, not to "psychologic" or "nonorganic".) As in Case 18E, stance and gait were much better than would have been predicted from the left leg examination. The normal nervous system, programmed to walk from an early age, is not very good at not walking! "Hysteric" patients tend to resist trying, or to hop or shuffle in a way that actually reveals considerable function, or to limp as one does in pain, a common life experience. These do not simulate very well the ataxias from identifiable nervous system lesions.

A neurologic "nidus"

2 Consider the likelihood of an "organic nidus" for the deficit or symptoms – an anatomic crystal upon which symptoms grow. In present day practice, most cases suspected of being hysteric conversions do not arise full-blown, but rather represent elaborations upon small symptoms or deficits that have triggered this reaction in the susceptible patient. A minor "pinched nerve" problem, for example, often presents with pain and a little tingling, but in the suggestible patient the symptoms may progress to local weakness and hemiparesis, as in Case 18E. As examiners, we are complicit in this process of elaboration, since our testing (or discussion) may suggest the possibility of more extensive or serious deficits.

Functional and observational examination

3 Because of this interaction of testing with the manifestation of deficits, repeated direct examinations may prove to be counterproductive. Certainly, it is essential to do at least one very good and thorough examination. Very objective tests such as deep tendon reflexes (DTRs), plantar responses, pupillary reflexes, etc. can be reconfirmed with impunity. However, as you sit and talk with the patient about life events, family, job, etc., watch for the small limb adjustments normally made while changing position in bed and observe sitting up, body language, etc. The entire care team can participate in viewing and recording functional performance. Take advantage of opportunities to view activity when the patient is not aware of being watched (including sleep and the onset of awakening, when much natural and spontaneous activity occurs). Note that true hemiparetic limbs may move dramatically during yawning!

You can rely more on close observation of functional performance than on direct examination in the following instances: (a) expert diagnostic assessment points to the likelihood of conversion; (b) appropriate noninvasive tests (such as neuroimaging by CT or MRI) are negative; and (c) the patient is stable or improving. Note that low output – relative absence of observable activity – makes any judgment more difficult; increased intensity of direct examination may be needed.

Utilize noninvasive tests

4 Because of the usual persistence of some diagnostic uncertainty, extra reliance should be placed on noninvasive testing, such as CT and MRI. These tests do not reinforce nonanatomic deficits.

Engage the patient

5 Stepping back from certain aspects of direct testing does not imply pulling away: the patient should not be abandoned as the symptoms recede. As the complaint ("I can't move my left side") is given less direct attention, the patient should be accorded more personal attention. As the symptoms are disengaged, engage the patient more.

Rapid "rehabilitation"

6 As briefly illustrated in Case 18E, a positive, nonconfrontational approach emphasizing "reeducation" and rehabilitation may be most efficacious. Improved performance empowers the patient to take control over return of function. Be aware, however, that the symptoms and signs of some pathologic processes (such as cerebral ischemia or chronic subdural hematoma) wax and wane. Transient improvement should never be taken as a signal that the diagnosis is necessarily one of conversion hysteria or some other psychologic disorder.

Nonmechanistic feedback

7 Unless you find a psychodynamic or other mechanistic key that promises to be effective in expediting the patient's recovery, do not offer the patient a detailed interpretation of your examination findings and diagnostic hypotheses. I often reflect back: "I can see that you're having some trouble walking," or "That seems to be difficult for you." The purpose of this open-endedness is to avoid confirming specific disabilities and to leave plenty of room for imminent improvement. If the patient asks why this problem has occurred, I might say, "I don't understand it completely, but your nervous system has had some kind of reaction that now seems to be subsiding. If I gain a better understanding later, we can discuss it in more detail."

Some final comments

You may have noticed that I have not specifically defined the term "hysteric conversion." It is often broadly used to describe almost any substantial deficit that is believed to be of psychologic origin and not due to malingering (conscious fabrication of symptoms). The distinction between a conversion symptom and other somatiform disorders is not easy to make. For example, many patients have headaches related to stress, depression, or other psychologic states, but these are not usually called hysteric conversion. Neurologic conversion states usually involve blindness, paralysis, loss of sensation, or inability to walk. The term hysteric conversion should not be used loosely, since psychologic mechanisms are difficult to confirm. "Hysteric" also bears pejorative connotations. Medical care-givers are quite prone to call a patient hysteric when there is some deficit that seems "improbable." Moreover, historically some practitioners have been conditioned to brand women with the hysteric label, with scant justification.

Parallel inquiries

Because cases of suspected hysteric conversion are fraught with such interpretive uncertainties, the ongoing diagnostic approach should comprise multiple parallel avenues: direct, indirect, and functional neurologic assessment; appropriate laboratory investigation (noninvasive insofar as possible); psychosocial inquiry, with formal or informal psychiatric input – not only for the patient and family, but also to help staff deal with a stressful and confusing case; and early "rehabilitative" intervention, the success of which carries both diagnostic and therapeutic implications.

SUMMARY

Four types of difficult examination situations have been exemplified by the agitated patient, the poorly responsive patient, the patient with an "unreliable," changing examination, and the patient suspected of hysteric conversion.

1 High, but uncontrollable output calls for observation, which can garner a good (but still incomplete) yield of neurologic findings.
2 In the low-output state any part of the examination requiring active cooperation is difficult, if not impossible. Obtain what information you can from passive acquiescence, but recognize the need for some

other form of intervention in most cases: neuroimaging, laboratory testing, or a trial of therapy.

3 In the patient with an "unreliable" or shifting examination evaluate factors (such as pain and fatigue) that may be causing variable effort. While remaining alert to an unstable pathologic process, apply indirect ways of assessing neurologic function. Learn from observations by nurses, aides, therapists, and other intimate care-givers.

4 In suspected hysteric conversion multiple avenues of assessment should be followed until the diagnosis is clear. This puts a premium on powers of observation, nonprejudicial thinking, and adherence to the maxim, "First of all, do no harm."

PROBLEMS FOR SELF-STUDY

Problems

1 Under what circumstances might you consider sedating an agitated patient for the purpose of obtaining more data?

2 A poorly responsive patient is found to have normal pupils, DTRs, plantar reflexes, tone, and no gaze deviation or papilledema. The physician orders the usual toxic–metabolic screen (of laboratory tests) and a CT scan, which are negative, and obtains psychiatric consultation. Evaluate this approach.

3 What explanation(s) would you suggest for the following changes in complaints and findings: a 34-year-old woman with a known psychiatric history presented to an emergency room with "headaches and tingling." She was found to be "sullen" but oriented and able to cooperate, and had a "nonfocal" neurologic examination. Plantar responses: "withdrawal". She complained of feeling very nervous. She vomited several times. Intravenous fluids were started. She said she was really scared; repeat strength testing showed "poor effort." She began to hyperventilate and stopped talking. Another examiner found her to be "tense all over." She started "shuddering" and her "pupils grew larger, as if in fright."

4 What laboratory test(s) or referrals, if any, would you consider in the following case: a 27-year-old woman was being treated for a right L5 radiculopathy with low back pain radiating into the leg. Because of increased pain codeine was added, but helped very little. Examination was made difficult by guarding. She had been under stress for years because of conflict with her father (a college president) who just 1 year ago had suffered a crippling stroke that left him confined to a wheelchair and incontinent. She returned the next day because of inability to void.

Comments

1 In general, sedation is avoided (unless there appears to be risk of injury to patient or staff) for fear of masking significant changes in level of consciousness, vital functions, or other indicators of pro-

gressive neurologic deterioration. However, at some point the information from neurologic imaging or lumbar puncture may be more critical than any additional examination data. Such decisions are forced when CNS infection, intracranial mass lesions, hydrocephalus, or spinal cord compression, etc., cannot otherwise be ruled out. Under circumstances like these, sedation to permit laboratory testing is warranted.

2 Some serious and progressive brain conditions may not be revealed by neurologic examination (especially when detailed mental status and behavioral examinations are unavailable). A CT scan will fail to show ischemic changes acutely, and some other lesions will be missed on a noncontrast scan. Certain types of encephalopathy and encephalitis will not be detected even by MRI, especially early in the course. Cerebrospinal fluid, electroencephalogram, and other laboratory testing should be considered. Parallel psychiatric evaluation may well be appropriate, in addition.

3 The vague report of a psychiatric history is prejudicial and should be excluded from consideration until something more specific is known that might contribute to the formulation. Headaches and tingling could represent tension and anxiety, but could just as well be due to an acute brain disorder; similarly for vomiting. A "nonfocal" examination (a usage that should be strongly discouraged) does not exclude bilateral, midline, or other pathologic processes without obvious right–left differences in signs. In the presence of an intracranial mass lesion, hydration can exacerbate the problem: in this case her verbal output ceased, and she hyperventilated, which occurs in upper brainstem dysfunction (for example, in some herniations). Simultaneously, her enlarging and less reactive pupils ominously suggested incipient CN 3 palsies, presumptively due to brain herniation (see Chapter 13). She was found to have bilateral chronic subdural hematomas, with superimposed acute subdural bleeding (probably related to a fall, that was not known at the time). Surgical evacuation resulted in complete recovery.

4 This patient apparently suffered from typical lumbar radiculopathy, which ordinarily would not lead to urinary retention. A background of psychodynamic material, suggesting some possible ambivalent identification with the father, raises the issue of a psychologic mechanism. Alternatively, could there be a more serious neurologic problem, such as spinal cord compression, leading to the urinary dysfunction? Actually, a disc or other pathology at the L4–L5 interspace (to which an L5 radiculopathy is usually referable) is below the termination of the spinal cord, so a myelopathy from a disc at this level can be ruled out. Compression of the cauda equina would need to be considered. The more mundane (and, in this case, correct) formulation postulated that she was experiencing a flare-up of her radiculopathy: her urinary retention represented a side effect of large

amounts of the opioid, codeine, as well as some effect from her pain. To be sure, spinal MRI neuroimaging was performed and did show disc protrusion at the L4–L5 level, but produced no evidence of cauda equina compression or spinal cord disease higher up. Her problem of urinary retention resolved (after initial catheter drainage) with rest and a change of medication.

FURTHER READING

The agitated patient

Lipowski, Z.J. *Delirium: Acute Confusional States*. Oxford University Press, New York (NY), 1990. Confusional states (agitated or otherwise) and their differentiation from dementia and psychosis are subjects of great importance in all of clinical medicine. (See also Further reading section of Chapter 10.)

The poorly responsive patient

Brazis, P.W., Masdeu, J.C., Biller, J. *Localization in Clinical Neurology*. 2nd edn. Little, Brown, and Company, Boston (MA), 1990. Clinicopathologic correlations, including the bihemispheric and brainstem lesions causing coma (Chapter 21).

Plum, F. Disturbances of consciousness and arousal. Sustained impairments of consciousness. In: Wyngaarden, J.B., Smith, L.H., Bennett, J.C., (eds) *Cecil Textbook of Medicine*. 19th edn. WB Saunders, Philadelphia (PA), 1992. Authoritative summaries in convenient form for users of this textbook (Chapters 443 and 444).

Plum, F., Posner, J.B. *Diagnosis of Stupor and Coma*. 3rd edn. F.A. Davis, Philadelphia (PA), 1980. The classic monograph on this penultimate failure of the nervous system.

Ropper, A.H., Martin, J.B. Coma and other disorders of consciousness. In: Wilson, J.D., Braunwald, E., Isselbacher, K.J., *et al.* (eds) *Harrison's Principles of Internal Medicine*. 12 edn. McGraw-Hill, New York (NY), 1991. Traditional concepts of the pathogenetic basis of depressed consciousness – the role of mass shifts and of diffuse metabolic impairment – are being increasingly informed by structural and functional neuroimaging (Chapter 31). Follow this subject in future editions!

The patient suspected of hysteric conversion

Barsky, A. The somatiform disorders. In: Hyman, S.E., Jenike, M.A. *Manual of Clinical Problems in Psychiatry*. Little, Brown, and Company, Boston (MA), 1990. Hysteric conversion placed in the context of other somatiform disorders.

Haerer, A.F. Examination in cases of suspected hysteria and malingering. In: *De Jong's The Neurologic Examination*. 5th edn. Lippincott, New York (NY), 1992. A repertoire of tests designed to expose nonanatomic, nonphysiologic deficits.

Keane, J.R. Hysterical gait disorders: 60 cases. *Neurology* 1989; 39:586–9. Diagnosis and treatment including the supportive, rehabilitative approach (known as "moral therapy" in the 19th century).

Lazare, A. Conversion symptoms. *N Engl J Med* 1981; 305:745–8. A brief, balanced overview of conversion hysteria and ways of studying it. One thing is sure: a significant number of cases are misdiagnosed.

Marsden, C.D. Hysteria – a neurologist's view. *Psychol Med* 1986; 16:277–88. A distinguished neurologist reviews part of the history of the subject and presents his experience and interpretations.

chapter 19

Selective Examinations: Screening and Problem-Oriented Assessment

Overview

There is no such thing as a complete neurologic examination. Even a seemingly thorough examination can be refined or amplified in dimension or detail. Selectivity is inevitable, but you can make choices rationally rather than haphazardly. Just as with laboratory testing, the testing of the neurologic examination requires planning. This process takes into account the individual patient, the clinical setting, and the time available.

Selectivity is applied for the sake of efficiency: go as directly as possible to "where the money is," that proverbial bank of the most relevant findings. Examination planning helps you to pare down the "standard" neurologic examination without a sense of guilt: omissions should be the result of choice, not neglect. On the other hand, the particular form of examination that you select for a specific patient may require augmentation of your usual examination. Your approach needs to be flexible. Once a clinical encounter is in process, you will modify the examination plan and format as the emerging data base demands.

THE SCREENING NEUROLOGIC EXAMINATION

Whether any routine neurologic screening can really be justified on the basis of effectiveness remains unclear. Neurologic screening in the absence of a neurologic complaint depends upon two principal rationales.

Baseline data

1 Baseline observations enable comparison with subsequent findings. You will often wish to know whether an observed pupillary inequality (anisocoria) is "old"? As in Case 5B, a patient may be brought into an emergency room with impaired responsiveness; knowing the baseline pupillary findings helps greatly not only in positive diagnosis, but in preventing unnecessary work-up.

Asymptomatic disease

2 Neurologic screening occasionally elicits signs of neurologic disease of which the patient is symptomatically unaware. For example, reflex and sensory abnormalities due to neuropathy can provide clues to undiagnosed diabetes.

Planning a screening neurologic examination (Table 19.1) should never proceed in isolation. It "stands on the shoulders" of a good history, a general physical assessment, and an observant approach to the clinical encounter as a whole. While the history usually provides the key to planning a neurologic assessment, reliance on the history alone is hazardous. Not only do symptomatically silent deficits occur, but some

Table 19.1 Screening neurologic examination in the asymptomatic patient

Key observations during history and general physical examination	Key tests of neurologic importance included with the general examination	Specific neurologic screening tests (bilateral)
Postures, deformities	Signs of trauma Neck mobility	Visual acuity Visual fields
Position and alignment of eyes	Carotid examination Funduscopic examination	Pupils Eye movements
Facial expression		
Phonation, articulation	Elevation of palate Tongue protrusion, bulk, (fasciculations)	Hearing
Adventitious movements Functional use of muscles	General muscle bulk, fasciculations	Limb tone (Proximal and distal strength)
		Pin, vibration in toes
Stance and gait Speech coordination		
		Ankle jerks Plantar responses
Mental status and behavior		

neurologic lesions mute or distort the ability of the patient to recognize or express symptoms (see Chapter 1). The less comprehensive the history, the more comprehensive the examination and ancillary testing need to be. Always be prepared to "shift gears." At any stage of the work-up, you may need to broaden or intensify your examination.

Clues on the general physical

The general physical examination provides numerous opportunities for making significant neurologic observations. By programming the goals of the neurologic examination into the general physical, you can capitalize upon the areas of overlap. For example, when you auscultate the patient's back for breath sounds, you may discover a winging of the scapula (usually due to a palsy of the long thoracic nerve) which otherwise might remain unnoticed. Conversely, in eliciting ankle jerks in the neurologic examination the finding of a possible "hung-up" reflex would instigate evaluation for hypothyroidism.

Screening for baseline and asymptomatic deficits

Visual acuity

Check visual acuity (with a pocket screener or newsprint) as a baseline. Test each eye separately, using corrective lenses, if any, since a decrease in acuity in just one eye may elude the patient's recognition.

Visual fields

Abnormalities of the visual fields are often asymptomatic, especially if the lesion is small or slow in development. Confrontation testing of all quadrants of the visual fields may elicit evidence of lesions anywhere in the extent of the visual receptive pathways from the front to the back of the brain. For quick visual field screening purposes, both eyes can be tested together, but the patient should be asked to report any visual change when each eye is covered separately.

Pupils

Pupil size and reactivity should be specifically documented. Estimating the pupillary diameter in millimeters reminds you to make precise observations and convinces the later reader that you had actually scrutinized the pupils closely.

Eye movements

A baseline record of normal alignment of the eyes and a full range of conjugate movement may well pay dividends in the future. The congenital origin of some cases of strabismus or nystagmus may not be obvious.

Palpebral fissure

A difference in the width of the palpebral fissures (separation of the upper and lower lids), is worth documenting. Asymmetry may be due to widening on one side or narrowing on the other (see Table 5.7). A slight ptosis, sometimes part of a mild congenital Horner's syndrome (Fig. 13.11), is an occasional incidental finding.

Hearing

Like testing of visual acuity, evaluation of hearing may fall in the gap between the general and specifically neurologic examinations. The history frequently fails to uncover a mild problem, or the patient may minimize a more severe one. Incipient deafness often contributes to a "silent" decline of function in the elderly. You may be alerted to any major problem with hearing discrimination by the patient's responses during conversation.

Strength

You can safely omit resistive strength testing in young people and fully active, asymptomatic patients who show no abnormalities of movements during the general encounter. However, in the elderly, in patients with other significant medical problems, or where any uncertainty prevails, screen proximal and distal groups bilaterally in upper and lower extremities. You can accomplish this quickly by checking dorsiflexion at the wrist, abduction at the shoulder, flexion at the hip, and dorsiflexion at the ankle. In combination, these tests are quite sensitive to the effects of upper motor neuron (UMN) lesions, proximal myopathies, and distal polyneuropathies. To expand the screening examination, assess the outstretched arms and hands for downward drift or pronation while testing the "Romberg."

Tone

Surprising as it might seem initially, testing for increased tone in the elderly is more productive than formal testing of strength. Test tone especially at wrist and elbows bilaterally. Even slight rigidity may provide the first inkling of Parkinson's disease (see Cases 8A and 11A). During the whole encounter, keep an eye out for resting or other tremor.

Coordination

Gait should be observed as a matter of course at the beginning or end of the encounter. Augmented screening combines simultaneous testing for the Romberg sign, drift, postural (action) tremor, and "flap" (asterixis); you can complete your observation of the outstretched hands by asking the patient to touch his or her own nose with each index finger.

Sensory

In the asymptomatic patient pin and vibratory sense testing in the toes screens effectively for most peripheral neuropathies and lesions of the ascending sensory pathways of the spinal cord. Finding impaired sensation can put you on the track of unsuspected primary neurologic disease and, more commonly, systemic problems, such as diabetes or nutritional deficiencies.

Reflexes

Tendon jerks and plantar responses (Babinskis) are important both as baseline observations and as asymptomatic findings. Despite a broad range of normal tendon reflex responses, baseline documentation (especially of the extremes of hyper- or hyporeflexia) is useful. Decreases occur early in polyneuropathies. Thus, you should include at least ankle jerks in your screening (see Chapter 16).

Head and neck

Funduscopic screening is more important to the general physical examination than to the neurologic specifically. However, the appearance of the optic disc and the presence of venous pulsations has some baseline value. In addition, optic atrophy, especially in one eye only, may not have been suspected because of lack of recognition of associated deficits, such as impaired acuity. Detection of a carotid bruit may influence management specifically, or only as a marker of general vascular disease (see Chapter 4).

Tests undone

Some tests which have been recommended by others for brief survey examinations have been omitted or deemphasized. Testing sensation on the face very rarely detects a significant asymptomatic deficit. Corneal and gag reflex testing yields little in the asymptomatic patient; baseline screening is fruitless. You can observe facial expression throughout the encounter, which obviates the need for specific screening tests. Like the corneal and gag reflexes, the superficial abdominal reflexes can be abnormal in either segmental disease or in long tract disease; however, the value in the asymptomatic patient is low and the chance of confounding factors high (see Chapter 9).

Recording the screening examination

When screening for baseline findings, the results of such tests should be very specifically documented. Recording reflexes as "physiologic" will spoil the confidence of a future examiner in relying on the "old records."

In summary, employ the concept of a screening examination flexibly. Take into account the specific context of the examination, general health status, epidemiologic factors, such as age, patient expectations, and any new data that emerge during the examination.

PROBLEM-ORIENTED NEUROLOGIC EXAMINATIONS

An example: lower back/leg pain

An otherwise well patient comes in complaining of back pain, radiating down the left leg (Fig. 19.1). You take a good history (see Chapter 16), including occupational and other environmental factors, and are about to begin an examination. Which aspects should you include in your examination? Is a thorough neurologic survey really needed? Is it feasible, given time constraints?

The presenting complaint determines the shape of a selective examination. It is problem-oriented, not diagnosis-oriented. Like the screening examination, the selective examination is not a static entity, but rather a flexible and realistic working plan. When embarking on a selective assessment you may, of course, also take the opportunity to conduct appropriate general neurologic screening.

Back pain and an approach to neurologic assessment of the spine

Local examination

A neurologic examination for back pain in general (or any spinal problem) should address three general issues: local or regional abnormalities, segmental neurologic signs, and evidence of myelopathy (involvement of the spinal cord itself). Local "neighborhood" findings in the back, such as tenderness, muscle spasm, limitation of range of motion, or skin changes may provide clues to causative disorders (such as an abscess); in any case, interpreting specific neurologic tests will depend upon the role of pain and guarding. The investigation of low back pain in general is not complete without consideration of an abdominal examination for

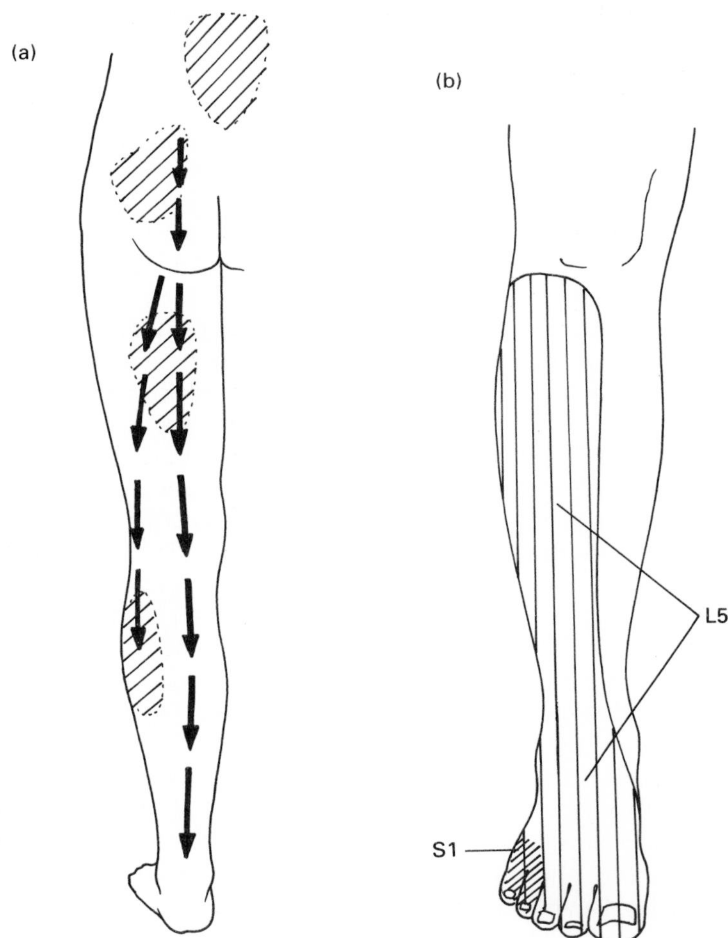

Fig. 19.1 Common distributions of pain and numbness in sciatica (L5 and S1 radiculopathies). (a) The arrows show pain radiating down the posterior or the posterolateral aspect of the thigh and leg. Pain usually does not extend into the foot beyond the heel. Pain often "settles in" to hatched areas shown in the low back, buttock, posterior thigh, and posterolateral calf. (b) The dermatomal distributions of the L5 root and S1 root are shown, as seen anteriorly. Numbness often occurs in the toes, usually in the 4th and 5th digits in S1 radiculopathy and in the first three or four digits in L5 radiculopathy.

aneurysm or other mass, pelvic examination, and rectal examination with prostatic palpation.

Segmental signs

Determination of segmental neurologic symptoms and signs will establish the neural level of the problem, such as the S1 segment. In this example, pain might typically radiate down the posterior thigh into the calf. Numbness would often be experienced in the 4th and 5th toes.

Findings might include mildly altered pin and touch sensation in the lateral foot and toes, an absent ankle jerk, and perhaps weakness in plantar flexion of the toes and foot, as well as atrophy and fasciculations of the calf (if the process is chronic). Note that the S1 neural level of involvement does not mean that the disease process is necessarily at the vertebral L5–S1 interspace or in the sciatic nerve itself (see Chapter 13, including Fig. 13.9, and Chapter 16).

Long tract signs?

The third area of concentration focuses on any possibility of myelopathy, in the form of long tract motor, sensory, or reflex signs, or bladder, bowel, or sexual dysfunction. Root involvement in sciatica (lumbosacral radiculopathy), caused by an intravertebral disc, occurs at a vertebral level below the end of the spinal cord (see Fig. 13.9). The most common interspaces are L4–L5 and L5–S1. No myelopathy resulting in long tract signs could occur at the level of exit of these roots (or at L3–L4). Even so, check for long tract symptoms and signs, which might signal a more extensive pathologic process or a coexistent lesion higher in the neuraxis. Certainly, with radicular pain at a thoracic or cervical level, the identification of coexistent myelopathy assumes critical importance. A careful examination includes assessment for UMN signs such as increased tone, nonsegmental weakness, hyperreflexia, and an extensor plantar sign. In the sensory evaluation the examiner should be certain that impaired sensation in the foot does not extend, even to a lesser degree, to the more proximal leg and thigh, or even to a sensory level on the trunk.

Bladder, bowel, and sexual dysfunction

As noted, always inquire about bowel, bladder, and sexual dysfunction. If symptoms or other signs signal possible abnormalities in S3–S5-mediated functions, then perform a perineal sensory and reflex examination (see Chapter 9). Urinary or fecal retention or incontinence, as well as impotence or other sexual dysfunction, can occur on either a suprasegmental or segmental basis, as well as for non-neurologic reasons. You should not count on making a definite distinction from the history alone (see Chapter 13), but must add examination, imaging, and/or physiologic testing data. Lax anal sphincter tone, often with diminished voluntary and reflex sphincter contraction, and blunted perineal sensation are most readily identified. These findings usually point to localization in sacral segmental circuits, but may be part of a more extensive deficit due to myelopathy (long tract) involvement at a higher level (even though the phenomenon of "sacral sparing" of sensation sometimes occurs).

Cauda equina syndrome

Segmental sacral dysfunction that is bilateral and involves more than one level usually can be localized to the cauda equina (see Fig. 13.9). In the cauda equina syndrome, a pathologic process, such as tumor compression or infiltration, affects lumbosacral spinal roots as they descend within the lumbar spinal column, before exiting. This syndrome would be suggested by a multidermatomal sensory pattern, lack of long tract signs in the legs, and abnormal perineal findings, as described above. Note that any lumbar as well as sacral, roots still within the spinal canal at the level of the lesion are vulnerable to involvement.

The autonomic control of bladder function is summarized in Chapter 13, and aspects of it are presented schematically in Fig. 13.12.

Testing for radiculopathy

The local and regional examination for lower back pain starts, as previously described, with checking for signs of disease in other organs; testing proceeds with assessment of spinal mobility in all planes, as well as palpating for tenderness, muscle spasm, etc. The next step directly addresses the issue of a specific radiculopathy.

Straight leg raising

Disease or injury of a nerve root may be revealed either in signs of inflammation of that root or signs of impaired function in its distribution (see Chapter 16). Stretching the nerve root, by means of straight leg raising, elicits signs and symptoms of inflammation. With the patient lying supine and the leg fully extended at the knee, raise the leg up gently (flexing the hip). Ask the patient to make no exertion, but to inform you of any pain or other symptoms. Depending on the suppleness of the patient's limbs, you may be able to flex the thigh (with the leg still fully extended at the knee) to a 90° angle. Whenever you perform the straight leg raising test on one side, do it on the other side as a control – although it may be truly abnormal on both sides. The term "crossed straight leg raising test" simply refers to testing the side opposite to the symptoms.

Interpretation

Many patients experience a normal tightness and perhaps mild discomfort in the hamstrings of the posterior thigh at some point between 45 and 90° of straight leg raising. If this resistance feels roughly symmetric, and the presenting symptoms of pain or numbness are not reproduced, you can regard the test as negative with respect to a specific radiculopathy. An abnormal (positive) straight leg raising test consists of abnormal resistance (including involuntary guarding) compared to the other side or to usual expectations, as well as reproduction of symptoms. Since the pathology can be bilateral, the latter is particularly important. (Compare straight leg raising with the Kernig sign of meningeal and root inflammation discussed in Chapter 4, and the Lasègue sign to be mentioned below.)

Crossed straight leg raising

In addition, an abnormal response to straight leg raising on the side opposite the presenting symptoms (crossed straight leg raising) is sometimes associated with a "free fragment syndrome" – a disc herniation in which extruded material has broken free and may be in a position to irritate a contralateral root.

Other tests

A variety of other direct and indirect tests have been devised to assess the same problem – abnormal sensitivity to nerve root stretching. One sign (Lasègue) is an abnormal limitation of ability to extend the leg once the thigh has been flexed: first, flex the thigh to 90° with the leg also flexed at the knee, then gently extend the leg, noting reproduction of symptoms or resistance that appear earlier than on the other side. The stretch of either the Lasègue or ordinary straight leg raising is further enhanced by your gently dorsiflexing the foot.

Since the lower lumbar and sacral roots that innervate the leg are all being stretched, these maneuvers do not specify one particular root (e.g. L5 or S1). Only when pain or numb sensations are reproduced in a particular dermatomal distribution will these tests suggest which root is more likely affected.

When you question possible elaboration of symptoms and signs, such as more impairment of straight leg raising than you expect, watch how well the patient bends over at the waist. Does one knee flex with bending? If the patient is seated, is there any difficulty in extending the knee (the equivalent of the Lasègue maneuver)?

Inverse straight leg raising, performed with the patient prone, extends the thigh. This stretches the lumbar roots placed anteriorly at the hip, as opposed to the posteriorly placed lower lumbosacral roots. Inverse straight leg raising not only evaluates the roots of the femoral nerve (mainly L3 and L4), but also the roots innervating the iliopsoas muscles (L2 and L3) and the muscles themselves, either retroperitoneally or across the hip joint.

Nerve tenderness

If you can apply pressure to a nerve derived from inflamed roots, you may elicit mild tenderness. This is the basis of pressing over the sciatic notch posteriorly at the gluteal crease. Palpation here is not ordinarily a very helpful test. In any case, remember that "sciatic notch tenderness" does not imply that the origin of the pathology is in the sciatic nerve trunk itself.

Sensory testing

In radiculopathies involving a single root, clearcut dermatomal patterns of sensory impairment are difficult to detect. Damage to an individual nerve root (especially if partial) causes variable and often only minimal sensory alteration (see Fig. 16.2). Patients may be able to express a sense of mild impairment of tactile or especially pin stimulation, but this is very hard to document by mapping areas of altered sensory threshold. Thus, failure to find a clear dermatomal pattern of sensory loss on examination in no way disproves the presence of a significant single radiculopathy. (Of course, even involvement of a single root, such as left L5, does not differentiate between the anterior and posterior roots.) Clinical diagnosis depends upon the distribution of pain and altered sensation, as well as motor and reflex deficits when present.

Motor testing

For examination of muscles innervated by a particular root, refer to Chapter 16, section on selective muscle testing. All radicular motor signs are of a lower motor neuron type. Like sensory changes, weakness in cases of single lumbosacral root disorders is often absent or equivocal.

Electrodiagnostic evaluation (electromyography and special forms of nerve conduction tests) can document denervation in specific limb and paraspinal muscles, and conduction delays. Denervation in an appropriate paraspinal muscle segment demonstrates that the lesion must be quite proximal. This localizing finding confirms that denervation in limb muscles innervated by that same nerve root does not result from a more peripheral nerve lesion. Paraspinal muscles react symptomatically (pain, spasm, and feelings of postural weakness), but clinical examination for localizing segmental signs is unproductive.

Correlation

The problem of incidental findings looms especially large in the arena of spinal diagnosis. "Degenerative joint disease" and disc bulging are very prevalent, even rampant! Without a firm bead on the clinical localization and probable pathology, irrelevant bony spurs and protruding discs will be diagnostically implicated and possibly even operated upon. With a characteristic pain pattern (that need not include lancinating pain actively shooting down the leg), radiculopathy should be suspected. In L5 root involvement (usually L4–L5 disc), numbness tends to involve the dorsum of the foot and medial toes, but usually no ankle or knee jerk depression. Dorsiflexion of the great toe may be diminished in strength. Disorders of the S1 root (as from an L5–S1 disc) may cause numbness of the lateral edge of the foot, sole, and 4th and 5th toes, as well as a decreased ankle jerk. Weakness of plantar flexion of the toes and foot is harder to identify.

SUMMARY

1 Screening and selective examinations are practical necessities. Use your limited time rationally, not in a rote or haphazard fashion. Not everyone will agree on the details of an appropriate screening examination in the neurologically asymptomatic patient, but that does not invalidate the concept.
2 The main rationales for screening are to provide baseline data for future reference and to detect significant neurologic deficits of which the patient is unaware.
3 The screening examination should be flexible, varying according to age and other general criteria and individual patient factors. At any point in the examination (or general encounter) indications may arise to broaden or intensify the testing.
4 Screening for baseline data is useless unless specifically recorded.
5 Selective examinations are problem-oriented; they include the relevant parts of a thorough neurologic survey and are often augmented by additional tests (such as straight leg raising for low back/leg pain).
6 Emergencies call for a compressed style of selective examination, as briefly described in the context of rapid emergency formulation (in Chapter 12); for examination of the comatose and other poorly responsive patients, see Chapter 18.

7 The problems of back/leg pain and neck/arm pain are the most common ones for which selective, problem-oriented examinations are appropriate. (See Chapter 4 for examination of the neck and Chapter 16 for information on the cervical roots.) In general, spinal assessments should address (a) local or regional factors; (b) segmental neurologic signs; and (c) myelopathic long tract signs, whether directly related, indirectly related, or coincidental. Bladder, bowel, and sexual dysfunction should be assessed in the history and, if indicated, by perineal sensory and reflex examination.

8 Lower back and lower extremity pain (the syndromes of "sciatica" or lumbosacral radiculopathy) are diagnosed mainly by (a) history of the pain and/or numbness – the quality, distribution, and exacerbating factors; (b) evidence of radicular irritation/inflammation, as in straight leg raising; (c) if present, reflex and motor signs; and (d) relevant abnormalities by neuroimaging and electromyography/nerve conduction studies.

PROBLEMS FOR SELF-STUDY

Problems

1 A 33-year-old woman undergoes a screening neurologic examination as part of her annual health maintenance physical examination. Her family doctor finds absent ankle jerks. What steps would you propose?

2 A 50-year-old man also displays an abnormality on a screening neurologic examination; vibratory sense is reduced in the toes of both feet. What additional information would you like?

3 A 27-year-old woman developed low back and right leg pain and is referred for "sciatica." A selective examination reveals substantial sensory loss to pin and touch over the middle and lateral dorsum and sole of the foot, heel, and lateral aspect of the leg. The ankle jerk is absent, and there is mild weakness in dorsiflexion of the great toe and foot, eversion, and plantar flexion. Straight leg raising is abnormally limited and there is gluteal notch tenderness. How would you analyze this situation?

Comments

1 Let us assume that the doctor was skilled in obtaining ankle jerks and that they really were not obtainable, even with further relaxation and distraction. The first step might be to try reinforcement. Next, check the other DTRs to see whether there is a general absence or extreme hyporeflexia, or whether there is a disproportion between the ankle jerks and knee jerks, or both of these and the upper extremity reflexes. Totally absent reflexes may be completely normal or may be a benign condition associated with "tonic" (very slowly reacting) pupils. New and progressive loss of all DTRs occurs with the Guillain–Barré syndrome of acute demyelinating polyneuropathy and radiculopathy (a medical emergency). The most common form of this condition is marked by weakness and thus should have been evident from the

history and the rest of the examination. Turning to possible reflex disproportion, if the knee jerks and upper extremity DTRs were brisk you might chiefly suspect an axonal polyneuropathy, and look for distal sensory (and motor) impairment and consider various causes, such as diabetes, vitamin deficiency syndromes, etc. Perhaps by now the "old" medical record has arrived and you can check a prior screening examination to ascertain the status of her DTRs in the past!

2 Symmetrically impaired vibratory sense is a common manifestation of polyneuropathy, as in diabetes. In this case checking ankle jerks and more proximal reflexes would be helpful. In addition to this, further sensory testing, especially for pain, would help to differentiate polyneuropathy from a process mainly involving the posterior columns of the spinal cord.

3 In this case presenting as "sciatica," the remarkable feature is the relative severity and extent of the neurologic findings. They surpass the degree of neurologic deficits expected for a single nerve root lesion, and involve the more extensive sensory and motor distributions of L5, S1, and probably part of L4. While multiple disc herniations are possible, the burden would be on ruling out other pathologic processes that affect multiple roots. In this instance, a tumor of the sciatic nerve trunk itself was found.

FURTHER READING

Adams, R.D., Victor, M. Pain in the back, neck, and extremities. In: *Principles of Neurology*. 4th edn. McGraw-Hill, New York (NY), 1989. The spine is both a protection and a trap for the neural structures contained within; Chapter 10 introduces relevant disorders.

Deyo, R.A., Rainville, J., Kent, D.L. What can the history and physical examination tell us about low back pain? *JAMA* 1992; 288:760–5. Draws together experience from an extensive literature on low back pain – a prime example of a presenting complaint that calls for a problem-oriented examination.

Frymoyer, J.W. Back pain and sciatica. *N Engl J Med* 1988; 318:291–300. Categories, epidemiology, natural history, diagnosis, and treatment.

Glick, T.H. *The Process of Neurologic Care in Medical Practice*. Harvard University Press, Cambridge (MA), 1984. Chapters 4 and 12 contain further examples of problem-oriented, selective, and enriched examinations appropriate for patients with common disorders, such as back and leg pain, dizziness, headaches, and seizures.

glossary

ABULIA Slowness; long latency of responses; lack of initiative; behavioral characteristics associated with certain frontal lobe syndromes.

ACHILLES REFLEX See ANKLE JERK REFLEX.

ACOUSTIC NEUROMA Schwann-cell tumor of CN 8 (8th cranial nerve).

ADVENTITIOUS Extra; unintended; involuntary (referring to movements).

AGRAPHIA Inability to write (language deficit).

AJ See ANKLE JERK REFLEX.

AKATHISIA A sense of restlessness or observed restless movements; side-effect associated with antipsychotic medications.

AKINESIA Lack of movement or difficulty initiating movement, despite having the neuromuscular capacity for movement; characteristic of parkinsonism.

ALEXIA Inability to read (language deficit).

AMYOTROPHY Wasting of muscle (in the context of denervation).

ANAL REFLEX Contraction of the anal sphincter in response to anal or perianal sensory stimulation.

ANEURYSM A bulging or outpouching of an arterial wall; most intracranial aneurysms are "berry aneurysms," occurring at bifurcations on or near the Circle of Willis.

ANISOCORIA Inequality of pupillary size.

ANKLE JERK REFLEX A deep tendon reflex (Achilles) elicited by striking the Achilles tendon and resulting in plantar flexion of the foot. The reflex is mediated mainly by the S1 nerve root (sciatic nerve).

ANOSOGNOSIA "Lack of insight" or "denial" of a neurologic deficit associated with a lesion of the nondominant (usually right) parietal lobe.

ANTERIOR APHASIA Motor speech disorders due to lesion(s) in dominant frontal lobe; typified by a Broca's (nonfluent) aphasia with effortful, telegraphic speech (dysprosody) emphasizing nouns; agrammatic; comprehension is virtually normal; associated with right face and hand weakness and dysarthria. Written language also affected.

ANTERIOR COLUMNS White matter in the anterior sector of the spinal cord.

ANTERIOR HORN Anterior (ventral) part of spinal central gray matter, including cell bodies of "anterior horn cells" (lower motor neurons).

ANTERIOR ROOT Axons of anterior horn cells up to the point that they join a mixed spinal/peripheral nerve.

ANTERIOR SPINAL ARTERY SYNDROME The anterior spinal artery is formed from the vertebral arteries and collateralized by branches from intercostal arteries; occlusion may produce infarction in the anterior two-thirds of the spinal cord over a variable number of segments.

APHAKIC Lacking the lens of the eye.

APHASIA Disorders of expression or comprehension of spoken language.

APRAXIA An inability to perform a learned act, despite demonstrated ability to perform all individual components of the act.

ARTERIOVENOUS MALFORMATION An abnormal tangle of blood vessels, presumed to be of congenital origin; may bleed, lead to seizures, or shunt blood past tissue causing ischemia.

ARTICULATION Enunciation of speech sounds; impairment is dysarthria.

ATAXIA Incoordination of limb or body movement; impairment of smoothness and accuracy of directed movement.

ATHETOSIS An involuntary movement disorder characterized by slow, sinuous, twisting changes of limb and body posture.

ATROPHY Wasting of muscle; due to denervation, muscle disease, disuse, or systemic wasting.

AUTISM Developmental disorder(s) affecting language and interpersonal relationships (etc.).

AVM See ARTERIOVENOUS MALFORMATION.

BABINSKI SIGN The (abnormal) extensor plantar response (upgoing toe); a hallmark of upper motor neuron dysfunction. The test itself (as opposed to the pathologic sign) is often loosely called "the Babinski."

BASAL GANGLIA Deep gray matter (nuclei) of the cerebral hemispheres comprising the caudate, putamen, globus pallidus, subthalamic nucleus, substantia nigra, and perhaps others, depending on the authority.

BELL'S PALSY Lower motor neuron type of facial palsy, due to involvement of CN 7 in its peripheral course; traditionally implies undefined cause (idiopathic).

BICEPS REFLEX The deep tendon reflex elicited by tapping the biceps tendon with consequent flexion of the forearm.

BJ See BICEPS REFLEX (biceps jerk).

BRACHIOCEPHALIC ARTERY A branch of the ascending aorta on the right; it bifurcates into the right common carotid and right subclavian arteries. Also called the innominate artery.

BRACHIORADIALIS REFLEX A periosteal reflex elicited by tapping on the distal radius with consequent contraction of the brachioradialis and extensor carpi radialis muscles, etc. (Usually grouped with "deep tendon reflexes" because it responds in the same way, as opposed to superficial reflexes, like the superficial abdominal.) Supinator reflex.

BRADYKINESIA A partial or lesser degree of akinesia; often used interchangeably.

BROCA'S APHASIA See anterior aphasia; Broca's area is in the posterior/inferior frontal lobe on the dominant side; lesions producing persistent Broca's aphasia are more extensive than Broca's area itself.

BROWN–SÉQUARD SYNDROME A constellation of neurologic signs resulting from a hemisection of the spinal cord; below the lesion deficits of upper motor neuron and dorsal column functions on the same side; deficits of pain–temperature on the opposite side.

BRUDZINSKI SIGN A sign of spinal meningeal irritation in which flexing the neck causes flexion at the knee and hip.

BRUIT A noise, heard over a narrowed artery, due to turbulence. Akin to a murmur from a heart valve. Pronounced "brew-ee."

BULBAR Refers to the medulla, but is commonly used to mean the brainstem more generally, as in "corticobulbar tracts."

BULBOCAVERNOSUS REFLEX A reflex maneuver to assess sacral segments (S3–S5) and nerves, in which squeezing the shaft or glans of the penis causes a reflex anal contraction.

CALCARINE CORTEX Primary visual cortex on the "banks" of the calcarine fissure of the medial occipital lobe; "striate cortex."

CALORIC TESTING A vestibular/ocular test utilizing cold or warm water irrigation of the ear (see ICE WATER CALORICS).

CAROTID ARTERY The common carotid artery and/or the internal or external carotid arteries; if unspecified, usually taken to mean the internal.

CAUDA EQUINA The "horse's tail" of lumbosacral nerve roots hanging down from their respective segments of the spinal cord to the level of the appropriate foramen of "exit."

CAUDAL Lower on the neuraxis; e.g. the spinal cord is caudal to the brainstem.

CHOREA An involuntary movement characterized by quick, flicking, or "dance-like" movements; slower than the lightning-fast jerks of myoclonus and faster than the twisting movements of athetosis.

CINGULATE The C-shaped gyrus of the limbic system, just dorsal to the corpus callosum (see SUBFALCIAL).

CLARKE'S COLUMN See NUCLEUS DORSALIS.

CLASP-KNIFE PHENOMENON A type of hypertonia occurring as part of spasticity in the upper motor neuron syndrome; with increasing stretch resistance increases, but then gives way.

CNS Central nervous system.

COGWHEEL RIGIDITY A ratchet-like, increased resistance to passive movement (hypertonia), characteristic of parkinsonism.

COMPUTERIZED TOMOGRAPHY An imaging technique based upon computer processing of data from differential attenuation of an X-ray beam by tissues of varying density. An earlier, synonymous term, was "CAT" (computerized axial tomography).

CORTICOBULBAR TRACT A descending cortical motor tract destined for a brainstem motor nucleus.

CORTICOSPINAL TRACT A white-matter tract which includes fibers of neurons in the primary motor cortex (and elsewhere), destined to synapse mainly on anterior horn cells (or interneurons) in the spinal cord.

CT See COMPUTERIZED TOMOGRAPHY.

DEEP TENDON REFLEX The most widely used clinical term for a monosynaptic "stretch" reflex, elicited by tapping a tendon, with resultant muscle contraction.

DEMYELINATION Primary loss of the myelin sheath of axons, (or secondary loss consequent to axonal damage).

DOLL'S EYES In the Doll's Head maneuver, the eyes tend to roll in their sockets away from the direction of head turning in the stuporous or comatose patient, if brainstem mechanisms are preserved.

DOMINANCE As in cerebral dominance, each hemisphere is specialized for principal control of certain functions.

DORSAL COLUMN NUCLEI Nuclei gracilis and cuneatus in the caudal medulla; contain cell bodies of 2nd order neurons in the dorsal column–lemniscal ascending sensory systems.

DORSAL COLUMNS White-matter sector in the posterior part of the spinal cord; traditionally used to designate collectively the fasciculi/tracts conveying fine touch–vibration–position senses. These modalities and their pathways may be referred to as the dorsal column–lemniscal system, although tracts subserving touch are more widely distributed, and much of joint position sense is conveyed in dorsolateral tracts.

DORSAL HORN Dorsal (posterior) part of spinal cord central gray matter; contains mainly neurons involved in afferent pathways.

DORSAL ROOT (Posterior root.) Designation of the central process (axon) of a dorsal root ganglion cell (up to the point of entering the spinal cord), as well as its peripheral process to the point of joining the anterior root to form a mixed peripheral nerve. These individual fibers aggregate into the entire nerve root on each side at each level.

DORSAL ROOT GANGLIA Cluster of cell bodies of 1st order sensory neurons, at each segmental level on each side, located approximately at the intervertebral foramen.

DTR See DEEP TENDON REFLEX.

DYSARTHRIA Impaired articulation of speech.

DYSKINESIA A general term for nonrhythmic involuntary movements; most often used in the context of chorea-like movements complicating antipsychotic therapy (tardive dyskinesia).

DYSMETRIA Missing a target, as on finger–nose or heel–shin testing, due to limb ataxia.

DYSPHASIA Partial aphasia – impaired expression or comprehension of spoken language.

DYSPHONIA Impaired production of voice sound.

DYSTONIA Increased muscle tone causing a persistent (but not fixed) abnormal posture and impaired movement.

EDEMA Swelling; in the brain, edema occurs most prominently in white matter and is due to cellular damage (cytotoxic) or to vascular damage (vasogenic).

EOM See EXTRAOCULAR MOVEMENTS.

EPILEPSY A collective term for a group of syndromes characterized by recurrent seizures, due to abnormal electrical discharges in the brain.

EXTRAOCULAR MOVEMENTS Movement of the eyes, affected by extraocular muscles, as opposed to the intraocular muscles which govern the iris and lens.

EXTRAPYRAMIDAL Referring to nonpyramidal (noncorticospinal) motor pathways; extrapyramidal disorders are associated with the basal ganglia.

FALX CEREBRI Rigid dural fold in the midsagittal plane, separating the cerebral hemispheres.

FASCICULATION The contraction of a fascicle of muscle fibers, innervated by the branches of one anterior horn cell; a fasciculation appears as a rippling or twitching in part of a muscle, usually insufficient to move a body part except for the digits (slightly).

FINAL COMMON PATHWAY The segmental motor outflow from an anterior horn cell to muscle. All suprasegmental and other segmental mechanisms affect muscular activity by way of anterior horn cells.

FLACCID Limp, showing no discernible tone.

FORAMEN MAGNUM The large opening at the base of the skull allowing continuity of the medulla above and the spinal cord below.

FOVEA Central portion of the macula in the retina of the eye.

GANGLIA Clusters of neurons grouped together for some particular function; for example, in the peripheral nervous system: the dorsal root ganglia, or the sympathetic ganglia; in the central nervous system: clusters of neurons are usually called nuclei, but the term ganglia has been attached traditionally to the large gray matter masses deep in the brain, known as the basal ganglia.

GAZE The axis or direction of the eyes, as a pair. A gaze palsy is a deficit of conjugate gaze in a given direction (usually associated with a gaze deviation in the opposite direction).

GENICULATE BODIES (NUCLEI) See LATERAL GENICULATE BODY; MEDIAL GENICULATE BODY.

GLIA Supporting cells in the central nervous system, serving many metabolic, reparative, and other functions.

GLIOMA The principal type of primary central nervous system cancer, derived from glial cells. The term glioblastoma was traditionally used to refer to the more malignant grades of glioma.

GRASP REFLEX An involuntary grasping of the hand when the palm is stimulated; a so-called frontal release reflex, which is present as a normal finding in infants, but thereafter is typically associated with frontal lobe or more diffuse cerebral pathology.

GRAY MATTER Central nervous system tissue consisting mainly of nerve cells (and glial cells) rather than myelinated fibers.

HEMIANOPIA Hemianopia (hemianopsia) denotes impairment in one-half of a visual field.

HEMIPARESIS Weakness of one side of the body, often taken to mean incomplete weakness.

HEMIPLEGIA Very severe or complete weakness on one side.

HETERONYMOUS Refers to a visual field deficit that is on opposite sides in the two eyes, e.g. a bitemporal deficit (heteronymous hemianopia) is in the left field of the left eye and the right field of the right eye.

HIPPOCAMPUS A specialized cortical structure in the temporal lobes, serving as a key component of the system for memory and learning.

HOMONYMOUS Refers to a visual field deficit occurring on the same side in each eye, i.e. right side (left eye nasal field and right eye temporal field).

HORNER'S SYNDROME A triad of ptosis, miosis, and decreased sweating, due to decreased sympathetic input to the eyelid, the pupil, and the sweat glands of the face.

HYDROCEPHALUS Pathologic enlargement of one or more ventricles of the brain. When the enlargement is passive, secondary to tissue loss, it is called hydrocephalus *ex vacuo*. Enlargement due to blockage of cerebrospinal fluid flow or absorption is termed obstructive. When cerebrospinal fluid from the ventricular system can communicate freely with cerebrospinal fluid in the spinal subarachnoid space, obstructive hydrocephalus is categorized as communicating hydrocephalus.

HYPERTONIA Increased tone or resistance, tested by passive motion at a joint.

HYPOTONIA Decreased tone; floppiness; flaccidity.

ICE WATER CALORICS A test of brainstem function in the comatose patient; horizontal gaze is induced towards the ear stimulated by irrigation of ice water.

INO See INTERNUCLEAR OPHTHALMOPLEGIA.

INTERNUCLEAR OPHTHALMOPLEGIA The simplest and most common form of internuclear ophthalmoplegia is disconnection between the horizontal gaze center/CN 6 nucleus in the pons and the CN 3 nucleus on the opposite side in the midbrain. This is due to a lesion in the connecting tract called the medial longitudinal fasciculus. The result is impaired movement of the adducting eye (ipsilateral to the lesion) on horizontal gaze.

JAW JERK A corticobulbar reflex elicited by tapping downward on the chin, causing masseter contraction; an abnormally increased reflex is associated with bilateral corticobulbar dysfunction.

JOINT POSITION SENSE A sensory modality tested at a conscious level by indicating, by feel, the direction of movement of body parts, or by designating their position in space.

JPS See JOINT POSITION SENSE.

KERNIG SIGN A sign of meningeal irritation in which there is pain or guarding with attempted extension of the leg with the thigh in the flexed position.

KJ See KNEE JERK REFLEX.

KNEE JERK (PATELLAR) REFLEX A deep tendon reflex in which the patellar tendon is tapped causing a reflex extension of the leg.

KORSAKOFF'S SYNDROME Part of the Wernicke–Korsakoff encephalopathy, this is the "amnesic–confabulatory" syndrome of loss of short-term memory and new learning, as well as a tendency in some patients, to "fabricate" answers.

LATERAL GENICULATE BODY (NUCLEUS) Nucleus of the thalamus that receives the optic tract and sends out the optic radiations (geniculocalcarine tracts).

LATERAL MEDULLARY SYNDROME Syndrome of infarction in the territory of the posterior inferior cerebellar artery (a branch of the vertebral artery), which supplies the dorsolateral medulla and inferior cerebellum.

LEMNISCAL Usually used in reference to the medial lemniscus, the brainstem pathway for the vibration–fine touch–position sense modalities.

LENTICULAR NUCLEUS Grouping of the putamen and globus pallidus; also lentiform nucleus.

LOWER MOTOR NEURON A segmental motor neuron: an anterior horn cell at spinal levels, or a neuron of a brainstem motor nucleus; a neuron that directly innervates muscle.

LUMBAR PUNCTURE Introduction of a hollow needle into the spinal canal at a lower lumbar intervertebral space to withdraw cerebrospinal fluid from the subarachnoid space (or to instill medications, etc.).

MAGNETIC RESONANCE IMAGING A technique (nuclear magnetic resonance) that utilizes the effects of a changing magnetic field rather than X-rays to image structures and blood flow. Magnetic resonance angiography is an adaptation to visualize the blood column within blood vessels.

MEDIAL GENICULATE BODY (NUCLEUS) A thalamic nucleus involved in the auditory pathways, receiving inputs from the brainstem and projecting to the temporal cortex.

MEDIAL LONGITUDINAL FASCICULUS Tracts running longitudinally in the brainstem, connecting vestibular and ocular nuclei.

MERALGIA PARESTHETICA Sensory impairment in the distribution of the lateral cutaneous nerve of the thigh.

MIOSIS Abnormal constriction of a pupil.

MLF See MEDIAL LONGITUDINAL FASCICULUS.

MONONEUROPATHY Lesion of a single nerve.

MONONEUROPATHY MULTIPLEX More than one coexistent mononeuropathy.

MRI See MAGNETIC RESONANCE IMAGING.

MULTIPLE SCLEROSIS An immunologically mediated disease affecting myelin, characterized by a relapsing and remitting or progressive course and neurologic signs referable to two or more sites in the central nervous system.

MYALGIA Muscle aches or pains.

MYASTHENIA Weakness of muscle; usually refers to dysfunction at the neuromuscular junction, as in the disease myasthenia gravis.

MYELIN The lipid–protein "wrapping" around axons.

MYOTONIA A general term for abnormal, intrinsic, high-frequency firing of muscle cell potentials, causing excessive contraction and/or delayed relaxation.

NEURAXIS The longitudinal axis of the central nervous system running from forebrain rostrally, to spinal cord caudally. The neuraxis bends at the midbrain (mesencephalic flexure).

NEURONS: 1ST, 2ND, AND 3RD ORDER In the simplest scheme of sensory connections, this terminology refers to sensory neurons, starting from the periphery: the 1st order neuron has its cell body in a dorsal root ganglion (or cranial nerve sensory ganglion); its central process (axon) synapses with a 2nd order neuron located at some level of the spinal cord (or brainstem). This neuron in turn synapses with a 3rd order neuron, located in the thalamus, which projects to the sensory cortex.

NEUROPATHY A general term for disorders manifest in the peripheral nervous system.

NOCICEPTIVE Describes sensory receptors that respond to painful or potentially injurious stimuli.

NUCLEUS DORSALIS Cell bodies of 2nd order neurons in the unconscious proprioceptive (spinocerebellar) pathways from the body and legs; also known as Clarke's column (of gray matter).

NYSTAGMUS A variety of oscillatory ("jiggling") movements of the eyes (usually abnormal).

OCULOCEPHALIC REFLEX See DOLL'S EYES.

OCULOMOTOR Specifically, CN 3 nucleus and nerve which provide innervation to certain ocular muscles. Oculomotor is sometimes used more generally to signify the entire eye movement system.

OD Right eye.

OPHTHALMOPLEGIA Paralysis of one or more eye movements.

OPTIC NEURITIS Inflammation of the optic nerve, as in the demyelination of multiple sclerosis.

ORIENTED TIMES THREE In the mental status test, oriented to person, place, and time.

OS Left eye.

PAPILLEDEMA Swelling of the optic nerve head (disc) due to increased intracranial pressure.

PAROXYSMAL Suddenly and episodically occurring, as in electrical seizure discharges.

PAST POINTING A type of dysmetria (missing a target) manifesting a consistent bias in one direction, due to dysfunction of the vestibular/cerebellar system.

PATELLAR REFLEX See KNEE JERK REFLEX.

PERIPHERAL NERVE A nerve that is formed from sensory and motor roots (including autonomic fibers), and hence is a "mixed peripheral nerve." (See PERIPHERAL NERVOUS SYSTEM.)

PERIPHERAL NERVOUS SYSTEM This refers to all neural structures that are outside of the central nervous system: spinal and cranial nerve roots, mixed peripheral nerves, and all peripheral ganglia.

PERRLA Pupils equal, round, and reactive to light and accommodation.

PET See POSITRON EMISSION TOMOGRAPHY.

PHONATION Production of voice sound.

PHOTOPHOBIA Abnormal sensitivity of the eyes to light.

PLANTAR RESPONSE The reflex reaction to lateral plantar stimulation (the Babinski "test"); the Babinski sign (abnormal) is mainly an extensor response of the great toe.

PLAQUE A plate-like lesion, such as an atherosclerotic excrescence within an artery; also refers to the focal demyelinative lesions of multiple sclerosis.

PNS See PERIPHERAL NERVOUS SYSTEM.

POLYMYOSITIS Inflammatory disorder of multiple muscles, usually proximal and symmetric.

POLYNEUROPATHY Abnormality of peripheral nerves (neuropathy) in which there is diffuse and symmetric involvement of nerves. Most polyneuropathies are of the axonal type, in which the ends of the longest nerves are affected first and most severely.

POSITIONAL TESTING Used to elicit vestibular symptoms and signs, such as vertigo and nystagmus, that are often dependent on position or movement of the head.

POSITRON EMISSION TOMOGRAPHY A physiologic imaging technique.

POSTERIOR APHASIA Category of aphasias based upon general anatomic localization. See WERNICKE'S APHASIA, which typifies the fluent aphasias with impaired comprehension.

POSTERIOR ROOT, HORN See DORSAL HORN; DORSAL ROOT.

PREFRONTAL The anterior part of the frontal lobes – anterior to the primary motor and premotor areas.

PREMOTOR Frontal cortical areas, lying anterior to the primary motor strip, that are involved in the motor system.

PROPRIOCEPTION Sense of position, both unconscious and conscious. (See JOINT POSITION SENSE).

PSEUDOBULBAR PALSY A syndrome of bilateral corticobulbar dysfunction in which speech articulation, phonation, and swallowing (under bilateral corticobulbar control) are especially affected. Affective (emotional) lability is often associated.

PSYCHOMOTOR RETARDATION Slowness of mental and physical behavior; does not imply mental retardation.

PTOSIS Abnormal droop of an eyelid (pronounced "toe-sis").

PUTAMEN Part of the basal ganglia. Together with the caudate the putamen forms the striatum; together with the globus pallidus, it forms the lenticular or lentiform nucleus.

QUADRANTANOPIA Also, quadrantanopsia. Impairment of vision in one-quarter of a field – the upper or lower part of a hemianopia.

RADICULOPATHY Any pathologic condition involving one or more nerve roots.

RINNÉ TEST Hearing test comparing air conduction with bone conduction.

ROLANDIC Refers to the Rolandic fissure or central sulcus that separates the frontal lobe anteriorly from the parietal lobe posteriorly. The pre-Rolandic or precentral gyrus includes the primary motor cortex, and the post-Rolandic (postcentral) gyrus the primary somatosensory cortex.

ROMBERG SIGN (TEST) The abnormal response (Romberg sign) is difficulty maintaining balance with eyes closed while standing on the narrowest base that affords balance with the eyes open. This test stresses the proprioceptive system by excluding visual orientation.

ROOT (NERVE ROOT) Designation of segmental motor and sensory axons between the central nervous system and the formation of mixed peripheral nerves. (See DORSAL ROOT; VENTRAL ROOT).

ROOTING REFLEX A so-called frontal-release reflex in which stimulation at the corner of the mouth or cheek causes a turning of lips and face toward the stimulus, as in the infantile reflex in which the mouth is turned towards a nipple.

ROSTRAL Position on the neuraxis towards the forebrain and away from the lower end of the spinal cord. Opposite of caudal.

SCIATICA Common term for radiculopathic symptoms from one of the lumbosacral roots that will form the sciatic nerve.

SEGMENTAL In functional neuroanatomy, segmental refers to a cross-sectional slice of the brainstem or spinal cord containing or relating to the input or output structures for communication with the periphery. This segmental organization is embryologically derived and is most clearly still manifest in anterior and posterior nerve roots, dorsal root ganglia, and dermatomes.

SHUNT A tubing that carries fluid from a ventricle or other cavity to a place where it can be absorbed, such as the right atrium of the heart, the peritoneal cavity, etc. Shunting is a treatment for hydrocephalus and occasionally for fluid in other cavities.

SINGLE PHOTON EMISSION COMPUTED TOMOGRAPHY A physiologic imaging system.

SNOUT REFLEX A corticobulbar reflex elicited by tapping the lips, causing them to "pout."

SPASTICITY Clinically, hypertonia in the context of upper motor neuron disease; classically described as a "clasp knife" quality of increasing resistance against increasing stretch followed by collapse of resistance.

SPECT See SINGLE PHOTON EMISSION COMPUTED TOMOGRAPHY.

SPINAL TAP See LUMBAR PUNCTURE.

SQUINT Common term for strabismus.

STATUS EPILEPTICUS Continuous or repetitive seizures for at least one-half hour without regaining consciousness.

STENOSIS Narrowing of the lumen of an artery (as in carotid stenosis) or of the cross-sectional area of the spinal column lumen (spinal stenosis) etc.

STOCKING-GLOVE Pattern of neuropathic sensory impairment associated with axonal polyneuropathies; the feet are affected first, then lower legs and hands.

STRABISMUS A lack of alignment of the two eyes, such that they are dysconjugate – abnormally convergent or divergent.

STRAIGHT LEG RAISING A test for lumbosacral radiculopathy; passive elevation of the thigh with the leg extended stretches the lower lumbosacral roots, reproducing pain along the course of an inflamed root or numbness in its distribution.

STRIATE CORTEX Primary visual cortex. (See CALCARINE CORTEX.)

STRIATUM Refers to the caudate and putamen (nuclei of the basal ganglia). The term corpus striatum also includes the globus pallidus.

SUBFALCIAL Beneath the falx cerebri, the midline dural fold between the right and left hemispheres; used in reference to right-to-left or left-to-right herniation of the cingulate gyrus under the falx.

SUCK REFLEX A "frontal release" reflex in which stimulation of the lips elicits a sucking response, as occurs in the infant stimulated by a nipple.

SUPERFICIAL ABDOMINAL REFLEXES Contraction of the abdominal musculature of any one of the four quadrants surrounding the umbilicus, elicited by stroking the skin in each of these four quadrants.

SUPRANUCLEAR Used synonymously with suprasegmental when referring to the brainstem (where segmental neurons are organized in cranial nerve nuclei).

SUPRASEGMENTAL Neurons and tracts from a higher (more rostral) level of the central nervous system that influence segmental neurons.

SYLVIAN FISSURE The major horizontal fissure separating the temporal lobe from the adjacent parts of the frontal and parietal lobes.

TANDEM GAIT Walking heel to toe, one foot directly in front of the other.

TEMPORAL Area of the temples of the head, as in temporal artery or temporal bone, or temporal lobe of the brain; also, time or time course, as in the "temporal profile" of symptoms.

TEMPORAL ARTERITIS An inflammatory condition of cranial (and other) arteries; a manifestation of giant-cell arteritis. The superficial temporal artery is accessible to palpation and biopsy.

TENTORIAL NOTCH The opening in the tentorium cerebelli that allows room for the brainstem to connect rostrally with the cerebral hemispheres.

TIA See TRANSIENT ISCHEMIC ATTACK.

TJ See TRICEPS JERK.

TONSILLAR HERNIATION Downward shift of the cerebellar tonsils below the foramen magnum; associated with mass effect in the posterior fossa; cerebellar "pressure cone."

TONSILS The most inferior parts of the cerebellum, adjacent to the medulla and normally extending down to the level of the foramen magnum.

TRANSIENT ISCHEMIC ATTACK Brief, focal neurologic symptoms or signs resulting from focal brain ischemia; may herald a stroke.

TRICEPS JERK A deep tendon reflex elicited by striking the triceps tendon just above the back of the elbow, with resultant contraction of the triceps muscle, extending the forearm.

UNCUS A medial part of the temporal lobe referred to in uncal (parahippocampal) herniation through the tentorial notch.

UPPER MOTOR NEURON A neuron of the motor cortex whose axon is a fiber of the corticospinal or corticobulbar tracts; more broadly, any suprasegmental motor neuron that synapses on a lower motor neuron.

VENTRAL ROOT Portion of the axons of anterior horn cells between the spinal cord and the formation of a mixed peripheral nerve; these motor fibers are grouped segmentally to form a complete ventral root. Anterior root.

VENTRICLES The fluid-filled spaces in the brain, consisting of two lateral ventricles which communicate with a midline 3rd ventricle, connected by the Sylvian aqueduct with the midline 4th ventricle in the posterior fossa. Spinal fluid is formed in the choroid plexuses of the ventricles.

VERMIS The midline structure of the cerebellum which is particularly associated with truncal balance and gait.

VERTIGO Illusion of motion, such as spinning dizziness.

WEBER TEST Hearing test for lateralization of sound from a tuning fork on the skull; the Weber lateralizes to the side of decreased air conduction.

WERNICKE–KORSAKOFF SYNDROME See KORSAKOFF'S SYNDROME; WERNICKE'S ENCEPHALOPATHY.

WERNICKE'S APHASIA A posterior (fluent) type of aphasia characterized by impaired comprehension and repetition, and word and letter errors (paraphasias). Reading is similarly affected. Wernicke's area is in the superior plane of the dominant temporal lobe.

WERNICKE'S ENCEPHALOPATHY Synonymous with Wernicke–Korsakoff syndrome, due to thiamine deficiency, and characterized by the triad of deficits in recent memory, ataxia, and ophthalmoplegia. The memory problem may not be apparent during the acutely lethargic, inattentive state and the ataxia may not be recognized until walking is attempted.

WHITE MATTER Central nervous system tissue consisting mainly of myelinated nerve fibers (and glia) rather than nerve cell bodies.

index